Coping with Dementia:
Memoirs of a Catholic Husband

Michael Peter Hornsby-Smith

Published by New Generation Publishing in 2024

Copyright © Michael Peter Hornsby-Smith 2024

First Edition

The author asserts the moral right under the Copyright, Designs and Patents Act 1988 to be identified as the author of this work.

All Rights reserved. No part of this publication may be reproduced, stored in a retrieval system or transmitted, in any form or by any means without the prior consent of the author, nor be otherwise circulated in any form of binding or cover other than that which it is published and without a similar condition being imposed on the subsequent purchaser.

ISBN: 978-1-83563-328-1

www.newgeneration-publishing.com

New Generation Publishing

FOREWORD

This book was conceived towards the end of my wife, Lennie's seriously deteriorating mixed dementia and was essentially based on the diaries of how I coped with the development of Lennie's illness over the last decade of her life. At the beginning of this decade, unlike all our children, I was in substantial denial of her illness so the book traces significant changes.

I am grateful to my children, Andrew and Gillian, who read the draft of my first chapter. As a result of their helpful comments at the time, I decided to shift the focus of the book from the experiences of our family to its effect on my life as it had been recorded for a decade in my daily diaries. Andrew helpfully checked the amendments suggested by Heloise Murdoch (New Generation Publishers) and has added his own editorial suggestions and clarifications.

A second aim of my book, which emerged unexpectedly was evidence of the sexual lives of a couple of octogenareans and some of the questions it raised were thought likely to contribute to Pope Francis's Synod. I am grateful to Andrew and Gillian for their suggestions to remove over-detailed comments about Lennie's and my sexuality which might have embarrassed our family. I am also grateful to our other children, Stephen and Richard for the loving support they also gave Lennie over her final year.

During the drafting of the book, I had numerous difficulties with my laptop and I am grateful to Ralph Wong for his very helpful support.

COPING WITH DEMENTIA: MEMOIRS OF A CATHOLIC HUSBAND

INTRODUCTION

I went to Sheffield University in 1950, when I was still only seventeen, to study Fuel Technology and Chemical Engineering. I graduated in 1954 and proceeded to complete a PhD in 1958. But I couldn't get a job in either the coking or steel industries at that time, but was offered a job in the Metallurgy Department at Battersea College of Technology by my brother's father-in-law in 1958. At that time, in Further Education colleges, it was usual to have General Studies courses and I was attracted by this and was persuaded by a colleague to take a London University degree in Sociology through night classes at Regent Street Polytechnic. I completed the degree and graduated in 1968.

While I was a postgraduate student in Sheffield, Maureen, a fellow member of the Newman Association for Catholic Graduates, introduced me to her visiting sister, Leonide, after Mass at St. Marie's. Very rudely, I told her to 'stick her bum in' as she walked up the hill outside. The Newman Association group used to meet weekly in Cavendish Square in London, and on 4 December 1959, Maureen invited me to make up a foursome with Leonide at a posh dance at Senate House. We 'hit it off' and arranged to meet again both before and after Christmas. Fairly early in the New Year, I proposed to Leonide. That night I was frightened at what I had done but my mother was very reassuring and I put Leonide's engagement ring on her finger at the Easter Vigil Mass in Berwick-on-Tweed. We were eventually married by the Sheffield University chaplain, Fr. Shannon, on 29 December 1960. I was responsible for simplifying her name to Lennie following the TV series *Lennie the Lion*. We have four children, Andrew, Gillian, Stephen and Richard, and six grandchildren.

I am the oldest of four children. My older sister, Ann, is eighteen months younger than I am and my brother, David, three years younger. My younger sister, Sue, was born when I was eighteen years old and a student in Sheffield. She later married an Italian, Mario, and has lived in Italy ever since. I am fortunate to have had happy relationships with my two sisters over the years but, unfortunately, I have had no contact with my brother for well over a decade.

The main purpose of this book is to examine the development of Lennie's dementia throughout this last decade and the way in which I have responded and coped with it. As will become clear, our children were a great deal more aware of it at a much earlier stage than I was and, indeed, I wrote a letter to our G.P. in 2014 saying I was as close to her as I'd ever been and didn't think she did have it and could he advise us. It is fortunate that I have kept a daily diary for practically all my life since my adolescence, and in recent years this has averaged about four or five hundred words each day. My own current carers assure me that it would be quite useful to offer an account of what it is like to cope with a wife, mother and grandmother who has suffered from dementia. I hope that it will prove to be helpful to readers, especially those who have a relative with dementia.

We were both Roman Catholics and so one of my main concerns was to see to what extent the development of Lennie's dementia and our inevitable decline in mobility might affect the nature of our religious lives. This was obvious when eventually I stopped driving and we sold our car. But it began to be an issue before that, after I'd had two operations on my hip following a fall and a right knee replacement, when we first employed carers for Lennie. Our lives began to change noticeably around this time and there were occasions when we were dependent on the assistance of fellow parishioners to drive us to and from Mass on Sundays.

There were also global issues which increasingly dominated our lives and which we had to cope with. The first of these was the global coronavirus pandemic, which led to a national 'lockdown', which Lennie was seemingly never aware of but which clearly influenced the way we lived our lives and inevitably how we coped with it and the conflicts about COVID-19 which emerged between us. The other global issues which affected our lives included the consequences of the Russian invasion of Ukraine and the increasing cost of energy.

Another matter became apparent to me as I was drafting the first chapter and that was the nature of our sexual relations, as we were both in or nearing our eighties. I've never seen these issues discussed before so it did seem to me to be an issue worth exploring. Relevant to that is the question of how a Catholic couple coped with such issues, given that when we grew up in the early post-war years, there was a particularly strong sense that the sole or primary purpose of sexual intercourse was to produce children. Any departure from the teaching of the Church was potentially sinful. One of the outcomes of this book, therefore, will be to explore how I coped with such issues in the more synodal Church advocated by Pope Francis.

This book sets out a chapter on each of the years from 2013 to 2022, the decade of my eighties. Each is based on my diary for that year. The final chapter will cover Lennie's thirteen months in Claremont Court Care Home until her death on 3 March 2023. Because the diary quotations are daily summaries, they may well be generally relatively rough compared, for example, with smoother summaries to avoid endless repetitions. But I hope they serve the purpose of illustrating the realities of the tensions and challenges I was living through during these ten years. What I hope will emerge is firstly, a growing awareness of the fact of Lennie's dementia by me as well as our children, and secondly, a growing adjustment in the way that I, her husband, managed to cope with the changing demands on my life as a retired academic. The bulk of my life was still spent reading and preparing papers or talks on serious issues such as justice and peace concerns or changes in Roman Catholic thinking and practice in the light of the Second Vatican Council (1962–5) and Pope Francis's stress on discernment and synodality.

Part of the reality of our lives was that we experienced and had to cope with various ailments over this period. Lennie had a number of accidents including a broken arm, a fall outside Sainsburys, and severe problems and pain with her knees and back. I experienced the unexpected transfer of my pacemaker from the left side to the right and then a hip operation and knee replacement just before the two-year responses to the COVID-19 pandemic. It is something of a blessing that the Lord allowed both Lennie and me to survive the whole of this transformative period of our lives. When I was in hospital, we decided Lennie needed regular carer assistance and the Everycarers remained afterwards. But when I came out of hospital, I was given no special care or assistance to cope with my quite serious immobility.

This points to another aspect of this particular study, which is how my Catholicism contributed to the way I responded to the challenges we were facing. What is helpful is that my account is based entirely on my diaries which are in turn based on daily accounts and not written with the aims of this book in mind. It is worth recalling that this book was only conceived early in 2022, so the pleas for help from God were not conceived at this time but are genuine reflections of the way I attempted to respond during the whole of the ten-year period. I just hope and pray that this book will serve as a useful and helpful account for those faced with similar problems.

CHAPTER I

THE YEAR 2013

Lennie and I entered the year 2013 in the fifty-fourth year of our married lives together. She was seventy-seven years old, and I was three years older, entering my ninth decade. When we were married, life expectancies were up to nine years lower than they are today and we would have been regarded as very old and approaching the end of our lives. But actually, in spite of various ailments, we were still fairly well and active, as indeed were many of our fellow parishioners in the same generation. I'd had a pacemaker inserted in 1997 and upgraded ten years later. Early in February, my diary recorded that "Lennie and I have become more aware of my shaking hands, which makes carrying cups of coffee a risky business. I notice, too, that my writing is becoming more erratic as readers of my diary might note." In general, as we shall see, we both had health problems during the year but the evidence for Lennie's dementia was not strong and I tended to resist the suggestions which were mainly coming from our children.

Our second son, Stephen, has suffered from schizophrenia for three decades and has coped with it well with his medication, stopping smoking and drinking alcohol, and managing his finances aided by housing benefit. In 2012, Lennie and I bought him an apartment in a Georgian house in Cranleigh, which was his preference. We set up two trusts with his three siblings as fellow trustees to manage the apartment, the proceeds of which after Stephen's death are to be shared equally among all our grandchildren. Stephen is a very accomplished painter and in October 2013 he held an exhibition of his paintings in Cranleigh, which was attended by the mayor and was generally regarded as a great success.

On the first Saturday of the year, I reported on the half-yearly meeting of the Trustees: Gilly arrived first having given up her Zumba class. Then Andrew arrived late in a temper but calmed down and prepared for the start of the meeting. Richard arrived cheerily, now completely unaware of Andrew's earlier anger. Andrew, as chair, asked me to make an opening prayer and the meeting then proceeded.

As can be seen, personal relations between Stephen's three siblings were not always great and this wasn't helpful to the running of the two trusts. We were fortunate to have invited Pat Jones to attend one of the meetings of the Trusts and she came and gave us some helpful advice. In due course, a general pattern emerged, with Andrew acting as chairman while Gillian took over the administrative, financial and legal aspects of the trusts with Richard agreeing to manage all maintenance issues.

We have been regular and fairly active parishioners at St. Pius X in Merrow, Guildford, since its foundation four decades ago in the early 1970s. Most of our fellow parishioners were strong advocates of the Vatican II reforms from the early 1960s, which stressed the notion of 'a People of God' Church. This emphasised the role of the laity in the Church and advocated the use of the vernacular in place of the older traditional Mass said in Latin. The priest now says the Mass facing the congregation, who now more obviously participate in the Eucharist around the altar. The role of women was also promoted, and they are not only welcomers but are also servers, special ministers for the distribution of Holy Communion and readers of the liturgy.

At this point of time, Lennie and I used to start our day with a mug of tea, then read the day's Mass readings and the commentary in *Bible Alive*, ending with prayers for the living and dead relatives and friends. We were still active as ministers of Holy Communion at Mass, though I was getting shakier and concerned about my ability to come down the steps of the altar safely without spilling the chalice. Lennie continued to take Holy Communion to a sick parishioner. I was still on the rota of readers at Mass. Lennie was also a regular driver of elderly people to and from the women's lunch at the Merrow Methodist Church Hall. She continued to attend the weekly U3A keep-fit class on Mondays, after which a group of Catholic women friends went into Guildford town centre for a coffee.

Lennie and I were both members of the Scripture Reflection Group, which discussed the Thursday morning Mass readings, usually for twenty to thirty minutes before Mass. In mid-March my diary recorded: "We picked up Jill on the way to St. Pius. There were only five of us at today's scripture reflections. I'd spent quite a long time yesterday preparing for it but both Lennie and Norman were not enthused by Ezekiel's stream from the Temple. When I waffled about allegories, Lennie wasn't impressed. She and I were both eucharistic ministers, because at the start of Mass we were the only recognised ministers."

I continued to participate in a range of monthly activities. I was a member of the monthly U3A Opera Group and usually made a presentation once a year. I also participated in a lively monthly U3A discussion group, again probably leading the discussion about once a year. I also continued to be a member of what had originated some time before as the West Surrey Pastoral Development Group. Following the deaths of some members, our numbers fell to four or five and we used to take it in turns every few weeks to discuss some theological, scriptural, or social justice issue in what I then called the 'Bookham Group'. For several decades I had been a member of the parish Justice and Peace Group.

At the end of our busy days and after supper, we used to watch a bit of television. In 2013, Lennie was still hooked on *Eastenders,* which she used to watch regularly. I tended to be disappointed by the TV options available. One of the few programmes we used to watch regularly was *Downton Abbey,* which I found a fascinating account of how Grantham aristocrats coped with the social, economic and political changes resulting from the First World War. And, of course, after Lennie had bought me Sky TV as a birthday present, I used to watch every Chelsea game, usually with Stephen, and occasionally a visiting Richard.

One indication that we were both quite active was that in 2013 we went on three continental holidays. Shortly after Easter, Lennie and I went on a week's tour of Seville, Cordoba and Granada in Spain. An indication of Lennie's declining memory was the fact that she got lost coming out of the toilet at Gatwick. I recorded that: "when I went to look for her after twenty minutes or so, we eventually found each other but she was really frightened, and tears welled up in her face. She really does not have any sense of right from left, etc. Without me she wouldn't go on holiday. So, help us, Lord, to make the best of the opportunities left to us. And help me to be kind and thoughtful to her this holiday."

On our free day, we decided to go to the *Musée de Bellas Artes* and were particularly impressed by the room devoted to Murillo, which was quite the loveliest chamber we have ever been in any art gallery. It was a stunning room. On the day we returned from Malaga, Lennie's nervousness became obvious. In my diary I wrote: "The nervous and apprehensive Lennie asked me, I think, at 2 a.m., 3 a.m. and 4 a.m. what time it was. At 5 a.m., she got herself up and washed in the bathroom. At one stage after we'd had words, I told her to 'go to hell' which wasn't very nice, but a slice of irritation."

Our second overseas trip was a long weekend in Prague, one of our favourite cities. We took Stephen for his first flight for a couple of decades – probably a holiday in Malta was the previous one. We were booked into a small hotel within walking distance of Wenceslas Square and the Charles Bridge. During our visit we saw a rather stolid performance of *Carmen* at the State Opera House. Sadly, the weather was awful over the weekend with almost continuous rain, but we'd also been to a couple of concerts. As I wrote in my diary, I suppose Prague really is my favourite city, though I added later that I had a fairly strong sense that this was my last trip to the city.

Our third holiday was a fortnight Lennie and I enjoyed in the Cevennes, near the town of Le Vigan in August. I'd arranged to book a car, but we found it a nightmare getting out of Montpellier and in the end, I drove to the west towards Millau. But we eventually managed to find the little gîte, rented out by an English owner in a lovely little hamlet. We went to Mass several times in Le Vigan, where all the major responses were in Latin. On a couple of occasions, we attended an evening concert in the church. We visited the mountains not far to the north and I wouldn't be far wrong in saying I fell in love with the Cevennes and even hoped we might return again. But halfway through the holiday, I noted with regret that we weren't thirty years younger and able to do far more walking and extensive day trips than I felt like at that moment.

On one day when the weather was not great, we went to see the famous bridge at Millau, some three decades after we had taken Richard there on a camping holiday. We had difficulty finding our way back and not for the first time I observed that Lennie: "is lovely, but she is the world's worst map reader! She doesn't know right from left or north from south! The Languedoc is such a fascinating area ... yet we have only scraped the surface." Our neighbours at the gîte were charming and wondered "if we'd return next year but I pointed to my knees and implied it was unlikely!" It was a relief to manage to return the car at Montpellier, having driven 800 km in our two weeks' holiday.

I suppose it is about time to offer some reflections on our personal relationship after fifty years of married life together. I suppose all couples have disputes, but in January, after we had had "hard words", I noted that "Lennie has a tendency to define any suggestion I make as 'nagging'". Later in the month I noted that "Lennie sometimes drives me up the wall when she mixes up the plates ... after I've put them into a clear sequence". At the end of January I acknowledged: "The great love and care Lennie has given me over fifty-two years" and I asked the Lord "to help me show my love in return by not being so irritable when she seems to get things wrong. I recognise that we are both getting more forgetful these days and our memories are going. But I don't think that we are suffering from Alzheimer's. I know we are both, a little apprehensively, dreading the day when one of us is left on our own and, on the face of it, that day seems to be getting ever closer."

In February we were again both "more aware of my shaking hands which made carrying cups of coffee a risky business and wondered if it was the early stages of Parkinson's." At this point in time Lennie was still using her mobile phone but we were never successful in keeping in touch with each other in Guildford. "Lennie dropped a bottle of tomato bolognaise, a messy business – and one or two of our cups." At this point in time, I think I was seen as the most vulnerable special minister; for example, I was unsteady when carrying the chalice with the precious blood down the steps of the altar. One of the difficulties I had with Lennie was that "she loves gossip ... but on the whole, I am not a gossip ... and get irritated when she talks when I am writing, reading or thinking!"

In late April my younger sister Sue and her husband Mario visited us from Italy, and we arranged for all our children to come and see them and have a meal. These extra cooking demands put pressure on Lennie. I noted that "I also detect elements of forgetfulness in Lennie – last night she forgot to put the filter in the coffee machine with the result that it spilled all over the place. She is angry with the children not informing her in advance of their plans." But we had a very pleasant visit to Wisley Gardens. Early in May, we had another "fierce but trivial spat over opening the cupboard door under the stairs. Of course, I said 'sorry' again while also accusing Lennie of being a model ... in passing the blame. All verbally. For the first time we seem to have bought pants in the pharmacy brazenly put under the sign 'Incontinence'!"

At the celebration of our grandson Will's fifth birthday, I recorded that "what surprised and alerted me was that Richard, Carol and Stephen all thought that Lennie was becoming quite forgetful and was repeating things. They rather took me aback. They seemed to think I ought to ask the G.P. and ensure appropriate action was taken now to slow down the process. This morning, she forgot where she'd put the presents for Will and Iris and this evening, she'd forgotten she had an appointment at the Jarvis Centre (a breast screening clinic). She tells me she couldn't remember what pills she was on, her address or [the] name of her doctor. The children all suggested my memory, loss of words, etc., is quite different. This agreement among Richard, Carol and Stephen has shaken me a bit. I hope the Lord will guide me as to what I ought to do."

Around this time, I noted that it was one of the disappointments of our married life that we didn't have the same intellectual interests. For example, I watched an interesting documentary about Anne Boleyn whereas Lennie was still regularly watching *Eastenders*. My diary records: "Lennie has worked like a slave today, cleaning the house this morning in the absence of our cleaner, on holiday, putting out a load of washing on the line and later ironing it!"

Lennie also required help with our laptop and printer. Inevitably, I got frustrated, angry and impatient. But we coped and survived. The following morning, I added: "I was very conscious about Lennie's <u>possible</u> loss of memory and general vulnerability. I was impatient with her last night when she just didn't seem able to do straightforward things on the computer. This morning I've felt sorry about my impatience and have asked God to help me to be kind, gentle and patient with her as we both age. She was very apprehensive about driving to Cranleigh, where she is going to pick up our granddaughter, Iris, from nursery school with Stephen as Carol is on a school trip with Will. But it worried her that she'll remember the right street and house number. Whether or not this is the first signs of Alzheimer's, help me, Lord, to be totally understanding, patient, gentle and helpful. After all, she has looked after me faithfully and with absolute commitment for over fifty years of married life together. I love her dearly and wish to support her in our declining years as best I can."

What seems to have emerged in the first half of 2013 is that I was gradually becoming aware of Lennie's memory loss, even if it had not yet been medically acknowledged. Parallel to this was my own awareness of my own declining abilities. What is also interesting is the fact that, on several occasions, Lennie expressed anger "with Gillian for planning to contact her by email and not face-to-face". She elaborated at some length and on other occasions regretted never having the opportunity to go on a "girlie" shopping trip with Gillian.

Lennie expessed worries over preparing a meal on a Sunday which included our grandson, Douglas. I pointed out that "she'd been preparing family meals for fifty years, so why was she so worried? She said because she was lacking in confidence. That prompted me to try and be a bit more helpful. Earlier, in the hall, I was amazed at my own inability to remember names and words. Help me, Lord, to cope gracefully with our ageing."

Another potential sign was that Lennie seems to take an eternity getting ready to go out. Another indication of the approach of dementia was the note that "both Lennie and I are struggling to remember words these days. Often, I remember the first letter and then go blank. Natural loss of memory with old age or early signs of dementia?" Later in the month I added that "Lennie is showing signs of stress and a busy life".

Lennie and I regularly attended a brief twenty-minute scripture reflection before Mass at St. Pius' on Tuesday mornings. On a week when it was Lennie's turn to make the initial presentation, I recorded that "I thought her presentation was very good, in spite of the fact that she is getting a bit careless over keeping a place in the missal. She is also getting a bit forgetful in other areas – leaving her bag in the car, etc." After a Thursday morning Mass, Lennie drove me into Guildford, and I recorded that "at the top of Horseshoe Lane she would have had an accident with a speeding motorcyclist if I hadn't shouted".

On one afternoon in August, I noticed "signs of ageing – such as the somewhat uncoordinated nature of my writing; going both downstairs and upstairs one step at a time; having increasing difficulty putting on my socks". I took Lennie to a hospital appointment "following her recent tummy scan. The consultant decided Lennie needed another scan and a second visit." When I told Stephen that evening he asked if it 'was about her dementia.' I was a bit shocked, really, but it reminded me that two or three of the children recently asked if she was suffering from it."

Just before the Bank Holiday weekend, Lennie and I drove down to Southsea for the day. But when we went for a swim

"Lennie was genuinely frightened that she wouldn't be able to get out again. I could see that this was real, a product of her experience last year on the Normandy beaches", where she had had a frightening fall and been rescued by a kindly young lifeguard.

Early in September, I was having problems with my leg, thigh, back and knee. My leg was becoming more persistently painful. I noted, "I'm getting close to doing what Lennie and friends advise – go and see my doctor. My leg is aching pretty well all the time." Later in the month she told me at supper that I was a bully when trying to help her in computing!

In October, I saw Dr. Barnado, my G.P., who told me he'd "had a look at my recent X-rays and my problem had to do with 'wear and tear' on my back". Later in the month, I wrote that Lennie "is nagging me to tell the physio how painful my leg is" when he comes. "I am in danger of exploding with irritability! I've told her jokingly that she is a bloody nuisance. Thank you, Lord, for giving me such a loving and caring wife." Two days later I added that "I was irritated with Lennie when for the second time in a couple of days she declined an invitation to be a special minister. My leg wasn't good enough for me to volunteer."

Early in November I noted that "sometime before or around midnight I had a slight chest pain which made me use my nitrospray. This upset Lennie a bit, but it is also a sign, perhaps, of approaching end time. It is interesting that for some time Lennie has been looking after me by giving me breakfast in bed with severe back and knee problems with little sign of her dementia. She cheered me up with Sky Sports TV as a birthday present, but I was surprised she didn't know how to read her debit card ... I think her eyesight is getting bad." When taking Stephen to the bus station later in the month, I "told him briefly about Lennie's fear of sounds at the door in the middle of the night and I think he is aware that he may have to give Lennie (or me!) more time in our older years".

Towards the end of the month, I recorded that when Lennie seemed to be delaying irritatingly before we set off for Mass that morning, I probably raised my voice in exasperation as Lennie is always supersensitive to my shouting at her "in front of the neighbours". This time, her anger took the form of refusing to hold hands as usual during the 'Our Father' and even refusing to give me the 'sign of peace.' I was staggered and have felt numb ever since, even though she has tried to make peace with cups of tea and pleasantries. Of course, we must forgive, and I do, but I still shudder when she tells me that shouting at her 'in front of the neighbours' is a 'mortal sin' as far as she is concerned.

In December I noted aspects of Lennie's irritations. "Firstly, Lennie was furious to see a car parked outside our kitchen window. It really fires her up! I tried to joke about it but she wasn't having any of it!" The following day I noted that Lennie couldn't fix a brooch and messed around finding a substitute for twenty minutes or so! ... Later I wrote that my right knee suddenly gave way on my way to the altar. Thirdly, ten days later, I wrote that "both Lennie and I are increasingly conscious that our memories, particularly of people's names, are failing. To me it also seems Lennie is becoming increasingly forgetful – for all the good things she does." On occasions I got irritated by Lennie's interruptions when I was busy or reading or writing. Just before an Advent Group meeting in December, I recorded that Lennie kept gossiping away. This did rather annoy me as it seemed insensitive to my desire for space and quiet. Lennie has frequently interrupted me when I have been working and especially writing. Why can't she talk at other times like during meals? But the other side might be, why don't I make space to discuss, chat and gossip with my wife?

This book provides an opportunity to reflect on some aspects of the sexuality of a couple of 'oldies'. It is interesting that it is mentioned at least four times in my 2013 diary. In March, after a busy day, I noted that "before midnight Lennie and I made love, enjoying the closeness of each other's bodies ... and, in Lennie's case, achieving a climax. Sadly, it is years since I was so lucky. But it is good to still enjoy the intimacy at our ages." But it wasn't always so successful. In April I wrote: "naughtily, but unresisted, I undid Lennie's blouse and caressed her breast. Would the Lord be cross or treat it as a loving intimacy?" In May I wrote that "shortly after midnight I initiated love-making. Lennie seemed to be satisfied, but as soon as she was satisfied, she left me, and I felt irritated and frustrated. At the age of eighty, who am I to complain? But I did make a mental note not to initiate love-making again. If Lennie does, I'll respond as best I can, but ...!"

The changing nature of sexual relations among oldies was also clear in a note written in August: "Before midnight we flirted around and caressed each other, which led to attempted love-making. However, whichever position we tried, our weight and weakness led to failure. Yet I know we love each other, in some respects more than we have ever done. It is just part of the sexuality of people of our age." My guess is that our attempts this August are quite exceptional for people of our age. This diary may "simply point to a single case. I think we are only just coming to terms with the notion that sexual love is normal, not sinful. We are the products of a pre-Vatican socialisation."

When we were on holiday in the Cevennes, I recorded that at 2.30 a.m., "Lennie came for a cuddle, and this eventually turned into attempted love-making. It began to seem to me that for about the first time in my life I wasn't enjoying attempts at sexual intercourse. Here I am recording the fourth attempt in seven days. I try to respond to Lennie's invitations, which this week have been quite explicit." I recorded, that I enjoy opening the buttons of her nightie and arousing her interest by caressing her. Why am I recording this intimate stuff? I think because it may give a flavour of the life of an eighty-year-old ... We are very different in many ways, but the Lord has given us over fifty-three years of loving each other. "Help me, Lord, not to nag but try to be humble enough to satisfy her various needs even if I feel a bit fatigued at times."

"It is difficult to write about this because it seems to be a completely new phase in our lives. Lennie encouraged me, almost instructed me, how to stimulate her breasts – something she's never done before. She half complains that I've not paid enough attention to our sex lives and that I've been too bogged down in reading ... this new surge of sexual activity has come as quite a surprise. I've tried to please Lennie as best I can but my eighty-year-old body can only do so much. How am I, an eighty-year-old unable to achieve a realistic erection, meant to satisfy a wife who is so aroused? Into your hands, O Lord."

Later in the same month, I wrote that "I don't think that it is just self-indulgent if I ponder again the quite remarkable shift in Lennie's and my love-making over the past month. Around 2.30 a.m. for a good half-hour we just enjoyed the closeness and the curves of each other's bodies. We doubted that we would have done the same in our early married years when 'two in one flesh' meant literally erection, penetration and ejaculation, then probably an immediate and exhausted withdrawal ... In our near-eighties, there are few erections, I can't penetrate, and there is no ejaculation. But we have enjoyed just caressing each other – I play with Lennie's breasts, and she excites me down below. Strangely, we feel closer together than I think we have ever done!"

Reading my diary for 2013 has opened my eyes to our lives nearly a decade ago. It was a pleasure to recall the facts that we'd had three very enjoyable holidays in Europe and that at home we were both still active in our social lives and in the parish of St. Pius X. We were both still performing as eucharistic special ministers and I was also a regular reader of the scriptures at Mass. My records showed that we attended Mass more than four times each week and the scripture reflection once a week. What has surprised me is how strong and persistent our sexual lives were despite our ageing. The diaries record that Lennie and I made love on average once a week But there was persistent evidence of declining health and mobility in both our cases. Because this book is largely based on my personal daily diary, an unexpected aspect was the quite persistent extent of the children's warnings about their mother's dementia. Yet in spite of my diary's recognition of changes in Lennie's behaviour, I was still strong and persistent in my denial of dementia. In the following chapters we shall see to what extent the children's predictions were realised and how we coped with the development of Lennie's dementia over the rest of the decade.

CHAPTER 2

The Year 2014

I am starting to write this chapter on a key year, 2014, in the development of Lennie's dementia, having this morning received emails from Andrew and Gillian which were very critical of my first chapter's draft but also quite suggestive and helpful in some of their comments. In this chapter, I'm going to try and take on board their helpful suggestions. In particular, I am taking seriously the idea of changing the title of the book to *Coping with Dementia: Memoir of a Catholic Husband* rather than *A Catholic Family*. I will continue to focus on how Lennie's and my relationship responded to the changes taking place in our lives as I, Lennie's close partner and husband, interpreted it at the time in my daily diaries. I admit that I was largely in denial about her dementia, but so was Lennie, and I had to cope with her quite angry opposition to going to see our G.P.

This was quite a busy year for me, and I had to prepare two presentations to make in Rome in June and October and Lennie wasn't always very understanding about my need for peace and quiet while I was doing the necessary study. It seems that during the year both Lennie's and my health declined and we did eventually consult our G.P. But we managed to slot in three holidays in Provence, Verona, Berwick and the Edinburgh Festival. Early in the year we changed our car, and in March bought a new Seat Ibiza.

During the year, we averaged four Masses each week with scripture reflections just under once a week, and it seems we made love about every nine days. Otherwise, our lives carried on much as before. Around this time, we started our day with a routine which included reading the day's Mass scripture readings and the *Bible Alive* commentary, followed by a series of prayers for our family and parish friends, living and dead. Lennie and I continued to be on a special ministers' rota and I was on the readers' rota. But after a "chest twinge in the middle of the night, I decided that today, Pentecost Sunday, would be my last day of formally being a eucharistic minister. I asked to be taken off the formal list, even though I will still be commissioned for weekday Masses. Even so, quite a milestone."

Both Lennie and I continued to participate in the twenty-minute scripture reflection before Tuesday morning Mass. Lennie continued to take Holy Communion to a sick parishioner and to drive three elderly or disabled people to and from the Merrow Methodist Hall for a regular lunch. She continued to attend the U3A keep-fit classes and join a group of fellow parishioners for coffee afterwards. She continued to do all the shopping at Sainsbury's. Meanwhile, rather to Lennie's annoyance at times, I continued to participate regularly in a number of group activities, including the parish Justice and Peace Group, the U3A Opera and Discussion groups, and the group which I later called the Bookham Group, which met around every six weeks. I was also a volunteer for the Merrow food bank.

The Trusts, which Lennie and I set up some years ago, continued to be managed by Stephen's three siblings, Lennie and me. The June meeting was the eighth and I recorded that "the meeting went quite well. It seemed to revolve around the theme of how to run the trusts when I am no longer able to do it. Gilly made it quite explicit she was too busy to take over as trust secretary and I think we all understood that. But in the end, she offered to write the minutes and sort out one or two things. Richard, too, offered to be responsible for maintenance issues including the buildings insurance and BG Homecare and Insurance cover."

There is a fair amount of evidence from my diary that we felt our health was declining during the year and this certainly made me sense that the end of my life was approaching. For I felt "puffed and tired" having walked a quarter of a mile to post some letters in March. At the time I noted "another sign of ageing. Lord, I take it that You are telling me to get ready and put my house in order ASAP." In September, when my back and knee were giving me some trouble, I wrote that "Lennie is nagging me to stop committing myself to things such as the food bank ... We'll struggle on!" Early in March I drove Stephen to the hospital, where he had a growth near his right eye removed.

It is interesting to read about an accident I had on 11th March. "We'd been to St. Pius' for Mass where I led today's scripture reflection. Afterwards Lennie said it sounded 'professorial'; was that good or bad? After Mass, Lennie dropped me at Boxgrove [some shops about a mile away from our house], where I had my scheduled hair appointment. I then started to walk home via the underpass at George Abbott School, but tripped as I came to Merrow Copse. I ended up falling flat across the pavement into the road and bashed my nose, forehead and left hand. Within ten seconds, two cars had stopped, and the ladies got out to help me. One was a nurse, who stayed with me until an ambulance arrived." A fellow parishioner who lived in an adjacent house "brought out a chair. How kind and thoughtful people are. God bless them." The ambulance staff then drove me home and Gillian was phoned to contact Lennie. "We managed to arrange to see our G.P. In 17 days' time!"

That same evening, we went out for a meal with two friends from the parish, one of whom "obviously feels aggrieved by the attitude of the former Anglican priests who see themselves as 'the bosses', so continuing struggle in the parish seems inevitable since four of the five priests in the Guildford area are former Anglicans. But where would we be without them?" At this point in time, five years after the publication of my *Parish Still Alive?* there were significant "tensions which have built up between authoritarian priests and at least older generation parishioners". For example, planned arrangements for celebrations after Mass on Pentecost Sunday were changed and our two former Anglican priests "have decided to erase surnames from the bidding prayers for the sick. Why? There has been a fair amount of grumbling about this. People resent the dictatorial omissions." One of the priests, who defiantly wore a biretta, "was furious and even threatened to do away with bidding prayers, which he claimed didn't fit in with any liturgical rule book. Plenty to think about. Do the clergy take on board what [Pope] Francis is saying in *Evangelii Gaudium*?"

Issues such as love-making in our eighties continued to concern me in 2014. As I mentioned in the previous chapter, "our love-making ends with Lennie on top of me and is usually successful from her point of view. I can't say I enjoy it; she is heavy and I'm glad when it is over but pleased if she is satisfied. Perhaps an extraordinary reflection on the sexuality of eighty-year-olds." Other reflections during the year suggested typical pre-Vatican concerns about the sinfulness of sex were being challenged by our flirting and caressing. I'm sure the Lord doesn't mind such activities, even among the near-eighties! "Later in May, Lennie encouraged me to make love but as soon as she reaches a climax she stops and I feel rather frustrated." A few days later I observed that "Lennie seems to be going through a phase of heightened sexuality – as last August in the Cevennes". Then in early July I noted that Lennie initiated love-making and was clearly "up for it". It was at this stage that I wondered guiltily if what I was doing by using my finger as a surrogate penis was masturbation and sinful. So I broke off then, though my thinking was: why would it be sinful if I was giving my wife sexual pleasure, which, if I understand Vatican II properly, is perfectly legitimate?"

A diary written just a few days before the end of the year helps put things into perspective. I was still busy writing the odd articles and I frequently complained about not being given sufficient time and space to do the necessary work. This, no doubt, contributed to my irritability, which generated Lennie's anger. "I am aware that Stephen is currently seeing me as the cause of irritations between me and Lennie."

For nearly fifty years we had been a member of what we then called a 'Family Group' in the parish. We were six couples and we used to meet in each other's houses every month. Thus, we were hosts for twelve of us about twice each year. Early in February, it was our turn and "after an initial prayer from Lennie" I led the discussion of around an hour on Pope Francis's encyclical *Evangelii Gaudium*, particularly on Chapter 4 "on Francis's critique of liberal capitalism. One member, Maureen Martin, a headmistress, did more than her fair share of commenting and mainly stressed the need for better education to sort out inequalities. Another member, Mary Comerford, was the only one who agreed basically with the need for a structural change in our economic relations. Lennie's tuna meal went down OK, and we had a pleasant enough evening." But after everyone had left and we'd tidied and washed up, Lennie and I both "went to bed exhausted", another sign of our ageing.

When my Auntie Pat, three times a junior minister in Tory governments, died in 1985, I filed away many of her files and records in a suitcase. Another sign of my ageing was the realisation that I ought to do something about them. I noted that "I'd been disappointed to find that most of them relate to her time in the House of Lords and very little to her time as an M.P. Also, I've only found one thin file relating to S.O.E. [Special Operations Executive, a precursor to the SAS]." Later in the year, in September, I discovered additional box files which included "quite a rich source on

S.O.E., including letters from Lord Selbourne, her boss, a fair bit of early political drafts and a draft autobiography". Over the next few months, I contacted the National Archives and the Royal Historical Society and, eventually, I think some of them were archived in the Conservative Party archives in the Bodleian Library, Oxford.

Life still seemed to be very busy, in spite of our ages. For example, my diary for a Tuesday in late April records that after scripture reflection and Mass on the Feast of St. Catherine of Siena, Lennie drove me home and then took Holy Communion to a sick parishioner. I then printed choir sheets for Lennie and did some proofreading until she returned, and we had lunch. In the afternoon I drove to our parish hall for an ecumenical 'Together in Christ' for Merrow meeting. There were about twenty-five people present, probably over half from our parish. "Our session was superbly led by Pat Jones, who cajoled, suggested, hinted, prompted and guided us in ways which encouraged conversation and sharing and prompted some ideas along the lines of where ecumenism might be going, especially in Merrow. There were some interesting, informative contributions, too, for example on the productions of the Anglican-Roman Catholic International Commission (ARCIC) over the last thirty years. I helped clear away the chairs and tables afterwards, so I didn't get home until 4.30 p.m." After tea and a quick skim of the *Guardian,* I drove us off to the Yvonne Arnaud Theatre where we both enjoyed a performance of *HMS Pinafore* which Lennie had performed in at school. After returning home I "just managed to finish my proofreading before going to bed". This gives some idea about how busy we were at this stage in our lives.

Stephen and I often had 'spats' and I often got irritated by his non-stop talking. This was another reality of my life. I was always delighted to see him because he assisted me in so many ways. It seems that my best strategy was simply to 'shut up' during one of his rants and remember that he was suffering from schizophrenia. But one example of our spats occurred on our return from Oxmarket in Chichester, where he had a lovely exhibition of his paintings. As I wrote in my diary: "Stephen and I were still a bit cross with each other so while he ranted on about his illness in the car, and what M.I.5. *et al* were doing to him, I drove him to his apartment in Cranleigh."

On the last Sunday of the year, I added the following note, which says something about generational changes in the Church. I noted that Gillian and her husband were not at Mass with us and my diary noted "they seemingly went to Holy Trinity (C of E). Until recently we would have regarded this as sad and non-Catholic. Rather suddenly – and the Synod has promoted challenging new perspectives – we are inclined to think it is better to go and worship God in a C of E Church than not at all, like our four oldest grandchildren. I no longer believe missing Mass on Sundays is a 'mortal sin', though it does worry us that so many young people just opt out. We are no longer a fortress Church held together by strict conformity to clerical regulations."

In 2014, I was invited to attend two conferences in Rome promoted by the Vatican on the theme of 'The Idea of a University: Investing in Knowledge in Europe and for Europe'. On the first visit, I gave the first talk, challenging new perspectives based on lectures given in the mid-1880s by Cardinal John Henry Newman, which emphasised teaching and learning but failed to recognise the significance of research and the discovery of new knowledge and understanding as important elements in the work of a university. Secondly, I offered some reflections on scientific research on religion based on my own research on changes in English Catholicism, particularly from the 1970s to the 1990s. I suggested this might be relevant to current surveys of lay opinions on sex, marriage and the family. Thirdly, I reflected on a clearer, sustainable and socially inclusive strategy, as promoted by Europa 2020, for the growth of the university system and research. I considered the consequences of the increasing proportion of students going to universities for university staff in a period of globalisation and liberal capitalist hegemony. I was given the impression that it went down quite well.

The first visit over four days in June was a bit uncertain, as I was given no clear information about where I was staying or whether or not I would be collected and taken to the university and to and from the airport. In the end it was fine and I was given time to explore Rome from Santa Francesca Romana in Trastevere. I managed, in spite of my limited mobility. I noted it wasn't so easy on the second visit in October, when I had to make my own way to Santa Emerenziana near the Lateran University, from where I "was due to be picked up by bus to be taken to Campidoglio where the opening ceremony of the Symposium was being held. To my consternation, there were dozens of steps to be climbed." The opening ceremony included a welcome from the Mayor of Rome. There were a number of interesting points made in the following series of speeches, including "the stress that universities had social and moral dimensions and were not solely concerned with developing work skills; innovation should also include ethical principles and the purpose of universities was not just to train workers". There were some interesting research seminars and I made points, for example about climate change, which two students later came to thank me for. On my second visit I noted that "there is a strong element of disorganisation about Italian conference arrangements". But I felt very tired and that I would not be fit or mobile enough to go again.

As I mentioned earlier, we had three holidays in 2014. The first was a week's trip in late June to Provence. Richard kindly drove us to St. Pancras, where we caught the Eurostar to Lille. There we took the train to Avignon, where we were taken by coach to the Hotel Bristol which we thought was 'very basic.' We were with a fairly large group so it was not before the end of the week that we began to make friends. But my diary recorded that our guides were very friendly and helpful. It seems we largely had to find our meals outside. But we managed and kept within our budget. We went on a series of trips: to Aix-en-Provence, "the magnificent Roman world heritage site at Pont du Gard," Orange, Châteauneuf du Papes, Arles and the Camargue and Roussillon, "which had changed a bit since we had a holiday there with Stephen, possibly around thirty years ago". I thought I'd lost my wallet there and the group were very friendly and supportive, and it was eventually found on the floor of the coach!

Our second trip abroad was a brief four-day trip to Verona to go to the opera in the Arena only about 100 yards from our hotel, Hotel Torcolo, which was very friendly. We saw *Turandot*, which we quite enjoyed, and *Carmen*, where "I think we were both a bit disappointed by the performances". On our second day, we were taken by my sister Sue and her husband Mario to Lake Garda, where they had prepared a delightful picnic lunch. They were, I think, staying with relatives nearby but had taken the trouble to drive all the way from Ivrea, near Turin, to see us. In the evening the four of us had a very pleasant meal in the Piazza Bra opposite the Arena "before saying our final affectionate farewells and returning to our room". Before the end of our trip, I managed "to photo Lennie against the background of Juliet's balcony!"

In August we went to the Edinburgh Festival for the first time. We spent a couple of days first in Berwick, where we visited Lennie's parents' grave. "Lennie tried to scale the gravestone a bit but Andrew, on a previous visit, seemed to have done a good job before us. Lennie and I prayed for her parents, who have now been dead for nearly thirty years. I guessed this might well be our last visit." We enjoyed walks along the pier and the cliffs over the sea and Lennie was stimulated to "wish and imagine we might come back here on holiday". The following day I added that "I'm afraid my knees don't seem up to it and I hope she doesn't push for us to come for a longer stay, for example next year". We went out for an evening meal with Rosemary Dorse, Lennie's longest-living friend from Berwick and her husband, Ian.

From Berwick we took a train to Edinburgh, where we were joined by Stephen in a pleasant bed-and-breakfast apartment not far from Princes Street. They cooked us splendid breakfasts and were very friendly. We aimed to attend a variety of events at the festival, including the Tattoo. This "was an experience worth having, with the magical sound of the massed pipes and the evidence of the distinct Scottish pipes and dance culture but also the strong Commonwealth links; I particularly enjoyed the exuberant Zulus from South Africa. We also enjoyed *Imala,* a lovely and unique combination of African dance and ballet. Interesting fringe events included *The Jungle Referendum* performed by five girls who gave an interesting and critical appraisal of the arguments for and against the Scottish Referendum next month. It was humorous and took the mickey out of monkey Cameron and wolf Salmond." Another fringe event we attended was *Forever Young,* unexpectedly presented by a group of young actors from the Yvonne Arnaud theatre group from Guildford, who recalled "the reality of the young generation of W.W.I, and felt that there were themes that shouldn't be forgotten". Stephen frequently went off on his own to visit some of the fringe events. He also "spent the day visiting art galleries and exhibitions". On our last evening the three of us went to the Usher Hall, where "we saw a performance of Britten's *War Requiem* – a magnificent piece which I doubt I will ever see again". During the day Lennie loved to go shopping in Princes Street. But my knees were causing me a lot of trouble because "there were no seats for me to sit on in the stores and eventually I sat in a bus shelter for the best part of three-quarters of an hour while she looked around for a pair of summer shoes." On our final morning, Stephen left us to visit John O'Groats while we caught the train back to Kings Cross, where Richard kindly met us and drove us home.

The major focus of this book is intended to be the development of Lennie's dementia and how I, her husband, and to some extent other members of the family, coped with it. In mid-February I recorded that "Lennie has increasingly expressed concern about her loss of memory. Today for the first time our cleaner commented on her forgetfulness; the children have observed this over the past few months. Please help me, Lord, to watch over her and keep her safe." Later in the month when Gillian, our daughter, joined us for coffee after Mass she "tactfully but bluntly suggested that Lennie ought to consult her doctor about her memory loss and what she ought to do about it and whether medication would help".

In mid-March I noted that Lennie was "deeply hurt by the repeated suggestions from the children that she should consult a doctor about her memory loss and she angrily replies she doesn't need instruction from them and is perfectly capable of making such decisions herself. She feels very angry and hurt and it will take some time to ease. Whatever I say is dismissed. I pray for her hurt to be eased ... I am not aware of acute issues though it is interesting that all our children have commented on it to me." At the end of March, Lennie and I did in fact go and see our G.P. My diary noted that "Lennie raised issues about her back and stomach and then reported some loss of memory, etc., and should she be worried?" Strangely, my diary has no reference to any comment by our G.P., though Lennie was having difficulty again printing attachments from emails so I often had to take over this task from her. But early in September there was the unexpected note that "for the first time Lennie wondered if she should go to see our G.P. about feared Alzheimer's".

One day, when we were at the Edinburgh Festival and we were wandering around fringe events, "Lennie couldn't see me because of the crowd until it disappeared after the acrobat and comic act. She really was frightened – another sign that she seems more dependent than I've ever known her." Gillian was quite persistent in mid-August, several times "expressing a concern that Lennie seemed to be showing early signs of dementia. She urged early advice from our G.P., perhaps as part of the over-75s care plan ... I confess I'm not aware of Lennie's repetitive questions, which the children seem to notice, though we both have memory loss of people's names and words and I was aware of how dependent she was on me in Edinburgh ... There is a lot where we don't see 'eye to eye'!" It was in mid-August that I finally wrote to our G.P. expressing the children's concerns and saying that I didn't see it that way and asking for advice.

In due course, Lennie did see our G.P. in early October. She returned "rather disturbed that he'd subjected her to some memory tests and apparently is putting a specialist colleague in touch with her to pursue a more professional investigation ... Poor lass! I hope the outcome is successful." She had another memory test in early November. Afterwards and "until lunch Lennie expressed her anger at the nature of the test, which she felt would have been fine for bright seven-year-olds but was not appropriate for her. She senses, I guess, that she 'failed' the test and feels angry and hurt; let's hope the result was better than she thought."

Around April, I was quite busy self-publishing *Letters to my Grandchildren,* which was intended to be a simple introduction to Catholic Social Teaching, but also drafting my paper for the Rome conference. I expressed my irritation at non-stop TV and observed that "I became increasingly irritated that I had no 'space' to read ... But I do have a nagging sense that I am not behaving patiently, kindly and lovingly. Please Lord, forgive my irritability." In mid-June I expressed uncertainties: "Life at the moment seems strange: morning work; afternoon reading the papers; evening being lazy. But I am not happy with running out of energy by lunchtime. Today we celebrated St. Richard of Chichester and prayed his prayer at the end of Mass. Great prayer."

There were times when Lennie seemed to lose control of her cooking. For example, in late February she "managed to leave a blackened pea pan and overcooked her treacle pudding; the smell of burning permeated the whole house ... Lennie's inability to use the new microwave oven she asked for irritates me ... Lennie drops things on every surface around the kitchen. She doesn't tidy as she cooks. But she is still lovely!" Early in March, "Lennie came upstairs to tell me how bad-tempered I'd been at various points throughout the day. Lord, I pray for patience." A couple of days later I noted that "Lennie had problems with the grill when cooking fish fingers and I had to help. I guess I'm going to have to take over some of the cooking not using the oven or hob."

One day in mid-March, on my return from a U3A Opera Group, "Lennie expressed annoyance that I had had so many meetings this week so that she had hardly seen me". In mid-July, and in the spirit of trying to keep my "diary for archival purposes, hopefully to be of help to future generations, I'd better record my impression that Lennie is becoming less self-reliant. She repeatedly asks for dates when she could have a perm; eventually I get frustrated and point out that I've told her three or four times already. This leads her to complain about my being wrapped up in my books and angry exchanges follow. Again, she doesn't pick up instructions such as the printer's on-off button in the bottom right-hand corner or can't switch on kitchen equipment. All this shouldn't be exaggerated, but it is part of our lives together. We both love each other and thank

God for His gift to us. But it is part of the 'background'." In early October, on a day when we had three spats, I noted that "it is sad that Lennie and I are at loggerheads; she often complains about my 'lecturing' her". On the following day, Andrew, who'd been for a swim in Bournemouth, phoned for a long time and "Lennie was furious I'd nattered for so long and complained about my ignoring her – which I thought was unfair".

By the end of October, my diary suggested that life was changing, slowly but surely. I recorded that in the mornings I "helped Lennie take her pills. She is not systematic over them, so I have to insist. Poor lass, she was in real pain with her knee." I'd never seen her cry like she did "till she settled down". Early in November, Lennie "was in a lot of pain with her leg ... and decided she couldn't cope with Sunday Mass" but she was brought Holy Communion that afternoon by one of our Family Group. My general impatience was reflected when "I then expressed irritation with Lennie when she couldn't find the place in today's readings for All Souls. She burst into tears and told me how horrible I was; this adds to her accusations of bullying and now 'shallow' religiosity – a new one."

Another example of the difficulties Lennie and I were having was when I asked her if she'd like to go to a concert. My diary records that I "lost my cool when Lennie wouldn't answer the simple question. As she went on and on about it being tomorrow, I got more and more angry as she failed to answer my question. So, Lord, please forgive me for my impatience and irritability which Lennie put down to my being overtired with too many commitments." A couple of days later I recorded that "Lennie again expressed concerns about her memory test and was angry because I, as her husband, didn't agree with her as husbands are supposed to!" A couple of days later I added, "Lennie is still very worried about the memory test and what she will say to our

G.P. This morning she feared she wouldn't be allowed to continue driving!"

Towards the end of the month, things got worse and one evening, "Lennie wanted help with emails and almost immediately drove me mad. When she got up to leave the laptop, I forcibly pushed her back and she has just told me she's never seen me like this and it's the first time I've ever been physically rough with her. Dear Lord, please forgive me. I find her so terribly frustrating. It just isn't her gift. But help me develop the gift of patience." The following morning, Lennie reminded me it "was the first time I had used physical 'violence' against her. I was a bully. Well, I think that is overstated but it is a reminder that I very soon get exasperated when she doesn't respond to suggestions when checking emails. It is just not a gift she has, and I find it very frustrating but occasionally realise that I am pretty incompetent technically myself. It is also a reminder that we are both ageing, possibly quite rapidly, and I worry about how Lennie would cope when I'm not here to deal with correspondence etc. or ... how she would order shopping from Sainsbury's."

Early in December when I returned from lunch with the Men's Walkers' Group, "I couldn't hear a sound from upstairs so sat and read for half an hour before suggesting it was time to go to the Advent Group. To my surprise and eventual anger, Lennie berated me, accused me of never enquiring after her, and she just wouldn't listen to my defence. She was so angry she refused to go to the second Advent Group, which was attended by six of us." On her birthday, I noted that "Lennie has received a rather unsatisfactory letter from her physio, who has sent it to our G.P. ... she is still upset about the physio's letter to our G.P." Later in the month, I noted Lennie's suggestion that we decline an invitation to go for an evening meal with an old friend now living some way away on account of her leg, our ageing and driving late on mid-winter nights.

In retrospect, 2014 was the year I first took on board the possibility that Lennie had dementia, although all our children had interpreted it at least a year previously. My diary that year suggested that though we were still close together, life was still rather busy. I became increasingly irritated when my times of study, reading and writing for conferences, etc. were so frequently interrupted. Lennie also frequently complained about my workload and failure to give her adequate attention. So, my thinking was that it would be interesting to see how I coped with increasing tensions in the years ahead. Otherwise, our lives were still full with holidays abroad and being active in our parish. What also became more obvious during 2014 were our increasing health problems. I had a painful leg and limited mobility and could no longer walk far. Lennie was still busy but there were signs of declining competences in the kitchen and so on. It will be interesting to see how things developed in 2015.

CHAPTER 3

The Year 2015

In August, 2015, I tried to explain what my diary was about. I noted that "my diary takes roughly half an hour per day, say three hours a week, which is equivalent to four to five weeks of work a year. So, readers in future years: this is my attempt to explain what life is like for an octogenarian in the second decade of the 21st Century. Later on the same day, I noted that I had sent "apologies that I wouldn't be attending the Caritas reception in the House of Lords on 8th October. Two decades ago, I would of course have attended, but now I feel it sensible to focus on what I am physically able to do in the parish, especially Justice and Peace and in preparing talks or papers." During the early part of the year, I spent a lot of time writing a paper about 'Religion and Politics', which I think might have been intended for The *Tablet,* but which came under a lot of criticism from colleagues and fellow parishioners.

My diary for New Year's Day gives an interesting overview of what 2015 might be like. At this stage of our lives, we were still reading the day's Mass readings from the Missal before getting up. We went to St. Edward's, Sutton Place, for 10 a.m. Mass, which was said by a frail and ageing former Anglican priest. There were a good number from our parish of St. Pius X's and also a former member of the Burpham parish of St. Mary's, "one of those embittered by the closing of St. Mary's, I think, in 2003". I noted that "it was nostalgic to be in the church where Stephen and Richard were baptised and where the then parish priest was so supportive when we were so desperate after we'd had four children in under six years, and where at Mass he'd cuddled Stephen as a toddler while I read the epistle and where he'd joked 'it is a venial sin to be late but a mortal sin to be early' and reassured Lennie by joking about Bridget, who'd crushed her pill and put it in Paddy's tea!" My sister, Sue, phoned from Italy. "I told her that we'd not yet booked for Verona because of the uncertainties of our knees and general health." The day ended with our moaning over Chelsea's defeat by Spurs, Lennie watching *Eastenders* and Stephen and I watching a rather disappointing, "shallow and not very convincing" Wallander on Stephen's laptop.

What seemed to be clear is that we were both still living pretty busy lives. We were attending Mass on four days each week: on Thursday, Saturday and Sunday mornings and Monday evenings at St. Pius X church. During the rest of the week, I was busy on my laptop writing papers. I was still attending two monthly U3A groups: Opera and a discussion group. I also attended the Catholic Bookham discussion group. Lennie and I were both regular special ministers at Mass and I used to drive Lennie into Guildford, where she used to take a disabled parishioner Holy Communion and also every Monday morning for her U3A keep-fit class. Both of us had aches and pains – Lennie with her knee, and me with a dodgy knee and also a weak and sore back. Occasionally, I used to do a bit of gardening, but my diary points out that my weakening back and legs left me exhausted after only twenty minutes or so.

In March, it looked as if life was going on as normal. We attended the funeral of Mary Comerford, a member of our Family Group. The group had been meeting monthly for over forty years. We visited Frances Allen, another member of the Family Group, when she was in a care home. We babysat for our granddaughter Iris and apart from my regular driving of Lennie to her U3A keep-fit class, I visited the Farmers' Market in central Guildford. In addition to my usual attendance at the U3A Opera group, I spent a day with a group of former Battersea Salesians from the late 1940s at a restaurant near Waterloo Station. Lennie kindly picked me up from Guildford mainline station in the evening. This shows that I was still sufficiently 'with it' to carry with me and use a mobile phone. During the month we also managed spontaneously to go to the Yvonne Arnaud Theatre on one occasion. Our evenings seemed to be often taken up with *House of Cards* on the TV. Apart from these normal, everyday events, I was asked to give a talk to a history group at the Guildford Institute, led by a former university colleague on 'The Catholic Church and the Family: Recent Developments'. There were only ten at the session. I took a quarter of an hour presenting my talk, but the discussion was quite lively.

In April, we seemed to be pursuing regular schedules. I attended both the U3A Opera Group and the Bookham Group, and we both attended the Family Group. After my Lenten reading, I continued reading another scripture commentary. I was disappointed that no Catholic paper reviewed my self-published book, *Follow me: Letters to my Grandchildren,* which was intended to be a simple version of my book on Catholic Social Thought. Another event bringing me down to earth was the notice from Bloomsbury that they had not sold a single copy of my edited *Catholics in England: 1950–2000* in the past year.

In May, there was the General Election result, which seemed to surprise most people and then the 70th anniversary of VE Day. We celebrated both Will's and Iris's birthdays. Gillian generally came to spend an hour or so with us for coffee after Mass on Sundays. I came to terms with the fact that The *Tablet* had rejected my article on 'Religion and Politics', though they had not informed me. The six-weekly Bookham group had a pleasant meeting and there was another at the U3A Discussion Group on assisted suicide. "I eventually gave my faith-based input based on the Catechism and Pope John Paul II in *Evangelium Vitae* and it was respectfully accepted, though I think it was one view out of eleven. I also got down to the long and slow business of clearing away those documents of Auntie Pat's which were not wanted, for archival purposes." On the Spring Bank Holiday, we went to visit the Surrey County Agricultural Show in Stoke Park. We also managed to go to the Yvonne Arnauld Theatre to see the excellent film, *Suite Française*. But "we seem both to have decided not to go to the diocesan jubilee celebration at Brighton Stadium. We feel we are both too old to cope with the coach travel and a very long day."

June turned out to have quite a few problems, which again consumed a great deal of time and so limited the amount of reading and study I could do in preparing articles or discussions. Lennie continued to take three or four elderly people to the lunch at the Merrow Methodist Hall, with volunteer support from the other churches. Early in the month I recorded that "today we had the tenth meeting of the Trustees of our two trusts (set up to support Stephen, who has schizophrenia, and provide him with an apartment in Cranleigh as long as he lives). A cheerful Richard and Gilly turned up; Andrew had sent apologies because of an ACTA (A Call to Action) meeting in Winchester. Gilly chaired the meeting and very professionally outlined the financial reports. Richard kindly offered to take the minutes. It was a friendly meeting. Gilly wasn't too pleased that it looks very much as if the main tasks will fall to her since Andrew doesn't live locally. Before he went, Richard gave us a flavour of the pressures of his work abroad and the difficulties of being expected to pay for hugely expensive meals in Finland. Gilly also told us of the pressures of her work with the NHS and that she had accumulated, I think, eighty hours of unpaid extra time. It was good to see and talk with her. I raised the worry that none of our grandchildren seemed to be committed Christians and she made the point that too much pressure on them would have been counterproductive."

The following day, "Richard unexpectedly turned up and immediately fell into my arms crying his heart out. He told us that his wife had had an affair with someone she'd met at work who was ten years younger than her. But she had said she loved him, and that she didn't love Richard." In the end he experienced a second divorce, but the sharing of care for Will and Iris worked out quite amicably.

Life continued to be pretty busy. In mid-June I again attended the Merrow Food Bank but again, nobody turned up. On a Friday we went to have lunch with two fellow parishioners, Norma and Ian, who also lived in our cul-de-sac, at the Clandon House Garden Centre and in the evening, with a large number of fellow parishioners, attended the Golden Jubilee celebration of our previous parish priest. "Afterwards I introduced myself to Bishop Moth, whose face lit up because I'd taught him at Wonersh. So, I can claim two bishops – i.e. including Archbishop Bernard Longley – whom I'd also taught at Wonersh."

In 2015, Armed Forces Day took place in Guildford, with a march due to go past Stoke Park. We sat and waited for the military marchers – all three services – to march past from High Street at midday. Stephen decided to return home quite quickly, but "Lennie and I continued to sit on our seats for a couple of hours, enjoying the gentle and friendly atmosphere and the six parachutists who came down in the main arena. For probably the last time, we therefore walked down about a mile to Stoke Park. We knew we had to walk home so decided to call it a day without the energy to go to the Fringe events. My knee was hurting quite a lot so it was a real relief to return home."

The following day, there was a parish picnic and I'd hoped to sell some of my books there. Unfortunately, it rained for a couple of hours, so this kept numbers down to around seventy, of whom about twenty had set up stalls, etc. "Fortunately, it stopped raining around 2.15 p.m. and I was able to put out my parish history and the two other books. I think I sold about five books." The following day, "I sat outside and read *Laudato Si*. My first reactions were of disappointment. It was a bit platitudinous and without much in the way of specifics for action at governmental or international level. Its dominant theme seemed to be the need to pursue and develop an ecological spirituality. We'll see; I must read it again."

In July it seems I first began to notice the dangers of hacking and cold calls. "I was phoned by someone claiming to be a Detective Chief Inspector dealing with fraud. When I asked him how I would know he was genuine, he said to phone 161 to confirm. Something made me phone the police. After Mass, I went to the bank to inform them of possible fraud. I was glad that there was no sign of anything wrong." Later, back home, "a policeman arrived to follow up my earlier call and took down the details of the first call, confirming it was probably an attempted fraud". This continued all day with another dodgy phone call and another policeman came. "Later, Surrey Police phoned to say that because I hadn't lost any money, I probably wouldn't hear from them again."

In July, we enjoyed a pleasant BBQ in the cul-de-sac. The pair of us were busy with regular tasks. In my case, I attended the Bookham Group lunch and discussion, the monthly Justice and Peace Group meeting, and the Food Bank, where I didn't feel I was being very helpful. In mid-month, Lennie "at midday, drove off to do her last ever chauffeuring of old people to lunch at the Methodist Hall. She says how much she gets out of it – the old people make a real effort to smarten themselves up and have smiling faces of enjoyment on this weekly social occasion." She was also still regularly taking Holy Communion to a disabled parishioner. I often had a sleep in the afternoon after lunch, outside in the sun when the weather was good. We went out several times this month. We had an evening meal at Jamie's before going to an excellent film in the Electric

Theatre. A couple of days later, we went out for a meal with friends in the parish, who drove us there and back. We had a nice meal. Conversation was fairly easy, but I had the sense that we didn't quite click that night and Lennie agreed when we returned home.

Early in the month, the Arundel & Brighton diocesan fiftieth anniversary was "celebrated at the Amex Stadium in Brighton. I feel guilty not being there with our new bishop, Richard Moth, but I/we feel we are a bit too old to have such a long day limited by bus timetables, etc. But I pray for the bishop and the diocese that they may discern the Lord's will and do it to the best of their ability." Later in the month we hosted the monthly meeting of the Family Group. Because of various ailments "there were only seven of us. I led the discussion, a little clumsily I suspect, on *Laudato Si* but there was a reasonable discussion." I was still regularly asked to be a special minister at Mass, though I "do wonder if I am getting a bit too wobbly on my feet. I use the rail on the wall beside the tabernacle to come down from the altar with the chalice."

In August, we had problems with our fire and security alarm and had to get it sorted out. We went for a walk over the Chantries and had a meal outside on a lovely day in Chilworth and we took Richard and three of his children for lunch at Carlo's, near Newlands Corner. We went out for a meal with friends to celebrate their birthdays and we went to see a couple of films at the Yvonne Arnaud Theatre. I noted for the first time how much I enjoyed watching on TV the various performances of the André Rieu orchestra. Lennie and I made our last long journey to Weston-super-Mare to attend the funeral of my cousin's husband. During the month we were concerned about the Labour Party leadership election, and I spent some time reading some of Jack Dominian's books, having been asked to make a contribution to his memorial later in the year.

Early in the month, I recorded that Stephen showed us his latest blog with its film of his paintings. We then coped with at least an hour-long near monologue about it, which I thought too intensely intellectual to understand, and then a prolonged discussion about why his Barcelona experience was so different from Andrew's in Lleida. At times the exchange became quite angry, and I eventually switched off, but Lennie was very good at explaining our uncertainties. On the last Sunday of the month, I tried, totally unsuccessfully, to respond to Stephen's series of three or four blogs on political radicalisation, etc. I found his language difficult and seemingly full of non-sequiturs. But it may be that I'm just thick!

September was another fairly busy month. I noted, in particular, that I seemed to be so tired that I slept for an hour or more practically every afternoon. We considered the breakdown of Richard's marriage and tried to encourage reconciliation, but with little sign of success. In the evenings, we watched practically every match Chelsea were playing and I continued to be interested in the *Downton Abbey* series, which gave some idea of social change after WW1. At weekends we watched sport, especially the Rugby World Cup. During the month we went to Wisley Garden Centre for lunch and out for meals with friends, and one evening with Richard and his four children. We spent a grandparents' day in Cranleigh at Will and Iris's school, though we wondered "at spending only twenty minutes with the grandchildren in five hours in Cranleigh!" Towards the end of the month, we drove to Royston for the marriage of our niece Emily to Stephen, the father of nine! "The couple seemed happy and in love and we wish them well. It was lovely to see Sue and Mario, both looking very well, Ann and Peter, both in fine form, and other members of the family who all seemed pleased to see us." Ten days into September, Lennie and I made our way to the St. Bride Foundation, where there was a celebration of the life of Jack Dominian. I had been asked to make a four-minute contribution. It was good to meet old friends. I talked "about Jack's contribution as a lay prophet. It seemed to go down quite well".

We were concerned "about the earthquake in the Labour Party, about Corbyn's election as leader". Later in the month, I observed that "basically the world of Old Labour, lifelong jobs and powerful working-class solidarity, has gone in the era of downsizing, outsourcing and globalisation". The issues of poverty and inequality dominated my reading and writing in September. "I was impressed by Alan Johnson's *This Boy,* which as a piece of social history reminded me of just how awful urban poverty was right up to the 1960s and 70s. Help me, Lord, to be genuinely and courageously fearless in opposing unjust, sinful social structures." My contribution to the Bookham Group was based on *Laudato Si.*

October was another fairly busy month. It was the month we finally got rid of the palm tree, which had deteriorated rapidly recently. During the month, I completed the task of ridding our garden of rats, but we were still adding our food waste to the compost bin behind the shed. Our Family Group meeting this month was in Croydon and I drove Lennie and me there and back. We went to the Yvonne Arnaud Theatre, but when a fellow parishioner invited us to join him at Glyndebourne, I noted that "the prices were up to £160 per seat and I'd have to hire a morning suit. Both Lennie and I feel uncomfortable with that; it's not in our league, so we declined." A lot of time this month was spent sorting out around 370 photographs and selecting those to put into albums.

In October, I attended, along with several former colleagues, the funeral service of my former head of department, Asher Tropp, who was very supportive of the research I pursued into post-war English Catholicism. "There was much emphasis on the way Asher encouraged many and influenced the development of empirical sociology with Master's courses in research methods, etc. One of the things which came out was evidence of the general commercialisation of academic life, which is no longer a pleasant communal exercise, but with uncertain jobs, no more pensions based on final salaries but increasing insecurity, etc." During the month, Lennie was cooking some Christmas puddings. I struggled to read Eamon Duffy's *The Stripping of the Altars* and did some work planting bulbs in the garden and tidying up the shed. As usual I attended the U3A's Opera Group and the Discussion Group, the Bookham Group and the Food Bank.

Sadly, we had quite a difficult row with Andrew, which lasted some time because we had not invited his partner Caroline's two children to join us in celebrating Lennie's 80th birthday celebration because we did not regard them as our grandchildren. He and Richard both failed to attend the half-yearly meeting of the Trustees, but with Gillian's help we managed to cope quite well. During this month, we in Guildford celebrated the first twenty-five years of the 'No.5' project to help the homeless. We also went to a classical concert in G-Live, saw a film at the Odeon and had a couple of meals out, and at Newman's and Elgar's *Dream of Gerontius*. I recognised that I was a 'sleeping member' of the Catholic Union and I continued to struggle to read Duffy's book.

In November, we had a meeting with our solicitor to consider Lasting Powers of Attorney. She was "charming and helpful. She talked us through the two types: (a) buildings and finance which we'd signed up to in 2006, and (b) the health and welfare type. She was helpful in explaining the safeguards and Lennie's concerns."

I have often felt uncomfortable that three of the four oldest grandchildren refused to participate in the confirmation programmes. In July, Katie challenged me and I recorded in my diary: "She says she is so tired with a 4/5 days/week work that she can't go to Mass. As a grandfather, what can I do except chide her and try to encourage her? But these days the response seems to be 'I'm old enough to make my own decisions' and I'm left with prayer as my only help."

The Justice and Peace Group arranged three 'hustings' in three of our Guildford churches in advance of the General Election. In mid-April, "Lennie and I went over to St. Mary's for the hustings meeting with the Liberal Democrat, Green and UKIP Candidates. It was quite good – about thirty-one there, eleven from St. Pius' and again Pat Jones and I tried to provoke serious debates, for example about aid, the E.U., and inequality. I noted that Lennie had done well to come with me. She is suffering with her knee." On a Thursday morning Mass where "I was a eucharistic minister. I was surprised at the large proportion who didn't receive the chalice. It seems to be growing."

Richard had kindly bought me two tickets for Fathers' Day to go and watch a Surrey vs Sussex cricket match at Arundel. He was unable to come so I took Stephen and we saw one of the most frightening accidents when two players attempted to make a catch and crashed into each other's heads. "Both players seemed to be unconscious and after three quarters of an hour, two ambulances came to take them away. We applauded them and it was a relief when both players lifted their hands. To my surprise, the match was then abandoned."

The monthly U3A Discussion Group meeting was attended by "about twelve of us and the weather was nice enough for us to sit outside in the sun ... We had reasonable shared food and I had plenty of wine! I ventured to suggest we use the occasion to frame next year's programme and suggested the theme 'Inequality', which I will work on during the summer for our September meeting." I had been reading Piketty and other sources such as Atkinson, which has the appropriate subtitle *What can be done?* I also planned to discuss it at the next meeting of our Family Group. Inequality was the prime focus of my reading and study for a large part of 2015.

In September, I managed to arrange a special welcome to national and ethnic minorities in our parish on Racial Justice Sunday. We gave a short welcome statement to people from seven or eight different nationalities to express in their own or original languages from the foot of the altar at the start of Mass, with the agreement of the priest. Unfortunately, only a week later, "the choir leader for the church as a 'People of God' director of music, had written a letter of resignation, having had a dreadful experience with the clergy over recent years. It is a sad reflection of clergy-lay collaboration in the last year or so, and the clerical authoritarianism of our former Anglican priests. Where has Fr. Brian's (our first parish priest's) 'People of God' post-Vatican parish gone? There was a huge proportion of new people at Mass this morning, a reminder that we belong to yesterday's generation and it's time for the new generation to take over." Two days earlier, the parish had celebrated how Fr. Brian was "always promoting the reforms from lay readers and special ministers to female servers, etc."

On the last Sunday of September, "the new head teacher at St. Thomas's Primary School was inducted. The church was packed, and the school provided a lovely and conscientious choir of forty or so children. The induction ceremony itself was a novelty and involved the diocesan education secretary and a highly inclusive set of commitments from the head, teachers, pupils, governors who stood up to identify themselves as they all made their commitments and, finally, the parents and then parishioners. A very moving and impressive religious commitment and occasion."

In October there was a meeting called by our ex-Anglican priest to discuss the Monday night services. "I felt obligated to go and express the views of a good few people of our generation. Help me to be blunt without being offensive. In the end the priest was ill and the meeting was chaired by a member of the Medugorje group, who promised to pass on our views to the priest. There were twenty-one present, of whom at least eleven objected to the Chaplet intruding into the Exposition rather than silence. I suspect the chair will give a rather watered-down version to the priest."

Our irritation with the former Anglican priests was promoted when in November there was no notice of our long-standing annual 10% collection for three charities (local, national and international) in the Newsletter and only a casual comment at Mass. Also, there was the first meeting of the Guildford Parish Council (of the formerly four separate parishes), where the members had been invited by the clergy without a parish meeting or election. I noted that "this is yet another issue about the rapid, clerical-led changes which have taken place in our parish in the past few years, which appear to have angered many members of the parish and which seem to have reversed the post-Vatican notions of the 'People of God' and 'collaborative ministries' which were built up until roughly six years ago". I led one of the seminars on the encyclical *Laudato Si*, which again had not been supported by the clergy. At the monthly meeting of the Justice and Peace Group, I noted that "there is no sign that there is a new generation willing to take over. Must the group die again?" But there was an evening meal in the parish hall which aimed to raise funds for refugees, which was very successful.

Early in December, on the Feast of the Immaculate Conception, Lennie celebrated her 80th. birthday. On the previous Saturday, we went to the Bull's Head in East Clandon with our four children, six grandchildren, one spouse and one partner. "The meal was excellent ... The service was unobtrusive, friendly and helpful ... In sum, it was generally agreed to have been a delightful family occasion." Later in the month we took Will and Iris to the pantomime *Jack and the Beanstalk* at the Yvonne Arnaud.

The rest of the month was pretty busy, and we went about a fortnight without a television until a new one was installed. We attended the AGM of the Oak Tree Gardens cul-de-sac, a pleasant opportunity to meet our neighbours. Rather to my surprise, all the active parishioners I contacted with a view to getting information which would facilitate an updating of the parish history were reluctant to participate and didn't want to create tensions between the clergy and laity. So, I wasn't able to follow up on this idea. The Amnesty International 'Write for Rights' campaign proceeded as usual. I visited one of our Family Group in a care home following a hip operation. Lennie attended the choir for possibly the last time. I took her to the G-Live to see a performance of *The Nutcracker* by St. Petersburg Classic Ballet. On our 55th wedding anniversary, we had a fun day down at Southsea before returning to go to the Odeon to watch a Cold War thriller. I was a special minister at Mass on Christmas Day when we went over to Gillian's for "a very pleasant five or six hours with them". The following day we drove over to Richard's, who had prepared "a lovely Christmas lunch. It was good to be with him and all his four children." During the month we also enjoyed two meals out with fellow parishioners.

Lennie continued to be "deeply hurt and angry and felt betrayed" when she heard me discussing an email from Gillian expressing concern about Lennie's memory loss and supposed Alzheimer's. Lennie was angered not only by what she saw as Gilly's stab in the back but also by what she saw as my betrayal of our 'oneness' in trying to defend Gilly and understand what I saw as concern that Lennie has treatment at an early stage. Lennie was also informed that her knee problem was due to arthritis. Her "memory is getting bad. She can't remember what day or year or month it is and spends ages looking at her diary. Help me, Lord, to be sensitive, gentle and patient."

The year started quite normally, though I was quite unwell for a while until unexpectedly, after attending Mass on the third Sunday of the year, "where I read some fine bidding prayers and was also an active collector for *Pax Christi* afterwards". But soon after returning home "I had a frantic dose of 'shivers' so badly that after twenty minutes or so Lennie phoned 111 and they sent an ambulance. In the end, I was put in the Royal Surrey Hospital and stayed in a cardiac ward with urinary concerns and antibiotics for a week." In April, my G.P. "told me my back X-rays confirmed I had numerous problems. He kindly demonstrated with a model and gave me the impression that I would have periodic problems with my back and could only control the pain. Thank God for the codeine tablets! While there I told him about my right knee. He said I wasn't too old to have a knee replacement, but we agreed not to pursue it at this stage since it wasn't keeping me awake at night."

In the same month, I seemed to lose my temper quite a lot and it seems possible that this was reflecting increasing difficulties I was having with Lennie and her dementia. There were times when "she accused me of never doing any shopping – more or less 'what do you contribute in this house?'" On other occasions she accused me of bullying, but her memory did seem to be deteriorating. For example, she "apparently forgot she was taking a couple to the Methodist Hall lunch today though she did take them home afterwards. Her diary keeping is pretty poor at the moment. But she is a great lass."

Similar sorts of issues also arose in June when we again had a couple of angry exchanges. On the first occasion she called me "an arrogant yob". I noted that I was less sure now about my 'denial' of Lennie's illness to our G.P. On the second occasion, I recorded that "I must learn to live with Lennie's almost infantile lack of capability about our finances. She didn't pick up the different account numbers and sort codes of 'our' two accounts (though both joint) and doesn't seem able to read accounts, e.g. hundreds from thousands, decimal points and so on. Very frustrating. It seems I've just got to live with such limitations. She is so good in other ways."

In the same month, after the Justice and Peace meeting, I recorded that "I had a coffee with Lennie, whose memory really is going. She doesn't know what day or month it is and whether she should find tomorrow's dental appointment in March or May. I hope there is no serious deterioration. Most routine things she manages perfectly well – shopping, car rides for the elderly and so on. Please help us in our old age, Lord."

In early August, I reflected on Lennie's and my increasing memory loss, particularly relating to people's names. "I can't remember names though I often recall the first letter. We are both experiencing it but I see now what the children said some months ago: Lennie does repeat herself and it sometimes irritates me. Please, Lord, help me to control my responses in order the better to follow You in our final and declining years." A couple of days later, after Lennie had three times asked me the same question, "I rather exasperatedly asked, 'Haven't you been listening to me? This is the third time you've asked.' To which she retorted that I was authoritarian and a bully. This is not the first time she's said this and I find it hurtful but also a reminder that I've got to be more patient, which I don't find easy. Help me, Lord."

Later in the month, I reflected that Lennie not only doesn't remember names, but also can't recall what month or day it is. She repeats herself over and over again and asks over and over again what day the funeral is or when are we going to

Alsace. Last week she went to check the front door in the middle of the night. We joke about her not walking down the street in her nightie – yet. If there was a chance, I'd have to remove the key from the door at night. None of this is currently serious, though it is probably an indication that we are ageing, and difficult times might be on their way. Each day we pray that we may discern God's will and carry it out to the best of our ability. Amen to that. Later I added: "The other day Andrew expressed concern about the steepness of our stairs. True, but we are not moving again and if necessary, will install a chair ride – hopefully."

In September, I noted that "Lennie is forgetting all sorts of things these days. It is difficult to identify closely aspects of her loss of memory, repetitiveness and general slowing down. For example, it took her nearly one and three quarters of an hour to do a forty-plus pounds shop at Sainsburys." More positively I recorded that "Stephen is a lovely lad and, very unobtrusively, he is adjusting to our steady ageing – preparing the vegetables for lunch; giving me a gin and tonic at midday; making coffee and washing up. Bless him, Lord and give him a good week." I was still being asked to be a special minister and I noted that "I can still manage it with a half-full chalice". Another sign of my awareness of my ageing was that "I made a very slow start to thinning the books in my library and started filling boxes for the parish, a charity, and a university. So, I started putting books into three boxes ... at least it was a start."

We weren't too well in October. I had a nasty nosebleed over several days and once had wet pyjamas early in the month. Lennie wasn't sleeping well and had chest pains once. "Lennie's teeth are paining her in spasms. She takes pills but gets them mixed up ... She spends more and more time going round in circles. She gets one or two charity requests each day and has to ask which day or month it is when writing a cheque. I'm becoming more aware of our ageing." Before they left us after a visit, Richard and his eldest son, Luke "tried to make me respond to what they see as Lennie's rapid memory deterioration. Perhaps, since I am with her all the time, I'm not so aware of a rapid deterioration."

In November both Lennie and I acknowledged that we were decidedly 'creaky'. Gillian, Stephen and Richard continued to express "concerns about what they saw as Lennie's apparent Alzheimer's disease. I reluctantly have to agree that Stephen was right to warn me to expect this increasingly and I must try not to get so frustrated and angry about it. Dear Lord, help me to show love for Lennie by walking with her through whatever difficulties we have to face in the years ahead ... Her memory loss or 'scatterbrain' has become more obvious to me, and I hope I am beginning to adapt to the changing reality and become more patient and understanding."

In the middle of the month Lennie and I went to a seminar on Alzheimer's which "wasn't quite what I'd expected and was mainly about the drugs expected to be on the market in four or five years. As someone said: 'Too late for our generation'!"

After a relatively small amount of gardening in December, I admitted: "sounds trivial but actually – and sadly – it is about my physical limit these days. My back and right knee are getting weaker. It is the reality of the ageing process." Later in the month, I again noted: "My right knee seems to be deteriorating quite steadily. I hope it is OK for our Italian Lakes holiday in four months' time." Lennie's dentist had said there was nothing wrong with her tooth. Later in the month I recorded, "Lennie has her memory test tomorrow and I made the bad mistake of saying her memory is going a bit. She was angry and it seemed like denial. Please Lord, help me be more sensitive and supportive even though it seems clear to me that her memory is going and she is repeating herself over and over again. Help me, Lord.

Lennie took the hated or feared memory test" and arranged to see her G.P. in a fortnight.

A few days later I recorded that "it does now seem clear to me that Lennie is becoming more forgetful but also repetitive. She keeps referring to the coming Easter festival, not Christmas, gets tied up in knots about days of the week, repeatedly expresses angry views about Andrew's protests that O and G [Oli and Georgie] aren't treated as his 'children', increasingly puts cutlery in wrong places, and so on. Sometime during Mass today, she asked if I knew she loved me. She is a love and I do hope, Lord, You will guide me so that I love her and give her all the care and understanding she deserves."

We managed to have three holidays abroad in 2015. Firstly, we had a week's holiday in Tenerife to celebrate Stephen's 50th birthday in January. We ended up in a hotel just opposite the church near the centre of Puerto de la Cruz. In some respects, it was quite a stressful week. In the first case I had to drive the car from the airport to our hotel in the north of the island and we missed a turning at one point but managed, in the end, to find it. There was no parking at the hotel, so we had to park in a beach car park and keep fingers crossed. Early in the week we discovered a scrape on the side of the car and I wondered about insurance cover and was amazed when on returning the car I was told it was perfect. During the week I read Thomas a Kempis's *The Imitation of Christ,* fifty years after I'd first read it. It was "full of guidance on humility, love of truth and dependence on the grace of God". Stephen "didn't want to go charging round Tenerife in the car – for which I was relieved – but really seemed to enjoy just sitting in the square sketching with pens. And Lennie and I were grateful to have been able to attend Mass every day in the lovely church with its humble priest." We also enjoyed swimming in the small pool on the roof of the hotel.

Our second break was a brief visit in July to Verona, where we stayed in the Hotel Milano, not far from the Arena, where we saw two operas, *Tosca* and *Don Giovanni*. My sister Sue and husband Mario came all the way from Ivrea to see us and we had a very pleasant time together and a couple of meals in the Piazza Bra just outside the Arena. "I kept ensuring Mario was kept involved in spite of our language difficulties." We also met for an hour or more in the Piazza Bra after *Don Giovanni* and chatted away over ice creams for over an hour before going to bed around 2 a.m. During the day, because it was so hot, 30°C or more, we enjoyed just sitting in the park watching the world go by. On the trip I also re-read Graham Greene's *The Power and the Glory,* which I thought "gave a perfect reflection of true love, solidarity and Christianity and its underlying theme: the goodness of ordinary people".

Our third trip abroad was to Alsace for a week in September. We stayed in an hotel in Obernai and had to climb forty-two steps to get to our room. But "over five days we saw something of the cities of Obernai, Strasbourg, Colmar and Freiberg, and were made aware of the differences between northern and southern Alsace and the beautiful valleys of the Black Forest. But it has been physically tiring. There are many friendly people on the trip and we've enjoyed their company ... We also attended two Masses while here and I thought the priest a lovely, pastoral man. But the world which generated the money, labour and skill necessary to build beautiful cathedrals has changed and these cathedrals simply remain lovely tourist attractions. The 'faithful' who still attend Mass are probably regarded as a bit freakish, oddities in a secular age." During the week, which was quite stressful with swapping trains in Paris, etc. and Lennie's obsession with shopping for gifts for Will and Iris and her obvious memory loss, I noted that "she hardly remembers where we have been. But we've had a good week and seen lots of things, even if we are not as mobile as other people. So, thank you, Lord, for that and for her. But I'm strongly inclined to think that this has been the last holiday of this sort we will undertake."

At one stage during our early morning prayers, Lennie said "'Richard, who is he?' I saw this as a sign that Lennie really is losing some parts of her memory. If this is the case, oh Lord, please help me to travel with her with patience and perseverance." At the end of May, I wrote in my diary: "What are the important things to record from the perspective of trying to record what life was like in 2015 for an eighty-two-year-old Catholic? One thing which I guess is not appreciated is the passion of sexual love even at this age."

An indication of my post-Vatican thinking was apparent in a comment I made about our love-making in January: "In the middle of the night Lennie encouraged me to make love. Since I'm no longer able to penetrate these days I genuinely tried to please Lennie and maximise her enjoyment of our love-making using my fingers, though I have mixed responses in respect of the Church's traditional clerical-led teachings on masturbation as opposed to more enlightened post Vatican II viewpoints ... I'm glad to say she seemed satisfied with our trying to express our love for each other." Just before we went on our holiday to Tenerife, I prayed, "Help me, Lord, during our holiday to do my best to be kind and loving to Lennie and Stephen".

In the middle of June, I recorded that "I must make this about the last time I reflect on our love-making ... Lennie observed that we have become more passionate in our recent years. This time I started caressing Lennie's breasts and she reacted very positively, so it was inevitable that we proceed to full love-making. But note our limitations. Lennie and I no longer ever have a climax. But Lennie seems to, so I try and respond." In July, "Lennie noted this morning that our love-making at the moment is more satisfying than it has ever been in all our married years".

The next day I noted: "There is so much love between us and tenderness that I can't feel it is wrong, yet we have both expressed concerns that we have sinned. Or are these concerns simply the result of an older type of Catholic education about sex? We are nearing the end of our attempts to make love, though I'm sure caressing will continue."

In mid-December I recorded, after trying to watch Chelsea in a Champions League game, that we went off to bed early and "in the end, I realised that a gabby Lennie was infinitely better than being alone. So we flirted with each other and I actively promoted love-making and to my astonishment we both achieved complete satisfaction for the first time for four or five years. The Lord is good and it was mutually enjoyed."

I have a sense that 2015 was a turning point in Lennie's and my married life together. Clearly, I came to acknowledge Lennie's memory issues and was open to her getting appropriate medical assistance. At the same time Lennie's effective denial was a fact which I had to learn to live with. But I wasn't a natural carer, and I frequently became irritated and provoked her anger. But I hope it was also clear that we loved each other. All our children kept pushing me to do something. But what? Even getting her to see our G.P. wasn't easy. In the meantime, we were both leading quite busy lives. We were both still involved as special ministers at Mass and Lennie continued to take Holy Communion to a disabled parishioner, though her chauffeuring of old people to the lunch at the Merrow Methodist Hall came to an end with her 80th birthday. She continued to participate in the U3A Keep-Fit Group but was getting more critical of the large number of groups I continued to participate in. But we were still going out occasionally for meals or the Yvonne Arnaud, Odeon films or G-Live concerts. We continued to go on continental holidays, though I think we were beginning to sense that our health and mobility were declining and were both aware that death might not be too far away. We prayed to the Lord to guide us through our final years.

CHAPTER 4
The Year 2016

The January diaries gave the impression that the lives of Lennie and I were carrying on much as usual. Both of us were busy. We went to Mass nearly four times each week; usually in the mornings on Thursdays, Saturdays and Sundays, with an evening Mass at St. Pius X's on Mondays. Before Mass on Thursdays, a small group of us met for about twenty minutes for a reflection on the day's scripture readings. For a couple of octogenarians, we were still active in our love-making, on average every five days. In January, we celebrated Stephen's 51st birthday. I also informed members of the Sociology of Religion Group about the funeral of Professor John Fulton, a long-term contributor to Sociology of Religion, and we both attended it. I tried hard to fit in regular reading or drafting of talks or papers, but Lennie wasn't always helpful. She was still a keen follower of *Eastenders* on the evening television. On the other hand, I preferred realistic dramas, such as Scandinavian and also French police dramas, and tended to avoid the bulk of TV "rubbish", so much of which "seems aimless and tabloid". I tended to fall asleep regularly after lunch and only managed short spells of gardening. We attended the monthly meeting of our Family Group and had a meal out with friends, and I still attended the Food Bank at Merrow. Of course, additionally, we watched practically every Chelsea match on television and other sports, such as rugby, most weekends with Stephen.

In the parish, Lennie was still taking Holy Communion to a disabled parishioner and she was angry when a coordinator suggested she might be replaced because of her memory loss. She reacted angrily when I proposed attending the annual diocesan Justice and Peace Assembly, so I withdrew.

I helped lead the Liturgy of the Word for Year 6 of St. Thomas's Primary School when they turned up but there was no Mass. Our ex-Anglican priest again annoyed members of the Justice and Peace Group by not allowing "Pat Jones to speak at the end of Mass for Peace Sunday ... and he only read the first paragraph of the Pax Christ prayer. Frances Allen challenged him on this but was more or less told to stop moaning and be a good girl!" Much of January I spent working on notes intended for the next Family Group and my Bookham Group on '125 Years since *Rerum Novarum*'. "Lennie was pretty critical about my notes, saying it was too academic and inappropriate for the Family Group; that I was showing off, etc". After she'd been to see our G.P., "to our surprise he'd said Lennie had done better in the test than expected for a woman of eighty. We were both delighted ... I get irritated every time Lennie interrupts whatever I'm doing but where would I be without her?"

Our daughter, Gillian, used to visit us for coffee and a natter nearly every Sunday after Mass. On the last Sunday of January, the former Anglican priest's "homily was organised round a 'pass the parcel' theme. Faith has to be passed on from parents to their children and then to their grandchildren." When Gilly came for coffee, I asked her how she interpreted this, thinking that neither of her children seemed particularly committed. This led to a fascinating and almost passionate articulation of generational change. Whereas Lennie's and my generation were not allowed to speak unless spoken to, Gilly argued we had brought them up strictly to follow our decisions, while they had recognised the social reality that Britain was no longer a Christian society and that their children were being brought up in a secular society. So, at the age of sixteen, Katie and Douglas were allowed to make up their own minds whether or not to go to church and to choose where to go – they all prefer the more communal and friendly Holy Trinity (Anglican) atmosphere to the crowded and more formal St. Pius X. Interesting and perceptive, but also worrying from the perspective of passing on the faith. In March I added: "Gilly was impressed that when she went to Communion in the Anglican Holy Trinity Church, the priest said, 'The Body of Christ, Gillian'".

In February life went on as usual. But we went to our solicitor and signed up to legal powers of attorney. I spent a long time reading through a manuscript, but after a long discussion with a publisher, "I had a horrible feeling that I hadn't done much in the way of making suggestions which an academic supervisor might have made. But I did suggest the need for a clearer thesis and argument and our discussion threw up issues such as historical context – e.g. globalisation and post-war secularisation of the U.K." But I am glad to say that the book was subsequently published. A lot of my time was spent trying to find space to read the 900 pages of Tolstoy's *War and Peace,* which I saw as a "great novel about the triviality of so much of our lives and the reality of death and the love of God. Other themes included hypocrisy, the evil of war and the nature of marital relations in an aristocratic society where wealth was more important than love."

Lennie and I attended the funeral of a fellow parishioner, but "I was really quite glad that Lennie didn't want to go to the reception. There is something about the Catenians which puts me off or makes me feel uncomfortable, in spite of the great support they give each other at funerals." I attended a lecture at the Guildford Institute given by a former colleague on gender and ageing issues. I went for an appointment with my G.P., who told me that "my X-rays confirmed I have severe osteoarthritis in my right knee but I was easily talked into continuing the paracetamol, plus a gel treatment to see if I can cope. Physio treatment was also agreed." At the monthly meeting of the Family Group, "my introducing a discussion on Catholic Social Teaching 125 years after *Rerum Novarum* led to an interesting discussion, mainly about ways of tackling the refugee problem". The main item on the agenda of the monthly meeting of the Justice and Peace Group "was how to promote a 'live simply' parish over the next year".

Before the first Thursday morning Mass, Lennie led "today's scripture reflection – she did it beautifully, unpretentiously and sensitively". On Ash Wednesday, one of our former Anglican priests had "finished giving everyone a black cross on their foreheads with burned palm and water, and at the end he walked from the altar down the aisle and knelt before me and asked me to repeat the prayer and put on a cross on his forehead. I felt very humble and full of love for a priest I don't always agree with, but who is always prepared to dialogue. Be with him, Lord." Late in the month, Lennie and I both attended a Lenten House Group and noted: "We both felt it rather boring and that the York booklet wasn't helpful in suggesting leads for discussion". At the end of the month, after Mass with the other former Anglican priest, I recorded that "in spite of his tendency to clerical authoritarianism, he is genuinely trying to make us all more sensitive to our position in an increasingly aggressive secular and materialistic society".

March was a fairly typical month. Every morning before getting up, Lennie and I read the day's Mass with the help of *Bible Alive* before praying for family members, living or dead. We celebrated Luke's twenty-third birthday and had a pleasant meal with Richard, Luke, Will and Iris and enjoyed an evening out with Pat Jones and her husband, Patrick. During the month, we were concerned about Stephen's savings accounts and arranged that Gillian took over the managing of the British Gas account for his apartment. Every morning, I had to clear about twenty or more emails and I struggled to sell surplus tickets for the opera in Verona, which I had somehow over-booked. Most days, I worked on preparing talks broadly on Catholic Social Teaching. By lunchtime, I was typically exhausted and after lunch I nearly always had a sleep for an hour or so. We were beginning to get regular calls about our ten solar panels, and it was always difficult to discern how reliable the different companies were.

On a Monday in mid-April, I took the train from London Road station to Waterloo and then walked with difficulty a couple of hundred yards to a restaurant where a group of Old Salesians from the late 1940s used to meet every year. Several of us used to play in either or both the football and cricket First XIs. Two Relton brothers used to come down from West Hartlepool for the day and another came from Merseyside; another was over from Canada visiting relatives; another was a priest in Kent I think; and our coordinator came from Berlin to visit relatives in London. The two brothers "led us in a rousing version of the school anthem. This drew applause from three ladies further back and when we were leaving, they invited us to sing it rousingly again ... our coordinator gave a round-up of his memories of each of us. I felt this could quite easily be my last appearance at this group, so I took the opportunity to propose a thank-you to him, without whose commitment and coordination these meetings wouldn't take place."

When I asked Gillian "if she would consider becoming a eucharistic minister, she declined, saying she felt stretched as much as she wanted to be. She was going to have to look after the trusts because Andrew and Richard wouldn't. We have often thought that Gilly feels discriminated against in our family." In mid-April, Lennie realised she had been subjected to fraud and fortunately the bank agreed to refund her. The police came round to interview her. One of our parishioners, Neville Vincent, kindly passed on his copy of the *Observer* at Mass every Thursday. I continued to drive Lennie into Guildford every Monday morning for her U3A keep-fit classes and Lennie continued to take Holy Communion to a disabled parishioner. We had pleasant visits from Katie and from Richard, Will and Iris. We are grateful to them all. Meanwhile, environmental concerns were beginning to come onto the agenda of the parish Justice and Peace Group. I struggled to do regular gardening with my back and leg ailments. A lot of my 'work' time was spent preparing to present Beethoven's *Fidelio* to the U3A Opera Group and write an update of the parish history. Our youngest grandson's first Holy Communion was shortly after his birthday in May. We had a very pleasant day with them all. I gave what was probably my last talk at the Guildford Institute History Group on the Church since Vatican II. "It generated some interesting, though often tangential, questions." On the bank holiday, we went to Mass at St. Edward's. On the spur of the moment, we went to see *The Merry Widow* at the Yvonne Arnaud and we had a meal out with some friends. In May, I think we finally coped with the regular visits of rats in the garden. The local authority pest controller was very helpful. We also completed the process of getting Legal Powers of Attorney.

A lot of my time on the laptop was spent "editing and adding to my updated parish history, now calling it *Parish Suppressed*, focusing on three issues: (1) the shortage of priests and adjusting to that; (2) changing authority styles and (3) generational shifts". In mid-May I noted the anger which some of our active parishioners felt when "no mention was made of the evening ecumenical service 'Together in Christ'. I opened up my 'Parish Suspended' file and added five or six examples of irritating clerical authority which I wished to record." On the 31st May I recorded that "today is the last day of our separate St. Pius X parish status. Tomorrow we are 'suppressed'". We became part of the Catholic Parish of Guildford (C.P.G.) along with St. Mary's and St. Edward's.

On the first Saturday in June, we had our six-monthly meeting of the Trustees of the two trusts set up to look after Stephen to the end of his life. In particular, they acted as landlords, renting him an apartment, 'Penrose' in Cranleigh. One of the issues which had concerned the Trustees for some time was coping with damp in some of the walls. On this occasion I recorded that "Andrew chaired the meeting but was quite blunt about the trusts not being his top priority. As Gilly was taking on all the responsibility for the financial and insurance tasks, I could understand her feeling aggrieved. But she didn't aggravate the situation and in future we agreed to circulate notices about meetings about five weeks in advance to ensure a fuller attendance. Richard, for example, wasn't present today because he'd 'double-booked' a break to take the children camping. Hopefully, Andrew's minutes will reflect some of these issues."

One of the jobs I did in June was to accompany Benedict when he was accused of plagiarism with his dissertation at Chichester University. "But the interview panel was very relaxed and aimed at being constructive. True, he had done wrong, but it wasn't over-emphasised while requiring him to re-submit his Draft Dissertation Proposal and penalising his module to 40%." We had a visit from Katie the day before she went off to the U.S.A. for twelve weeks.

I continued to drive a couple of fellow parishioners to the weekly meeting for a pub lunch with the parish Men's Walking Group. In June we joined our neighbours for a BBQ around the central oak tree in our cul-de-sac. As usual, it was friendly, and we enjoyed it as we offered our best wishes to one of them leaving shortly before he was due to be ordained in the Church of England. We also managed to go to the Yvonne Arnaud Theatre, enjoyed a BBQ at Gillian's, a lunch with Richard, Benedict, Will and Iris, and a lunch at the Clandon Garden Centre.

The big political event of the month was the Brexit vote. A fellow parishioner brought me a couple of Labour Party red 'Vote Remain 23 June' T-shirts. I even wore them at a couple of Masses in the parish. One of our fellow parishioners emailed us on 'Black Friday'. We were devastated. After Mass on Sunday, our parish priest "told me he was surprised I wasn't dressed in black because of the Referendum result!" Towards the end of June, "I decided to go to the Labour Party meeting to discuss the implications of the Brexit vote and Jeremy Corbyn's leadership. I'm so pleased I went. It was far and away the best political meeting I've ever attended. There were sixty to seventy members present, including a sizeable number who'd only joined recently because of Jeremy Corbyn. I made about the fifteenth contribution, explaining that I'd joined over fifty years ago seeking the common good, solidarity and equality. But the working class had changed, for example millions fewer workers in manufacturing, and we needed to focus on the issues of globalisation, climate change and ISIS. But we needed to dialogue with workers and other political parties and be pragmatic to gain government to implement our policies." I did wonder if this would be my last meeting. During the month I also attended a retired staff tea party at the university, where we were "addressed by the new President and Vice Chancellor, Max Lu". He was followed by a fellow parishioner who "quizzed us how best to improve relations between the university and 'the town'. I suspect we were mainly too old to be useful with suggestions."

I spent a large part of the month working on an updating of our parish history. Sadly, some of the major figures, including the previous parish chairs and treasurer, declined to give me any evidence of their grievances, arguing that it was better to move on and avoid unhelpful splits between the clergy and laity. During the month I recorded fears about my laptop.

Occasionally, Stephen's concerns exploded, and we had to cope with them as best we could. For example, on one day I recorded that Stephen "before long, was getting oppressed by his voices, concerns about exhibitions and galleries and so on. We had to tread warily and at one stage I was told just to listen when he was going on and on about Nietzsche." I sent off an email for him and decided not to go to the Men's Group lunch. Lennie made us a great mushroom omelette. Stephen did the bulk of the washing up and I drove him down to the printers, and then I drove home. Lennie and I are both concerned at how near the surface Stephen's paranoia about how MI5 are controlling his life is and that we wonder who will help him after we have gone. As Lennie said, he was much more relaxed when he went than when he came. The important thing is to listen!

The following month, after Richard and Benedict had taken Stephen and I to watch a county cricket match, I told Richard that "Lennie and I were worried about Stephen after we died. Richard really doesn't appreciate the paranoia and MI5 voices which Stephen brings up with us most weekends. At the match I unexpectedly couldn't read the scoreboard one hundred and fifty yards away, or see the ball, only when I noticed the players chasing it. So, I'm not sure I'd choose to go to a county match again. But having said that, we all enjoyed a relaxing day together and the break from routine, stress and tensions."

I was given a lift to go to the monthly meeting of the Justice and Peace Group where "the main topic was initial planning for the 'car-free weekend' in mid-September. To be honest, I felt I'm slipping out of it these days and not contributing much. What value I am I'm really not sure." I was involved in the construction of the bidding prayers for the Sunday Mass at St. Pius X's, still under lay supervision. The Bookham Group, only four of us now, discussed 'indulgences'. "Interestingly, none of us was convinced by the notion of indulgences and I think we all saw it as some sort of attempt to reconcile permanent and temporary punishment and assert the threefold communion of the faithful, in heaven, on their way, and here on earth."

We typically relaxed in the garden after lunch and often slept for an hour or more. As I noted in my diary: "Obviously we'd both worked hard this morning! Lennie was totally disoriented, didn't know whether it was time for breakfast, tea or supper." I was still going to the Farmers' Market but was finding it very difficult to walk up to the top of the town from the car park in the bus station.

In September I had a growth on my arm removed. I also had a nasty wasp sting in the garden and had to go to the hospital for appropriate treatment. I spent a lot of time in the garden planting loads of bulbs. Lennie had broken her wrist in the summer, after a fall in the road. A fact that was confirmed later in A&E (see below). Following this, I did the Sainsbury's weekly shop. Lennie returned after seven weeks and invariably spent a couple of hours there. We were concerned about Stephen's savings, which we were looking after with the aim of safeguarding him from a cut in his benefits. Lennie and I both spent some time in the study thinning files, mostly financial records, in anticipation of the approaching ends of our lives. In the evenings we both often felt there was nothing worth watching on the TV. At this stage I was quite enjoying *Outnumbered* while Lennie still usually watched *Eastenders*. We babysat for Richard one night and during the month had a meal out with him and his family.

The end of the Catholic development charity 'Progressio' led me to write a letter to the *'Tablet*. The planned closure of Heythrop was disturbing because the library there had been the depository of all my research documents. I went to the meeting of the Bookham Group on the theme of 'populism' and to the first meeting of the U3A discussion group. Lennie and I were both concerned about Donald Trump and I recorded that "I just hope Donald Trump does not lead to the sorts of bigotry and tyranny experienced during the McCarthy times". Gillian and Doug went down to explore housing in Dorset, where they eventually plan to retire. I noted in my diary that "these plans disturb Lennie, who thinks they are premature before Gillian retires and because she fears being left alone when I die. I expect I'll hear about it over and over again!"

The younger of our two former Anglican priests left to go to another parish. Having sent copies of my *Parish Suppressed* to all the clergy, I got a very nice appreciation of it from one of the deacons and a fellow parishioner. I managed to sell a few copies in the hall after Mass on a Thursday. I drove Lennie to the Women's Group lunch at the Golf Course. On the last Sunday of September, we made an "effort to walk or car-share. After Mass and the last hymn, I spontaneously went up to the microphone and thanked people for participating and added that it aimed to raise consciousness about how important it was to combat climate change and think about the world we were leaving for our grandchildren. Rather to my surprise and pleasure, this was met with a good round of applause."

Lennie continued to show signs of her illness throughout September. For example, "to my astonishment, Lennie apparently told one caller this morning that we had no solar panels. I pointed out that a few years ago we'd invested £9,000 in installing ten solar panels in addition to the two thermal ones in the original building. She doesn't refer to <u>anybody</u> by name, doesn't know the day, month, year, etc. I take it these are the first signs of dementia and pray its onset will be slow to develop and allow me to adjust to a more proficient and loving carer's role." Later in the month, I added, "I just hope she will never get to the state of two male parishioners' wives, who didn't recognise their husbands in their care homes". Gillian and I had a pleasant lunch at the Guildford Institute "discussing Trust issues and also Lennie's slowly developing dementia". Gillian visited us later in the month and "beautifully, lovingly and professionally raised the question of Lennie's deteriorating loss of memory. Lennie was quite critical of my 'nagging', but on the whole listened well, though still in denial. But I hope a useful starting point for future discussion and action." Lennie and I had a pleasant meal out at the Onslow Arms "which she saw as a bit of a peace offering, though her deep anger with her daughter remains".

Early in October I went off to a grandparents' day at the Cuthbert Mayne school in Cranleigh. "I bought some cake to bring home, but sadly I think I left it on the roof of the car, and then forgot it. Back home, I realise I've lost it!" At this time, we were still starting our day with a mug of tea, then with the help of *Bible Alive* reflecting on the day's Mass readings before praying for family and friends, living and dead. Our plans for a holiday in Benidorm were met with 'a loud guffaw'! Lennie has been rather disappointed that she hasn't been able to go out 'girlie' shopping more often with Gillian. "Please, Lord, help me set the alarm right ... It may well be our last holiday abroad." On our return from Alicante, "Andrew phoned, full of his activity for ACTA (A Call to Action) and the evangelical courses in his Reading parish. He really is a great activist, or, as he would put it, a polemicist."

November seemed to be another fairly busy month. We were a bit disappointed by *Room with a View* at the Yvonne Arnaud Theatre. I went to the U3A Opera Group presentation of *The Barber of Seville*. We attended the meetings of our two trusts and the Oak Tree Gardens residents. We also took our brother-in-law, Terry Dobson, out for lunch to celebrate his birthday; afterwards, I noted that I was finding it increasingly difficult to climb the hill to the car park. I was still being asked to be a reader or special minister at Mass, but I frequently wondered if this would be the last time because of my ageing. In the middle of the month, we were driven to Croydon for the monthly meeting of our Family Group. "There was a lively and angry exchange of emails about one of the former Anglican priest's insistence that charities for the 10% collection be

Catholic, something that has never been the case before now. Pat Jones sent him a very informed and punchy response. Who does he think he is? Boss or servant?" Lennie and I went over to St. Mary's, where the younger former Anglican priest celebrated his last Mass before going to another parish.

Lennie and I went to the Yvonne Arnaud to see *Dead Sheep*, "but I was disappointed the comedy wasn't all that great". Two days before my 84th birthday, I went to confession to the older former Anglican priest and "he was remarkably pastoral and understanding and said we are all 'flawed'". I arranged to pay £600 into all the savings accounts of our children and grandchildren for Christmas. I continued to work on a paper on eight decades of change, though I don't think anything came out of it in the end.

On the first Saturday in December, we celebrated three birthdays: Andrew's, Lennie's and mine, with a family lunch at the Queen's Head in East Clandon. All our children and grandchildren were with us, but we uncomfortably angered Andrew. We had a very nice three-course meal and afterwards returned home, where Andrew put on a "great firework display. I'd invited the neighbours' children to watch and they all went into the next-door garden and enjoyed a great display. We then called in the half-a dozen children for the sparklers."

We were given tickets to go to a Carol Service at Holy Trinity for the Mayor's Charity. "I found myself admiring the way Church of England churches are inclusive and involve 'everyman' and how impressive it was to hear so many people singing hymns about the birth of our Lord and Saviour." The following night, a member of the Justice and Peace Group was "very outspoken about the seeming lack of response of Roman Catholics to refugees compared to the Anglican Diocese, who are apparently housing five families but wish to keep quiet about it because of fears of intimidation, etc."

In the middle of the month, the Men's Group had a splendid lunch at Ewhurst. I enjoyed the U3A Opera Group's *Die Fledermaus* and a Saturday afternoon visit from Richard, Will and Iris to watch the Chelsea game. Lennie was still insistent on doing the Sainsbury's shop on her own. My preference for late night Scandinavian police dramas was not supported by Lennie or Stephen, so I usually disappeared and did some reading. Andrew came over with his presents for Christmas and told us about "his lovely experiences of warmth and friendship in Anglican Churches. He thinks clericalism is killing the Church and is fighting it through his involvement in ACTA." Lennie and I took Will and Iris to the *Aladdin* pantomime.

St. Pius' was very full at Mass on Christmas morning. Lennie was scheduled for her last session as a eucharistic minister, but when I noticed there was no seventh minister I went up, and so for me it was also possibly my last time. I volunteered to distribute the hosts because I felt less likely to spill them. After Mass, I thanked a fellow parishioner for his successful production of the *St. Pius in Print* magazine – a genuine lay initiative outside the veto of our former Anglican priest.

After a pleasant Christmas with the family, I took Lennie to a production of *Swan Lake* by the St. Petersburg Ballet, which she enjoyed. On the 29th, we went to Mass and "when nobody went to bring up the Offertory, I pushed Lennie into doing it because it was our anniversary. In the hall afterwards, a friend hinted to our former Anglican priest that it was our anniversary. Delightfully, he came over and gave us a lovely blessing in which all present were involved. Quite unexpected and appreciated."

We are trying to trace the development of Lennie's dementia in this book. In February, there were signs that I was becoming more aware and I wrote that "Lennie's forgetfulness is getting more and more apparent. She doesn't mention any friends or parishioners by name but says 'that woman'. And she sometimes forgets where to put things. But she still does all the domestic chores. This afternoon she did a big shop at Sainsbury's." In March I noted in my diary that "I now wish to record that there seems little doubt that Lennie's memory is deteriorating. She must have asked me several times how many times she has boiled the Christmas pudding. She keeps asking what day it is and has asked about our weekend arrangements about a dozen times. I pray that my growing awareness of this will help me not get irritated by her repeated questions. She is such a loving spouse, mum and nana, full of concern and help."

But let's be aware; memory loss isn't just Lennie, but also me. In mid-March I noted that "I'm aware that my memory is fading fast. I couldn't even remember the name of the town where we had our last cottage." Later in the month, at the Maundy Thursday Mass, I recorded that "I was one of the twelve volunteers to have my feet washed with a steadying hand from a fellow parishioner. It is quite possibly the last time I'll ever do it." On the following day, I took Stephen to the station on his way to see "the Wintershall demonstration of the Passion in Trafalgar Square. I had an hour to kill, which I managed sitting in the taxi shelter in the sun at the bottom of North Street until people congregated for the annual walk of witness led by the vicar of Holy Trinity ... It was a hard slog walking up High Street to Holy Trinity after the vicar had urged us not to mock and to help others like Simon of Cyrene (Mk 15:16–24). A fellow parishioner, whose name I couldn't remember, for three-quarters of an hour, helped me by giving me an arm all the way up High Street."

I had quite a heavy cold early in March and slept in the other room one night. Lennie let me lie on in bed for a while in the mornings and brought me porridge for breakfast. She had a nasty fall while shopping at Sainsbury's and she was suffering with a sore bottom and back afterwards.

Both Lennie and I had health problems in April. Early in the month, Lennie was "aching so much she. decided not to go" to the monthly meeting of the Family Group, but she declined my offer to take her to see our G.P. Early in the month, I was worried about Lennie taking the wrong pills and noted that "I do find myself wondering what she would do if I wasn't around". In the middle of the month, Lennie returned from visiting the bank in Guildford and "confessed she'd got her 'numbers' mixed up and had difficulty withdrawing money because she put in our phone number instead of her visa PIN".

I had a spell with severe back pains and "I'm seriously wondering whether the time has come for me to resign from the team" running the Merrow Food Bank. In May I was worried about our approaching holiday in the Italian lakes. My knee was so painful that I gave up kneeling at Mass. "Stephen told me, a bit ominously, that I must look after Mum. She has several times recently expressed the wish that she die first. Death seems not far away. The Queen is ninety this week ... will I make it?" To my surprise, our G.P. gave me an emergency appointment "possibly because I am old and have a reputation for not seeing him unnecessarily. He took me off the codeine pills but insisted that I had eight paracetamols each day and ended by suggesting that we'd have to look seriously at a knee replacement when we returned from Italy."

"Gilly is firmly committed to retiring at sixty and to moving, for example to Dorset, and will not be around to assist an ailing Lennie. So, part of my prayer is that I will have the grace to do everything I can to make life as easy as possible for Lennie." I noted that "her memory is deteriorating. She increasingly doesn't know where things are or puts them away in new places. But she has been a great spouse and I have been very blessed." After taking her out for lunch at the Clandon Garden Centre, I noted that "she seems so disorganised, buying two *Guardians* ... losing the card for a while, not having regular places for keys, driving licence, etc. It is frustrating but when I suggest a safe arrangement, she sees this as 'always nagging me'. I'm not sure whether she has early signs of dementia, but I pray that I may be always loving and supportive." After we'd had coffee with a neighbour, "when Lennie went into the kitchen, he quietly asked me if Lennie was losing her memory. I was quite taken back because I didn't realise that it was so obvious to other people."

On Referendum Day, I recorded "that in mid-afternoon Lennie came down after a deep sleep in her bedclothes, thinking it was time to go to bed". Later in the month I recorded that Lennie "is very frustrated these days with children playing outside and damaging our not very marvellous bushes. I'm surprised by how angry she gets (as a former infant teacher) but she definitely likes peace in our garden and road. I do wonder if she really is showing signs of dementia. She never refers to neighbours by name but 'the guy over the road' and has difficulty remembering our children's names. Help me, Lord, to be always patient and loving." Later that evening Lennie was outside with the neighbours and their children, and she fell and broke her wrist, as we found out the following morning in A&E. In my diary I noted that "I felt this morning was a preliminary warning that there will be increasing amounts of care time over the coming years. I think Lennie needed me this morning, not just over directions, but also over answering factual questions. Help me to grow in patience, sensitivity and love, Lord ... I must learn to drop everything when Lennie calls or needs me. Sometimes it is frustrating!"

The next day I added after a very busy morning at the banks, two pharmacies, and Sainsburys: "Lennie was driving me mad with her fussing but we both settled for a rest ...

Lennie's memory is deteriorating – she even asked how she'd broken her wrist two days ago and has difficulty remembering any names, including children and grandchildren and neighbours. Help me be with her, Lord." At Mass on Sunday, "loads of people crowded round Lennie to express their concern about her broken wrist".

An extract from a late Tuesday in August diary gives something of the flavour of a busy and sometimes stressful life. "Lennie observed that it would be better to put the camping table in the sun. Four times in five minutes or so, I'd said the sun would have moved where I put the table on the patio shortly. Eventually, I exploded. My patience is very thin, and I suppose I was tired after a domestic morning, which had seen me water the neighbour's flowers (they are on holiday) and our two flowerbeds; do a £20+ shop in Sainsbury's and paint wood preservative or teak oil on the water softening cover, bird cage and patio tables. I'd scratched my arm on the bushes and had blood all down my arm. Then we had our stupid spat and didn't speak to each other at all during lunch. Afterwards, I made the coffee and washed up. Lennie says I ought to go to bed because I am tired. I tried unsuccessfully to go to sleep outside in the sun. Then, when I was getting burned, I came in to try the lounger. But that wasn't successful either. Then there was a cold caller, and I gave up and went upstairs to check emails ... Lennie called me down for tea. We kissed and made up." After supper I was given a lift to go to the parish Justice and Peace Group, which, as mentioned above, was largely concerned with planning a 'car-free/share' day in September and considering possibilities of aiding refugees.

Generally speaking, life proceeded as usual. I was beginning to wonder if poverty and inequality should be my next project. We managed to go to the Odeon and have a couple of meals out. I also drove Stephen to the 21st birthday celebration of Andrew's partner, Caroline's two children in Reading. In the evenings we watched a lot of the Olympics and Lennie seemed to have stopped watching *Eastenders* so regularly. Stephen was coming to stay with us over the weekends and was very helpful. After I'd had a satisfactory annual pacemaker check-up, I called into the hospital chapel to find "a woman Baptist Minister saying the words of consecration. She invited me to receive Holy Communion but uncomfortably I declined and afterwards went up to her and asked for a blessing. Should I have received Holy Communion and not be intimidated by legalistic prohibitions? There is a bit of me feels I should have done, because Christ was at the centre."

"During August I had struggled to find the time to read Pope Benedict's *Jesus of Nazareth.* I found the chapter on parables demanding but more engrossing than I had found earlier chapters. He is so open to a dozen or more alternatives to the concept of 'parable.' He welds together Christological and eschatological interpretations and always seems to emphasise God as the doer; we are simply receptive or not. That may be far too simplistic. It shows my intellectual limitations."

It seems that with the combination of the four individual parishes into the Catholic Parish of Guildford (C.P.G.) there was some conflict over the future of their Parish Pastoral Councils (P.P.C.s). When talking to the "former chair of the St. Pius' P.P.T. (Parish Pastoral Team) in August, she revealed some of the details of apparently ferocious disagreements among the clergy over the announcement made at Mass about the dissolution of P.P.Ts, about which she had apparently been given a different message by the parish priest. It seems that our former Anglican priests, used to powerful parish councils, had assumed the reverse was true in Catholic parishes and had worked relentlessly to marginalise the P.P.Ts. I gathered both the St. Joseph's and St. Mary's P.P.Ts had been dissolved before that of St. Pius', which unfairly has the reputation of being an awkward parish, though it was, in fact, a pathfinder for Vatican II reforms."

For the first time, I noticed that I had a sore on my bottom which was a serious concern requiring treatment from every carer in 2022. After our return from Benidorm, "I spent a good half an hour going through Lennie's mail, making decisions about which charity requests to respond to at this time. She might not like my saying it, but it does seem she really does need my help more and more. But when after lunch I said her memory was really going – some of her comments about our holiday were wild exaggerations – she was very hurt. I must be more sensitive." On one occasion, she forgot her PIN number in the bank. Poor lass. The woman in the bank was charming, *Deo gratias*. Later in the month, after I'd expressed irritation, she "complained, not for the first time, that I bullied her into doing what I wanted her to do. She is hurt by what she sees as my persistent attempts to belittle her. Forgive me for all my faults, Lord." At the parish Justice and Peace meeting in early October, "we talked through quite a few things, including follow up of the 'car-free' day, the 10% Christmas collection for charities; the Write for Rights campaign; a day of prayer for peace in Syria; and the suggestion that the parish office might be adapted for use by a refugee family." I was given a lift to and from the meeting by a fellow member, John Williams. Later in the week, he drove both Lennie and me to a film night in the parish hall. After a tasty curry supper, we saw an excellent film *A Good Lie* about some Somalian refugees "and the good fortune of being accepted as refugees in the U.S.; then the culture clashes there and the goodness of volunteers. Pat Jones gave an excellent talk on her frightening experiences on a CAFOD (Catholic Fund For Overseas Development) visit to Somalia." At the monthly meeting of our Family Group, "I rather angrily challenged a member's seeming gloss of the British Empire's benevolence to former colonies, and it led to a lively discussion".

When Gilly and Katie visited us on a Sunday morning after we'd been to Mass, "Gilly, Stephen and I talked about the onset of Lennie's dementia – they both were convinced and were aware that I was far more conscious of it than I was a year ago. Gilly thought I ought to discuss it with our G.P and ask him to advise what I, and we, ought to do." Gilly came with me to see our G.P. "We then had a chat about Lennie's loss of memory, etc. and he said he wasn't surprised, but couldn't do anything until she agreed and ceased her denial. If she didn't, it usually took a crisis to get the patient to agree treatment. Gilly said she'd try and persuade Lennie to let her go to see the G.P."

Early in December, I drove Lennie in to see our G.P., "but she didn't want me to go in with her. She came out and immediately said our G.P. had said I'd raised concerns about her memory. To my surprise, she didn't berate me and seemed basically aware of the three alternatives: (1) just old age, (2) dementia treatable with medication, and (3) non-treatable dementia. Later, Lennie went off to do a small shop at Sainsbury's." But a few days later I recorded that "last thing last night and first thing this morning, Lennie angrily accused me of betraying her to our G.P. and said she was so hurt that it would be a long time before she could forgive me. So that shows a sort of 'up and down' of our relationship. She keeps talking about being sent to Brookwood, the former notorious mental health hospital, and I struggle to tell her that this is not the case and that all that our G.P. probably did was refer her to a dementia specialist in the hospital for evaluations." After Mass, Lennie took Holy Communion to the usual disabled parishioner, "who sounds a bit spiky at the moment. I agree with Lennie that it is time she ended this service of hers." After a deep sleep after lunch in mid-December, Lennie "came down totally disoriented. She didn't know whether it was morning or evening, whether Maureen and her mother had died, how long we had lived in this house and how long we had been on our own."

That the issue of Lennie's denial was raising temperatures was illustrated in this diary for two days before Christmas. "Andrew had challenged me to do something about Lennie's treatment and when I said it was my responsibility, his response was that it wasn't just mine but his, Gillian's, Stephen's and Richard's too. Peace, Lord."

During the year, we had several holidays. At the end of April, we took Stephen to the Italian Lakes for a week's holiday. My younger sister, Sue, and her charming husband Mario came over from Ivrea to be with us on one of the days. I am glad to say that the holiday was quite a success and that both Lennie and Stephen enjoyed it. I struggled with pain in my back and knee in Verona, where in July we attended performances of *Carmen, Aida* and *La Traviata* in the Arena. I had been helped at the airports by customer assistants and Easy Jet. We spent a few days in the same Hotel Milano as the previous year and were delighted that the staff remembered us from the previous year and were so friendly. Lennie's and my tastes were not identical, and I struggled with my limited mobility to wander around the town. I loved just sitting in the garden outside the Arena, watching the world go by and parents coping with unruly children. "It's all a delightful part of the Verona atmosphere and culture. It is good being here watching the world go round with a complete lack of conformity to dress style." At the Arena, a charming assistant kindly managed to sell the couple of tickets which I had accidentally double-booked. Back home, I noted that "I'm very conscious of ageing and vary between saying we'd be fit enough to go to Verona again next year and judging that we are honestly past it".

In August I booked a fortnight's holiday in Benidorm with Saga in October. Because of a lively TV programme about noisy Brits in Benidorm, this amused some of our fellow parishioners. We spent a fortnight in the Gran Hotel Delfin in Benidorm and enjoyed the break and swam regularly in the outdoor pool. Saga arranged visits to a chocolate factory and to interesting museums high up in the mountains and a very enjoyable visit to "the Benidorm Palace for their very professional cabaret with several acts that I would say were clearly world-class". We were lucky to find a bus which took us to Mass six times in the fortnight, including one on the day of the funeral of a fellow parishioner. To our surprise we met two parishioners from St. Joseph's, Guildford, at Mass. On our last weekend, "I slept soundly for two and a half hours until just after midnight when Lennie had one of her middle-of-the-night dreams. She said she'd showered and was getting up and came and sat on the edge of the bed and asked me if I was her husband. She was very disorientated and kept on about having to pack our cases. I managed to keep cool, and several times stressed that we didn't need to pack until tomorrow night. This morning everything is calm. At the end of our stay, I noted that I suspect that we both feel that in spite of the friendliness of the hotel staff, we are unlikely to go again. Thank You, Lord, for our break."

In early January, my diary recorded that "around 6.30 a.m. Lennie said she'd wanted to make love all night. I picked up the signals pretty quickly and we both stripped naked, cuddled, caressed and made love with pleasure and satisfaction. So, it was 'eros' but also I believe 'agape'. I would never have believed in the past that eighty-year-olds could have strong sexual drives but here we are, making love about once every week. I realise that we are called to live like Jesus. But Jesus never married (how did a thirty-year-old never marry in Israel?) and never made love, so how can we live like Jesus in all things but sin? How does an eighty-three-year-old layman explain sexual ethics to celibate male clergy? We just try and do our best."

On the following day, Lennie made similar approaches and I tried to respond. I noted that, "I tried to please her but these days my erection is not great and I can rarely penetrate her. As a substitute I use my finger and she clearly responds to this. As I have noted in previous chapters, the question recurred to me as to whether this was masturbation, and if so, is it wrong? As I am not the beneficiary, I really don't see it as sin, whereas sixty years ago it would have necessitated confession. I am simply trying to please her as best I can. I think Jack Dominian might have agreed. But given my generation's upbringing, which regarded submission to sexual urges as immoral, I do have a sense of guilt, though there is no way I can regard it as 'mortal' and a rejection of God. I do believe God gave us our sexuality, even in our eightiess, and that we are currently enjoying each other and trying to express in our sexual relationship our love for each other. I pray that the Lord will guide us." Two days later, Lennie made similar approaches at 3 a.m. "My first reaction was a grumbly 'oh heck' but I tried to respond to her desires for closeness, tenderness and love as best I could." In mid-February, I recorded that "shortly after midnight Lennie made a suggestive move and I responded and we ended up making love so passionately that for the first time for probably a year or more, I ejaculated".

In late May, after we had made love twice one night, "I thought I would reflect on this sexual couple of octogenarians. When I was younger, I never dreamed that old people made love. But we do and in many ways we have spells like now when we have made love every day for several days. I believe this is a gift God has given us. Because I only have a minute erection and cannot penetrate Lennie, I sometimes use my finger to respond to her needs, as discussed above. I hope the Lord is not displeased. I am grateful for Lennie's wandering hand and cuddling, which I enjoy, but more importantly see as an invitation to my caressing her breasts and then trying to 'make love'. Reading *Amoris Laetitia* suggests that I am in tune with what Pope Francis is saying."

In the last fortnight of July, we made love on average once every day. Lennie was invariably the initiator. Thus, I wrote, "To be honest, I've found it hard going when she climbs on top of me, but I've tried making passionate love five times in the past four days. Whatever is happening to the octogenarians? I'm trying hard to make sense of it – the most passionate spell I can ever remember. The initiative on each occasion over the past few days of hot weather has honestly come from Lennie, who has suddenly come to me with nothing on. I try hard to make her satisfied but it is not easy when my penis fails to get erect."

At the end of the month, I asked: "When will this crazy spell of sexual love-making be satisfied? It has now lasted nearly a fortnight and is quite unprecedented. As we observed this morning, it has been like a second honeymoon." In the second half of August, I added that "our octogenarian sexual honeymoon continues strongly". Two days later, I added that "I honestly can't remember having such prolonged sessions in all our fifty-five years together. Thank you, Lord, for the blessing of our relationship." But a couple of days later I concluded by writing that Lennie "is threatening to come down in her birthday suit! She did indeed do so at 9.30 p.m. I went upstairs and did my best. But I'm not enthusiastic anymore and am beginning to opt out and switch off." Unexpectedly, I noticed that in July and August we had made love thirty times while in November and December only twice. What an extraordinary shift. I'm not sure why this was, but I suspect it reflected something about Lennie's shifts of mood, etc.

At the end of the year my diary had a quite useful summary of 2016: "What are my memories of this year? Brexit and Trump and Syria and refugees must be top of the list, but also my somewhat delayed recognition of Lennie's steady loss of memory and indeed mine also, to be honest, but her possible slide towards dementia. I've tried to respond by being more patient and understanding but I keep failing and we have regular mini rows, always in time closed with a 'sorry' from one of us." What seems difficult to record is the way in which Lennie's illness intruded on the way I tried to live my life and concentrate on what I was trying to read or write. Something of this was reflected in this extract from the final day of the year. "I tried to get a few minutes to read the *Guardian* and its series of articles trying to 'look on the bright side' after the disasters of the year, such as Brexit and Trump. But Lennie kept interrupting with queries and repeats. Eventually, I gave up and joined Lennie and Stephen in the kitchen where the three of us prepared lunch."

CHAPTER 5
The Year 2017

I started the year trying to identify clearly what I ought to be doing. "Lennie keeps telling me that I'm stretched too far, though I often think I'm lazy: for example, not tidying up my study, files, etc. and the shed in the garden. I suspect Lennie's loss of memory will challenge me more and more this year. Please, Lord, give me the patience of love. Should I go to the J. and P. annual assembly at Crawley? Please guide me, Lord." A couple of days later I admitted that "I'd asked what the Lord wanted me to do so I tried to update my notes in the event of my death". At the beginning of the year, I suspected that "Lennie's loss of memory will challenge me more and more this year".

Lennie had an unfortunate fall at Newlands Corner, which led to our not going to Carlo's for lunch. However, we did go to a comedy film at the Odeon in the evening. The temperatures were low in January and the car frequently needed defrosting early on. On the Feast of the Epiphany, Gillian, Doug and Katie came over to celebrate Katie's 21st birthday later in the month. "We nattered a bit aimlessly. In sum, I think our attempt to celebrate Kate's 21st fell a bit flat." As I drove Stephen to the bus station that evening after he had kindly taken down the Christmas tree and taken it up into the roof, he "reflected on the fact that Lennie's multiple repeats tended to drive me mad and I guess he was suggesting that after our many good years together, the Lord was testing me. So, give me patience and love, Lord." That evening the two Durstons, friends from our Family Group, drove us to our meeting in Croydon and back. On the following Monday evening, Lennie and I "both turned down the chance to be extraordinary ministers, saying we had both retired".

When Lennie frustrated me one morning, "I confess that in my anger I gave her a mini slap on the cheek. *Mea maxima culpa*. Still, we made up later." The following day I added, "I'm not finding it easy to cope with her these days, even if she is lovely". In the middle of the month, for possibly the last time, we made our way up to London by train to see the political comedy *This House*, about the Jim Callaghan government. Before that we'd had an excellent meal in an Italian restaurant near the Coliseum. So my diary noted: "Thank you, Lord, for a lovely day". On Peace Sunday I ended the day noting that "I'm trying to adapt to the situation where, for example, Lennie doesn't know which card is her bus pass". I was spending much of my time in January thinning old files to make things easier for Lennie, and Gilly, in the event of my death. "We then had some words about Lennie's Fidelity ISA savings files. I talked her through them, but she was totally unknowing about what they were, how she got them, what she should do about them and so on."

The U3A Discussion Group focused on rural C of E churches while our Bookham Group reflected on an excellent paper on the Eucharist. "In sum, the Mass is both a representation of Christ's sacrifice on the cross and a fraternal meal and food for our journey in the world." The U3A opera choice this month was Act 3 of *'The Mastersingers*. Later I recorded that "Dear Lennie. She really does seem to be losing it. Earlier today she had difficulty at Sainsburys making payments and trying to withdraw cash from the ATM. I'm sure she'd angrily object to my interpretation. But I must anticipate more challenges to my patience and ask God to help me learn love and patience. She deserves it after fifty-six years of looking after me."

Later in the month I wrote that Lennie's "memory is quite dangerous at times! And she sometimes accuses me of making things up because my memory is declining. Help me, Lord." A couple of days later I wrote: "Lennie every morning expresses anger and hurt at my 'betrayal', talking to our G.P. behind her back. I just try and be quiet and occasionally say I was only asking for advice as to how best to help her." As usual, on Monday mornings I used to drive Lennie into Guildford for her U3A keep-fit session and after doing a couple of hours work at home, drove off to pick her up from the bus stop. During one of the Men's Walking Group lunches, one of the walkers "came and sat next to me and asked how Lennie was. To my surprise, but in a funny sort of way also relief, he indicated that he was aware that Lennie was showing signs of dementia and he recalled that he had had the same problem with his wife several years before she died. Lennie was ready to go off shopping but before doing so rehearsed with me how to get cash out of the ATM machine."

In early February I was busy preparing an article on secularisation when "a nurse came to see Lennie and spent a good two hours with her. She was so gentle and sensitive that Lennie kissed her as she left. I was relieved and delighted that Lennie's session with the Memory Nurse had gone so well that she hadn't felt threatened or intimidated at all. Bless them both. I hope it helps Lennie; she admitted she'd found she couldn't remember how old she is." After a weekend watching the Rugby Six Nations matches, when driving Stephen to the station, "rather surprisingly he confessed to having found Lennie very irritating at times". As usual on Monday mornings, I drove Lennie to the U3A keep-fit class. The following day a group of fellow parishioners and I contributed to a focus group at the university on the theme 'Nation of Sustainable Prosperity'. In the evening, I was taken to the parish Justice and Peace Group meeting where the main topic was another car-free day.

I was a bit worried about "managing Lennie's contributions to charities. I think she is a fairly vulnerable recipient of a dozen or so requests, often bribed with unwanted 'gifts' from charities every week. I've suggested she collects requests over several weeks before making a selection, say, around Easter." The choir leader celebrated her 70th birthday at the Golf Club and members kept us up to date with the Six Nations and Chelsea scores! Otherwise, I noted that "another sign of the times was Lennie's angry attack on my 'betrayal', 'going to the doctor behind her back,' etc., which lasted a good hour. Then suddenly she came up to me and said sorry for being so nasty to me. It isn't fun but I keep suspecting that the Lord is either testing me or punishing me for past failures." On Valentine's Day, "I got our first MOT after three years. having driven only 11,000 miles in that time. We enjoyed an evening out at Carlo's. The following day Lennie walked to the dentist and then Sainsburys and was later taken out by Gillian for a 'girly day' together. It doesn't happen often, and I'm delighted for Lennie." The Thursday morning Mass was offered up for Lennie's aunt who'd died recently, and we took up the offertory gifts. I was unsuccessful in trying to recruit two more members to the Justice and Peace Group and then a close friend "told me, with a knowing look, that Lennie had told her she'd been shopping with 'Maureen', Lennie's sister who'd died some years ago. So, the awareness is gradually filtering around without me saying anything."

The rest of the month carried on as usual, except that I forgot to go to the U3A Opera Group. On a Monday I drove Lennie to her keep-fit class, after which a group of fellow parishioners always took her for a cup of coffee. Making love was not so easy and I recorded that "these days I find making love a bit of a chore". A parcel was wrongly delivered to us, so I walked round to the next cul-de-sac and commented that "it was enough for me; my legs and back can't cope with much more". A couple of days later, Lennie and I rowed pretty much all day. I can hardly remember how it started and what it was about. She complained about my never doing the cooking and I flared up about her always complaining about me working upstairs and ignoring all the things I did do. I confess I was furious. Later we made up and I apologised. " Lennie made us supper and I did the washing up and laying of the table for breakfast. So, this has been a bit of a mixed day today. I must try and learn patience and self-control and learn to live with someone who occasionally drives me up the wall. Please, Lord, help me to be guided by your call to be loving and patient. I do love her and am so grateful to You for having given me such a lovely wife of over fifty-six years."

"Bishop Moth was at all the Masses and when our former Anglican priest said the second collection was for Lenten alms, I spoke up and said it was Poverty Sunday all over the country and that we usually collected for Church Action on Poverty, a national ecumenical charity. I wasn't shot!" On the last Monday of February, I wrote: "I can't get away from Lennie's problems. Around 3 a.m. I found her getting dressed, asserting that I'd told her to get up. Then, when we were having tea, she asked me if I still drove the car because I had to take her into Guildford. Most of my time I was preparing notes on 'The changing role of women in society and in the Church' for our next Family Group. Lennie and I had a meal out at the Onslow Arms to check it out before taking friends there."

Lent started with Ash Wednesday on 1st March. We managed to go to Mass most days that Lent. "Lennie's middle-of-the-night concerns were that I was introducing gas into the house". At the weekly Men's Group lunch, one of those attending "gave a brief outline of the parish representatives' meeting with Bishop Richard. My guess is that few of our concerns about clerical authoritarianism would have been raised. On Friday around 4 a.m., Lennie invited me to make love and I responded as best I could, which was rather pathetic. All day I've felt a sore bottomback after my potentially dangerous fall backwards in the kitchen yesterday, which I didn't even record in my diary."

It could have been disastrous, and I was lucky not to break anything. Apart from Lennie's frequent panics, for example preparing for the visit of the Family Group at the weekend which I led, Stephen sometimes stressed me with his non-stop talking. But on Sunday, I drove him to the bus station and wrote: "Bless him, he has been a great help over the weekend". The next day I took Lennie to the Queen's Head for lunch. But the following day I was exhausted after walking up from the Farmers' Market." That evening, I was taken to the monthly J&P meeting attended by representatives from the Arundel and Brighton diocese and the local Anglican diocese to "discuss what we could do as a parish about the refugee crisis and the Vulnerable Persons Resettlement Programme".

The next day I led the discussion of the Bookham Group on 'Eight Decades of English Catholicism – A Case of Secularisation'. That evening Lennie and I went to the first meeting of a Lenten House Group. The following evening, we went to the Yvonne Arnaud Theatre and the next evening we felt obliged to go to a Fairtrade evening attended by about fifty parishioners. I helped Gilly write a letter to our G.P. "in response to his letter expressing surprise at Lennie's denial that he'd discussed with her the proposal to involve the Memory Clinic". But Lennie hadn't realised that was why the nurse had visited recently. On the next Monday morning, I drove Lennie into town for her keep-fit class in time to drive to St. Edward's for Mass, so that with Richard I would be able to watch the Chelsea vs Manchester United match in the evening. A variety of jobs inhibited the time I had to work on my various papers. One was to help Stephen to write to return the very large carpet which he'd decided was inappropriate for his apartment. One morning, "Lennie was coughing badly, so I let her remain in bed and brought her breakfast on the tray. Sounds simple, but these days I find it pushing me near my limit." I went to the Men's Group at lunch time and in the evening to the second Lenten House Group. After having problems with my laptop and observing that "it's not my day" we went to the Yvonne Arnaud Theatre in the evening after having a meal with two fellow parishioners. At the end of a busy week, we attended the annual Men's Walking Group lunch with wives at the Golf Club. Lennie lost her Visa card "… then the cooking at supper went all wrong and I had to step in to try and work the oven and micro. But it was another reminder that I'm going to have to learn to cook for us both, learn how the oven and micro work and gradually learn how to cope with a wife with a rapidly deteriorating memory and possibly the onset of dementia."

At the Saturday Mass, Lennie and I were asked to take up the offertory gifts. Afterwards, we went down "to the NatWest Bank where a helpful lady, probably treating us as doddery old folks, ordered a new Visa card for Lennie. It is worrying, though, that she can't remember her PIN number and may have trouble again. I found the walk back to the car tiring and do wonder if our Madeira holiday will be the last time we go abroad." After Mass on Monday evening, both Lennie and I "went to confession and the former Anglican priest was delightful with us both. Lennie was put at ease, and he flattered me while warning of the slowing down of old age. We came home and opted to watch André Rieu in Dublin." The Wednesday was another busy day. We didn't manage to get to Mass because I was leading the first hour of the Peace Vigil. Lennie and I put out the peace flag on two chairs at the foot of the altar. Our parish priest unexpectedly came and put out the Blessed Sacrament in the monstrance. Later in the day, I drove one of our friends to the Men's Group lunch and in the evening attended the Lenten House Group. The next day Lennie "didn't know where the fridge was in the kitchen. So, something is happening and I'm trying to cope without getting too irritated. I arranged with Tony Clarke, a widower in our Family Group, that on Saturday week I'd lead the discussion on Church Unity, etc."

On the day before Mother's Day, Gillian took Lennie for lunch and in the evening, we set off to visit Richard, Will and Iris, who entertained us for supper, Richard's contribution to Mother's Day. On the Sunday we had a Lenten message from Bishop Richard. Later, Andrew and his partner drove us down to Wittering for a pub lunch with her parents. Afterwards, we had a walk along the beach before we were driven home. The following day we went to the Yvonne Arnaud Theatre to have a simple meal and then watch *Nell Gwyn*. The next day I drove two friends to the Men's Group and later I led the Lenten House Group before having problems with my laptop at home. On the last Thursday of March, we took two friends to Positano for lunch. It was partly as a belated birthday present and partly, on my part, to recognise their help to me generally. It was a pleasant occasion. The following day we went to see our doctor. He was actually quite amicable and understanding and took a lot of trouble to talk Lennie through the aim of the Memory Clinic to assess how serious memory loss was in order to, where possible, administer medicine to slow deterioration. Lennie, at this stage, still didn't want to go down this path, but I think she is more understanding of where we in the family are coming from.

In early April we flew to Funchal in Madeira with Stephen for another week's holiday. At the airports I was given a great deal of assistance and kindness and wheeled around in a chair. We had a pleasant week. Stephen clearly enjoyed his holiday with us, doing his own thing, going for walks along the coast, and so on. Lennie was still having memory problems: she doesn't know where our home is and when we are going home, why we are here and where Stephen's room is, etc. On Palm Sunday I was worrying about a week's accumulated emails. I even felt I just wanted to go home. Lennie had some part in this, and at one stage, in the middle of the night, asked if the door to the balcony was the way to the loo. "My chest cold isn't helping either. Still, we've had a reasonable week, though I think I'll need some persuading to go on another holiday. We managed to go to a very pleasant Mass in the Cathedral. I made some final reflections on our return from Funchal. First of all, Stephen was lovely, a great and undemanding help, appreciative of the 'Peaks and Views' trip and of the flexibility to go and do a couple of walks on his own. Secondly, I felt I was a bit of a burden on the others, and I was aware of how 'old' and limited I really am and I'm not at all sure that I will be enthused to go on another trip abroad. Thirdly, thank you, Lord, for the gift of our holiday."

Back home, we quickly had to get back to the usual busy life. There was a time when Lennie didn't know I was her husband. This year I didn't feel 'up' to go on the Good Friday walk up the High Street. I had a chest infection, but we went to the Easter Vigil Mass with half a dozen baptisms and three receptions into the Church. On Easter Sunday, we were invited to lunch at Gillian and Doug's. Most of my free time I was spending trying to draft papers, attending the monthly meetings including the Justice and Peace meeting, "agreeing dates for peace vigils, etc. and planning future concerns with water and 'living simply'". On a Saturday afternoon, after I had been digging in gladioli in the garden, "I had a nasty experience when my left knee suddenly 'went' and I fell onto the lawn. Difficult to explain. But both Lennie and Stephen hurried to pick me up and look after me. They must have been frightened and it was, perhaps, a reminder to me of my mortality." At a meeting with our G.P., who said he saw no reason why both of us shouldn't continue driving, I think I may also have confirmed that I did not want to be resuscitated. Towards the end of April, I observed that there is little doubt that in many respects Lennie is becoming less coordinated. She doesn't always put things in the right place. Where, for example, did she put her hair dryer last time she used it? Stephen and I are trying to cope with Lennie asking the same questions four or five times.

May continued to be a busy month and we started trying to book visits to go to the opera in Verona. Stephen phoned me with his passport details, saying he thought I needed specialist help to cope with Lennie's loss of memory, which he thought was becoming ever more concerning. We frequently had rows when I became irritated by her repeated questions and, for example, when she went out and didn't lock the front door. We were having difficulties with the Justice and Peace Group and felt there was a need for a generational shift of activists in the parish generally. Justice and peace issues are marginalised, not just in our parish, but probably nationally. So, I stepped in to chair the monthly meeting.

The following extract gives something of the difficulties of Lennie's dementia: "(1) She remembers no names of friends – refers to 'thing be' or 'that guy's wife'. (2) She is in total denial of things she has done, such as put my medication in the sewing box. (3) She doesn't pick up hints, e.g., when I make a list of shopping and note the name of a box of cleaning capsules. (4) Angrily, I drove to Sainsburys where two smiling men showed me the SEAT bag and Gillian's bag of presents for Will and Iris to take this afternoon. One guy grinned and said, 'Has she gone loopy?'!! No comment. I sense we can't do anything until Lennie is convinced she needs help and is no longer in denial."

Stephen and I went to a lovely concert at G-Live with the Bournemouth Symphony Orchestra and after a big Catenian funeral, a fellow parishioner whispered that it was the Catholic Mafia! At the monthly U3A Opera Group, I presented *Peter Grimes*. I am growing increasingly attracted by its haunting themes. Because of the First Communion children we went to midday Mass at St. Edward's. That weekend Chelsea became champions after beating Sunderland 5–1 at home. In the evening, I drove Stephen to the bus station. He seemed to have enjoyed his weekend with us. Later, I noted that to be honest, I think my declining years may need to be spent just caring for Lennie. The following morning practically the first words Lennie said to me were "You are a very angry man, and you are getting worse as you get older". After shopping at Sainsbury's, Lennie returned, remarkably, after a fall in the car park, and from that point on I became a 100% carer. She'd damaged her knees. At first, we thought she'd cope but it became clear later that she needed an A&E check-up. Fortunately, the X-ray showed no break, but a couple of nurses gave us two zimmer frames to take home and the following day two Hospital Outreach Support Team (H.O.S.T.) nurses came to support her. At the weekend, Andrew expressed fears about Lennie's memory loss. "Frustrating times, but I must remember all the good times over the past 56 years of our married life together. Thank You, Lord."

Early in June I recorded: "One of the things I have been trying to record in my diary recently is the seemingly steady deterioration of Lennie's memory. I suspect the onset of Alzheimer's. For example, both last night and a couple of times today Lennie has asked if I am her husband or my nickname, 'Nookies', and for how long we have been sharing the same bed. At other times, she has asked if this is our house and she has no idea what month it is, or day in the week. At a guess this has only been obvious to me since about Christmas, though I think the children were aware of her memory loss long before that. She likes a cuddle and caresses and I'm always one to undo the buttons on her nightie and caress her breasts. This usually arouses her and she in turn caresses me, and we make love. On the whole, she enjoys this more than I do because these days I can't achieve an erection, etc. Several times during the rest of the day Lennie asked where 'Mike' was, or 'my husband or Nookies', even when I was sitting next to her." At Mass this morning I asked the Lord for guidance and the dominant impression I got was that I gave Lennie pleasure and we both felt very much in love. A couple of days later I added:

"I hope and pray that I am slowly adapting to what is needed. It is difficult when most of the time Lennie is quite with it but is sometimes 'with the fairies' and totally out of step with what has been scheduled." On another day I wrote: "A naked Lennie came and is clearly expecting love-making. Give me strength and love, Lord!"

My uncertainties were perhaps indicated in the following extract: "At the back of my mind is the question: am I too out of touch to contemplate another article or even a book?" A couple of days later I observed how very pretty Lennie was at eighty-one, but in her repeated reflections on past events, a couple of times she wasn't sure whether I was her father, or Mike or her Nookies. Meanwhile, life carried on as normal, with much discussion about the election, which had left the Tories without an overall majority. Gilly pushed Stephen unsuccessfully to explain why he had voted Tory. For Gilly and me, there were Christian social principles and values which we felt should drive our concerns for others. And, of course, we watched football and rugby at the weekends. After Mass on Sundays, I pushed parish newsletters through the letterboxes of our Spanish, Portuguese and Italian neighbours! A sort of mini evangelisation! These days, I was driving Stephen down to the bus station on Sunday evenings. In the middle of June, I drove Stephen to his P.I.P. (ex-Disability Living Allowance, now Personal Independence Payment) assessment in Chertsey, only to find the health assessor was ill. The half-yearly meeting of the Trust was held on a Wednesday evening. It "was one of the friendliest and easiest we've yet had. The three children worked constructively together and expressed their gratitude, especially to Gilly, but also to Richard for his work on maintenance. Be with them all, Lord." The following day we went to the Yvonne Arnaud Theatre to enjoy *The Pirates of Penzance*. "Lennie was moved to tears by her reminiscences of taking part in the opera at the concert in Berwick."

At this stage in our lives, I was often working upstairs on the laptop. I was looking for the notes I had written ten years earlier for the fiftieth anniversary of St. Thomas of Canterbury Primary School. "It was at this point that Lennie and I had another flare-up. It annoyed me that she had to bring two corn-on-the cobs upstairs when I'd yelled down it would be appropriate for lunch on a Friday. As usual, our squabble escalated. Lennie was upset and called me a bully. Eventually, we made up, had lunch and shared the washing up. But it was another reminder of how Lennie's 'competence' is being eroded, but also how I'm having great difficulty not exploding in anger, although I'm aware that I'm having to do more and more things which Lennie used to do. Today, for example, I replied to the head of St. Thomas's about the celebrations planned for its fiftieth anniversary, on behalf of us both, since I was a Foundation Manager for the first nine years. Later on, I cooked our supper. For the first time in years Lennie and I weren't recommissioned as eucharistic ministers. Only one of the six servers at Mass was a boy!" These days I seemed to be doing all the shopping at Sainsbury's.

We celebrated Father's Day at Richard's, where "the children were very friendly. It was a lovely evening." I was having a lot of trouble with my laptop and particularly when trying to book tickets for our proposed visit to the opera in Verona. Our Italian neighbour was very helpful, helping sort things out. We were invited to St. Thomas's for an anniversary concert. We met quite a few old faces and sadly, Lennie forgot more than I did. The school put on a delightful show of pop songs to fit each decade from the 1960s to 2010s, including the topics of Margaret Thatcher, the Berlin Wall and the Millennium – quite an entertaining social history." Andrew was about to go off to Cornwall for a fortnight with his partner Caroline and her parents while Gilly and Doug went off to Dorset with their two dogs for a week. Lennie's knee was hurting her, so she decided not to go to the keep-fit class. On the following day, Bishop

Richard said the Mass at St. Pius', celebrating St. Thomas's 50th anniversary, where Lennie had taught for several years. "To our surprise, we were taken up to the front row. The church was absolutely packed, and two rows of the youngest children were sitting on the floor in front of us. Bishop Richard said the Mass and gave a very nice little homily, talking directly to the children as he does so well."

At the end of June, Lennie and I made what was probably our last train visit to London, where, after a frustrating delay we caught a taxi from Waterloo "to the Platform Theatre where we arrived only just in time for the start of our oldest grandson Luke's play *Herons*, only because it started late! It was an excellent portrayal of the bullying of two youngsters by a gang of boys on an estate of the marginalised. Luke was the main part and was excellent, as were all the other members of the cast. He was so delighted to see us and show us his affection. Bless him." At Mass the following morning, "it interested me that there was one male celebrant, but that the two readers, two eucharistic ministers and three ministers who took communion to the sick were all females. How long before women deacons, priests and bishops? Lennie seemed quite confused about Richard and Luke, son and grandson, and we had another silly row. Please God, give me the patience which is love and help me to learn how to cope with unexpected frustrations." The following morning Lennie's doctor "said it would take time for her cartilage to heal". Then, at the pharmacy, Lenny gave our previous address in Merrow. "Just as well I was with her, and I think she was grateful." From there we went to St. Joseph's for the Requiem Mass for a very prominent Catenian. At the end of that day I reflected that "I admire the support they give to their bereaved but I just can't imagine joining. I'm just not comfortable with them. They behave like a superior class."

At the start of July, the weather was hot and sunny, and we often had lunch outside on the patio and during the afternoon sat outside and often fell asleep. Gillian unexpectedly returned a day early from Dorset and joined us at Mass on the first Sunday. When the priest again failed to draw attention to the Peace Vigil on the following day, I managed to get a video put up and "I went to the lectern to draw people's attention to it". In the evening, we were driven to Richmond for the monthly meeting of the Family Group. The following morning, "I drove Lennie into Guildford for the last keep-fit class of the academic year." I ended by noting that "things have changed rapidly in the last couple of months. People are beginning to notice. Help me be a patient carer, Lord." On the Tuesday evening, we "watched the magnificent last episode of Jimmy McGovern's *Broken*. I was in semi-tears near the end and thought it the most sympathetic drama about the Church I'd ever seen." I led the final hour of the Peace Vigil.

On the following afternoon, after the Men's Walking Group lunch, we attended a funeral Mass. "The Guildford Vox Choir ... contributed to a lovely service. I read the 1 Cor. 4–7 quote about love being patient, etc. Very appropriate! I also read the bidding prayers – I think this is my last remaining ministry." That evening we went to the Yvonne Arnaud to see Arthur Miller's *Death of a Salesman* and had a meal outside beforehand. The following morning, "Lennie decided not to go to Mass, but to try and rest her painful knee before we go to Verona. I found it quite oppressive in church and during the night had again been struck by pains in my chest, as I had been last night walking to the car park from the Yvonne Arnaud. It reminded me to face the reality that I am ageing and sooner or later I will die, possibly with heart failure. In the meantime, please help me to do what You want me to do, Lord." In the evening, we babysat for Richard as he went to the first night of the parents' First Holy Communion class. On Gillian's 54th birthday, we were invited to join all their family in the evening for a BBQ. "We had a very pleasant supper with them all and Katie and Douglas were very warm and affectionate." During the day the Lions had drawn 15–15 with the All Blacks in New Zealand.

On the following day, "They were short of a eucharistic minister unexpectedly so I went up to offer the hosts and the former Anglican priest very kindly offered me an arm to descend the steps before distributing the hosts". In the afternoon, the neighbours in Oak Tree Gardens met around the oak tree and chatted with each other around a BBQ, although some were in dispute about the attitude of the chairman to children playing in the cul-de-sac. On the Monday, Gillian and Doug drove to Canterbury for Katie's graduation while we looked after their dogs and one of Lennie's friends brought over the stick Lennie had left behind. Pity that Stephen had bought her a replacement! On the next day we enjoyed a lunch at Clandon Garden Centre with two of our neighbours. That night there was a heavy downpour of rain "for which the lawn and flowers are truly grateful". Nearing midday, I was given a lift to Bookham, "where we had a pleasant lunch and a stimulating discussion" on the theme of post-truth. The business of our lives continued with a Requiem Mass without great support from Catenians, after which we made our way to Waterloo and by taxi to Southwark Cathedral where Maureen Martin, one of our Family Group, was celebrating twenty-two years as a very successful headmistress of a renowned Catholic school with great success. And she is an inspiration to other local schools. So, it has been a very full day."

Booking for our four days in Verona was not easy but we managed, just as my diary recorded. "The process at Gatwick was a bit of a nightmare. Since we used it in April the process of booking in has been speeded up and made more 'consumer friendly' – a joke! Booking online is recommended but now there are machines to check in cases etc., rather than human assistants. It all seemed a bit difficult. It really began to feel like our last holiday out of Gatwick." But Verona Airport was easier, and we caught a taxi to the Hotel Milano, where the staff were very friendly. In the evening the three of us had a very pleasant meal in the Piazza Bra. Then we went to the Arena where we enjoyed *Nabucco*, which ended at 12.30 a.m. The following morning, Sue and Mario turned up and we went to the Piazza Bra, where we had an appetiser before lunch and nattered away about our families. "I think Mario's knowledge of English was a bit better than mine of Italian. But I tried. In my view, Sue and Mario looked as well and happy as I've ever seen them. I warned Sue it might be the last time but we both hoped it wouldn't be." Sue and Mario left around 2.30 p.m. and in the evening we went with Stephen to the Arena for a production of *Rigoletto*. I didn't have "a bad night's sleep though at 7 a.m., I became irritated at Lennie's repeated (at least three times) questioning about where we were, Douglas's 18th birthday, was this our home, what were we doing in Verona, and so on. I hope Stephen will use this day and opportunity to explore Verona before this evening's performance of *Aida*." We didn't have the easiest of days. "I am more and more thinking that this is or will be our last holiday, at least abroad, given our lack of mobility. Dear Lord, help the next twenty-four hours before we fly out from Verona to be happy for Lennie. The performance of *Aida* was very unusual, with indications of colonial exploitation before the opera. Lennie was most uncomfortable about the twenty-five-minute intervals between acts and angrily felt the opera had gone on too long. I definitely had the feeling that this really was the very last time we'll come to the Verona Opera. It was still dark when I woke to find Lennie packing and getting dressed. I managed to calm her down." We said some unusually affectionate goodbyes to the staff in the hotel restaurant and had long delays in the airport, arriving over an hour late at Gatwick. But our taxi was waiting for us and drove us home.

Back home after Mass on the Saturday morning, I went to do the weekly shop at Sainsbury's, and I was annoyed that "Lennie didn't help me to unpack the five shopping bags. I irritated her by making suggestions about lunch, for example finishing the old salad before today's lettuce." Stephen and I watched Chelsea beat Arsenal 3–0 in Beijing before Richard arrived with all his four children to celebrate Benedict's birthday the next day. "It was lovely seeing Richard and all his children. Luke and Benedict, in particular, cuddled up to Lennie, bless them. They are a lovely family." After Mass on Sunday, I was asked to "organise a campaign by CAFOD (the Catholic Fund for Overseas Development) to put pressure on the World Bank. Later we all watched England's Women Cricketers beat India in the World Cup." I'd driven Stephen to the bus station. He later phoned "to tell us he'd had a letter saying he was no longer eligible for Disability Living Allowance and that his bus pass would run out in August.

"For the first time since her accident nine weeks ago, Lennie did a small shop at Sainsbury's. On the following day, we discussed Stephen losing his Disability Living Allowance (DLA) and afterwards I phoned him and suggested he went to his doctor to discuss it with him and get medical advice ... Be with him, Lord." I mowed the lawn but found it hard going and suspected that "Stephen will have to do it next year". A lot of my time was spent managing our finances and negotiating insurances and I also drove two or three men to the weekly Men's Walking Group pub lunch. One gave me a phone number for Action for Carers to hopefully help Stephen with his problem with DLA. I was doing a lot of the cooking but recorded that "I don't enjoy cooking but I need to since my lovely wife isn't sure who I am; doesn't know we have been married for fifty-six years; that all our children live elsewhere and that her sister died some years ago. This is the largely hidden reality of my life. I'd love to have some free time to read." We went out for an evening meal. "It gave Lennie an opportunity to go over the difficulties she'd had at Hexham and then during the first few years of our married life, with little support from our parents and the five years of night classes I had. Lennie did wonders and it is only right that I should be giving her loving support now."

The following morning, "Lennie complained about her knee. So, I went off to Sainsbury's to do a £50+ shop. During and after supper, Lennie repeatedly asked me where Mike was and where the rest of the family was and if I was her husband, and when we met. Later, gently, I responded to her question that her memory loss began to be apparent about six months ago, though the children had been aware of it long before then. But she is still very resistant to going to see the doctor about it." Early on Saturday afternoon, I went upstairs to escape from a verbal battering from Stephen before and after lunch as I/we try to come to grips with and advise him how to budget following his loss of his DLA/PIP of £310 per month. His assessor's review later seemed to me very comprehensive, even if Stephen has a point about one particular assessment relating to contact/communication with others.

Interestingly, a worried Stephen "argued strongly that when Lennie and I died his three siblings would have an interest in pressurising him because of their children's benefits. It suggested to me that he was deeply suspicious of the potential concerns of the three trustees with respect to his rights and safeguards, etc." On the Saturday evening, "I drove off to St. Pius', put up a CAFOD poster on the church door and distributed about eighty CAFOD cards around the church. At the end of Mass, as promised, our former Anglican priest called me up, where I gave my brief support for their appeal for more renewable energy financing from the World Bank. The priest, bless him, said something like 'He's a bit of a pain in the neck, but let's thank him' and the congregation clapped me." On the Monday morning, I drove Lennie to her keep-fit class and then posted about 108 CAFOD cards.

I started August with a busy domestic day emailing our three children, our trustees, suggesting we reduce Stephen's rent for 'Penrose' to £700 per month, which he gets in Housing Benefit, since he has just lost £310 per month. During the morning, I managed to park near the Grammar School and walked down High Street to visit both NatWest and Nationwide before struggling to return up through the monthly Farmers' Market. "I regret that these days I just don't have the mobility to explore the local offerings. I should have done so more thoroughly in previous decades." On Wednesday, while Lennie went shopping to Aldi, I had a long session tidying my desk and clearing away unwanted documents. The following day, we enjoyed lunch with our near neighbours at Carlo's and in the evening, "after washing her hair, Lennie confusingly asked where Mike was and whether we slept in the same bed". The following day Lennie asked "which house we'd stayed in last night and more of the uncertainty about whether I was Mike or her husband and if we'd bought our house, etc. ... Her last question was 'are you married?'" That evening, I watched "Mo Farah win the 10,000m race at the World Athletics Championships in London in what I think was the greatest race I've ever seen". On the Saturday, we were driven to the 90th birthday celebration of one of our Family Group, Frank Comerford.

On Sunday, Richard and Ben came round and we went to the local pub to watch the Champions Cup because we had no BT Sport. "Lennie was unsure who Ben was and what relationship he had with Richard! Talking to Richard later, he expressed concerns that we were not doing enough to ensure that Lennie got the help she might need. But when I later raised this with Lennie, she was hurt that we were all talking about her; in other words, she is in complete denial and there seems no way she will agree to go to see the doctor for advice. When I get frustrated, she tells me I'm always shouting and why don't I help her? Sadly, she is in denial, and I see no chance of her admitting she has a problem which <u>might</u> be treatable with medication. Help me, Lord, to be a good husband." On the next day I took Lennie to keep-fit and later picked her up from the bus stop. "Lennie again had problems distinguishing 'you' from 'Mike'; she seems to think there are three of us ... Stephen phoned about his session with his doctor today and his loss of PIP. It seems the doctor was very sympathetic and helpful and encouraged him to go to C.A.B. and seek voluntary work. He remains very wary about employment and working with others because of gossip and ganging up against him, as he feels happened at St. Pius'."

On the Tuesday morning Lennie asked, "Where's Nana? Was she with me last night? Was Nana here this morning?" It is difficult to keep up with how things are changing. It seems to me that many of the household jobs that Lennie used to do automatically, she now needs my involvement or advice. On Wednesday, I drove two friends to the Men's Walking Group lunch and on Thursday took Lennie out for lunch at the Queen's Head. On the following Saturday, there was no Mass because the priest was ill. Later "for a good hour I listened to Stephen explaining his problems with his 'voices' and 'those controlling him' (i.e. MI5, etc.). Whenever possible jobs are discussed, he warns of potential conflicts with fellow workers, etc. He also argues that he already works hard at his paintings and blogs and sees these as his contribution."

Then on the Sunday "it was good to see Pat Jones on her birthday. Pat was conscious of Lennie's memory loss and always relates well to her." The next day I drove "Lennie into Guildford for her final keep-fit session". Later that evening we watched an André Rieu Gala concert, which is always good fun – populist classical music. "On the following Tuesday, Pat Jones came over to talk about her research into five Catholic charities. What seemed particularly interesting was the fact that there seemed to be no differences between the motives of Catholic and non-

Catholic staff and that few had heard of 'The Common Good' and practically none had any awareness of Catholic Social Teaching. Pat said polite things about how helpful it is to talk to someone about her research, but I suspect I didn't have much to offer her."

On Wednesday, Lennie felt "she would be lost without my monitoring her prescriptions every day". She had lost her front door key. "By a bit of luck, we had a spare which I gave her so she could go out today." We took our brother-in-law, Terry, out to lunch at Cote. "Conversation was quite easy, mainly about grandchildren. Terry has eight, but he also revealed some quite interesting facts about his work life – not just Phillips but also with National Coal Board for ten years, and teaching." When Lennie returned from a brief shopping trip on a Friday "she again said she thought Nana, her mother, had made out the shopping list this morning". Nana died in 1985. "She is quite aware of her strange memories … Lennie has given me permission to watch the Eroica from the proms."

On Monday morning I noted "I forgot to record heart pains in the middle of the night – I used the spray. I drove to Sainsbury's to do a middle-sized shop." At the evening Mass at St. Pius', "I interrupted the bidding prayers on the feast of St. Pius X and prayed for Fr. Brian O'Sullivan, our first parish priest, whose anniversary I understood to be today". On Tuesday I recorded, "Occasionally I shout, and Lennie tells me off for doing so! But we are coping with things at the moment, and she repeatedly tells me she loves me and is grateful for my care. Bless her." On Wednesday I noted, "I continue trying to document the difficult times I'm having to try to cope with Lennie's strange memory loss. Last night around 3.30 a.m., I woke to find the light on and Lennie frantically working through her various prescriptions. She took her various pills and I made sure she didn't replicate this when we later woke at 7 a.m. Later I drove three 'oldies' to join the Men's Walking Group at the pub at Puttenham, where I was wisely advised to avoid conflict." On the Thursday after Mass, I did a spot of gardening. That evening, Patrick Jordan kindly gave us a lift to his and Pat Jones's home for an evening meal. "On the whole, the conversation was quite easy. But I do feel a bit intimidated by Pat's huge range of experience with bishops, synods and even a pope. I'm not sure I contributed much to the conversation. Pat kindly draws Lennie into the conversation. Bless them, Lord." On the Friday, "Lennie's memory confusions were obvious". I helped with registrations for U3A's next academic year during the day at the Royal Grammar School. I also managed to do a weekly shop at Sainsbury's.

It is difficult to recall the process of Lennie's illness/memory loss. She has just asked me if I know Stephen and was surprised when I said he was my son. In the evening, she was bothered about whether we had enough beds for this 'woman' if Stephen came for the weekend. Help me, Lord, to be patient, to do what is right. The All Blacks beat the English women in the Rugby World Cup. On the next day " Richard came to tell us about his lovely holiday in Puglia. How difficult it is to make space to read. Lennie was full of worries about cooking meals for the family (all fantasy) around 3–5 a.m. which drove me to shout 'you are a selfish Madam' three times. As usual we sort of made up afterwards. Because it was a Bank Holiday and there was no evening Mass at St. Pius', Lennie and I drove off to St. Mary's for 10 a.m. Mass. Stephen is lovely to us and has done so much to make the bank holiday weekend so pleasant. I did a spot of gardening, not much really but as much as I can cope with. But I was the only observer of Lennie's continual asking when Mike was coming home, or where the 'other' person was who'd been here last night; and so on ... But she keeps asking about Nana or the woman who was here this morning. There was more ... Nana died thirty years ago."

After driving two 'oldies' to the Men's Group, I drove Lennie to Mt. Alvernia for her appointment with "physio treatment for her knee. I sent the strongest email I've yet sent to Anne Milton, our M.P., about refugees." In the evening, we went "to the Mill Theatre to see *As You Like It*. It was a good choice." On the final day of the month, "after Mass we went into the hall for the shared lunch for retired parishioners. There were about thirty to forty people there and at the end I took it upon myself to give a brief thank you and best wishes to our former Anglican priest and then all those who had helped over the years." At bedtime Lennie "strangely offered me either to join her or sleep. I led the final hour of the Peace Vigil in the single bed".

"On a lovely first day of autumn, after doing a medium shop at Sainsbury's, we had coffee outside on the patio, where our chatty conversation included questions like 'When will Mike be back?' and endless repetitions about our past lives. I'm not sure such behaviour is at all obvious to people outside the family. Over the past twenty-four hours, she has been concerned about the 'extra pressures' of Richard coming tonight to watch the England match; arrangements to pick up Stephen tomorrow and Douglas joining us for lunch on Saturday. These anxieties of hers are all new. I will have to take more seriously the role of a carer ... I had just settled down when a sad-looking Lennie on the verge of tears came out thinking that her 'Dad' (husband) was dead. I cuddled her and reassured her I was still alive and her husband. Be with her, Lord. There are other issues such as Lennie not realising that this is our home." I led the final hour of the Peace Vigil.

Stephen was a great help to us both on the first Saturday of September. As Gilly and Doug are on holiday in Skiathos, Douglas joined us for lunch on Sunday before going off to Gloucester University in two weeks' time. "Lennie has been struggling with increasingly painful knees and legs over the past few days. Unless there are signs of improvement, I'll have to take her to see the doctor. Lord, please guide me." There followed "another middle of the night passionate union – as far as we octogenarians can manage it. Again, I let my fingers explore where my penis is unable to these days. I have tinges of guilt as discussed earlier, and then wonder why; Jesus never had sexual intercourse, so we have no specific guidelines and what we do is love-making." Later I did a shopping trip to Sainsbury's.

I phoned and made an 'urgent' appointment at the surgery. When I took Lennie there, she "started by saying something like 'this is my mother' and a quizzical doctor caught my eye and I said 'husband'. Basically, there was nothing seriously wrong with Lennie's knee which time and careful exercise won't ease." While there I asked the doctor about my pacemaker scar and was astonished to find out that she had asked the pacemaker clinic to bring forward my next appointment. "The Tuesday turned out unexpectedly. I went to the Royal Surrey County Hospital for my pacemaker check-up, which apparently is still working well. But he took a photo of my chest lump and consulted a cardiology registrar. They agreed I ought to be called in immediately, perhaps for up to two weeks. Wow! What a surprise. I was worried about Lennie, so I phoned Stephen who agreed instantly to come and look after her. When I returned home, she was almost in tears." I took a taxi back to the E.A.U. (Emergency Assessment Unit) where "I had various assessments made by charming staff. In due course I saw a registrar and was taken up to the Merrow Ward." Later, Stephen brought Lennie in a wheelchair to see me.

The following day the cardiologist "more or less confirmed that they are likely to take out my pacemaker and then take me up to London to implant a new pacemaker, probably a few days in between to check that I have no infection. Then, unexpectedly, Sr. Theresa came to see me and later brought me Holy Communion. Bless her and thank You, Lord. Stephen turned up, wheeling Lennie in a wheelchair" and then we suddenly realised that the patient two beds down the ward was the fellow parishioner who sat in front of us at St. Pius'. I gave Stephen instructions about Lennie's prescriptions and the need to buy several anniversary cards. Later, I was visited by Katie and Douglas and then Richard. The surgeon at the Royal Brompton Hospital was abroad so the next day I was driven home by Katie and Stephen and a tired Andrew drove over from Reading to see me. "I have been truly humbled and gratified by the love and support shown me by my children and grandchildren over the last couple of days."

The next day, after Stephen and I had done a week's shopping at Sainsbury's, we went to the pub at Whitmore Common with Katie and Douglas, and we watched an England cricket match and had a cuddle. Later that evening Lennie was unable to respond to the Prayerline phone requirement. "I think her name ought to come off the list if she is so confused about it." When I drove Stephen to the bus station on Sunday evening "we agreed that Lennie's memory loss has accelerated in the last couple of weeks. Stephen doubted he would be able to cope as Lennie's carer without frequent breaks." The next couple of days saw plenty of evidence of Lennie's memory problems, now not putting dishes away in their usual places. "Mgr. Tony Barry phoned and discussed arrangements for tonight's 'Anointing of the Sick'. Bishop Richard had kindly sent his best wishes and prayers." Later at Mass, "Mgr. Tony Barry gave me the anointing of the sick".

Stephen was very good and patient with Lennie's repeated questions about the next few days. I was taken to the first meeting of the Justice and Peace Group of the academic year. Richard very kindly drove me to the Royal Brompton Hospital for my pacemaker operation to switch sides. Luke kindly and unexpectedly came and spent two hours with me in the morning and Andrew drove down from Oxford to see me; bless him. The next day I was taken into the surgery and seven hours later I woke up from the anaesthetic having had my pacemaker removed from my left side and replaced on my right side. The day after my operation I was subjected to a constant series of tests until I was told that one of the three wires connected to my new pacemaker wasn't working. I had a couple of days having a whole series of tests and being given antibiotics. Eventually, after a week in hospital, Richard drove me home to a very pleasant reunion with Lennie and Stephen.

Getting back to normal happened very rapidly. My diary reflected this: "Lennie started 'faffing' around in the bedroom looking for a handkerchief and I found it very frustrating and irritating. In time I began to see it as the cross which Jesus promised. Lennie had a terrible chest cough and I thought I didn't come out of hospital to be a carer for my wife. It irritated me that I didn't have space to read more than one page of the *Guardian*. When there were more interruptions, in frustration I went upstairs to delete no fewer than ninety-eight emails. Stephen was excellent." The following day I continued: "Lennie was cross I didn't go to bed with her at 9.30 p.m. last night. In the middle of the night, she was wandering all over the place for pants and I had to get up to show her where the Benylin was. She was saddened that I hadn't talked to her more yesterday ... In the end, we stayed at home and didn't go to Mass because Lennie had a heavy cold ... but I'm afraid Lennie's problems emerged again and again. She thought a couple was staying with us yesterday; she didn't know where her keys were; our G.P. is a permanent 'devil'; total denial of memory loss; repeated questions over and over again; arguing about shopping tonight or tomorrow; where is Mike going? ... Help me to grow in strength, Lord, so that I can learn to cope with the probability that my cross is going to be coping as Lennie's carer. One can only pray for God's guidance. Help me, Lord, to follow You."

The following day, I was exhausted simply climbing the stairs, so when Stephen and Lennie had driven off to shop, "I explored on the web about chair/stair lifts. To my surprise, one company contacted me later and arranged to come and consider our needs as soon as this afternoon and next Monday for the walk-in shower. I confess I have been rather taken aback by my physical weaknesses since returning home from hospital. Ideas of behaving normally were clearly unrealistic. I'm being told to 'take things easy' for another week or so. The salesman duly came and seemed pretty convincing, and he even hinted we could bargain down the price. During supper on the following day, I challenged Lennie as to why she no longer did the things she used to do such as cooking meals. Not surprisingly, this generated heated exchanges. I was sorry to have provoked the issue but it does illustrate the very real change with Lennie's memory which has accelerated over the past month."

On the Sunday, I was irritated that our Polish priest's homily was all about Walsingham and Our Lady and paid little attention to today's Gospel reading about paying hired workers the same for widely different hours of work. If such teachings are not discussed in Sunday homilies, when will parishioners ever get serious teaching? Before lunch Lennie and I had the angriest exchange for a long time. She was 'banging away' upstairs in every drawer in the bedroom and was ranting on before I found a pair of knickers in the bin for washing. I was angry she'd put both clean and dirty knickers there and wasn't careful in using her numerous drawers in the sideboard in a systematic way. Late in the afternoon, I irritatedly put out a load of washing with six of Lennie's knickers ... Stephen and Gilly seem agreed that Lennie's illness had developed very rapidly and that I needed help.

On Monday I wrote: "Last night Lennie was much as usual: angry to have been left alone much of the evening and then woken every couple of hours during the night as she got dressed for a fanciful day of teaching". Later, Gillian and I saw our G.P. and he arranged for me to see one of the nurses to patch up some bleeding near my pacemaker scar and arranged to see him about Lennie's illness. "Then about 9 p.m., Lennie had one of her crazy spells. Two or three times she came down half-dressed and enquired what she ought to wear. Stephen went upstairs and put her in touch with her nightie. I was then pulled upstairs to clear away piles of other clothes and, for example, put away two or three bras." The following evening "Lennie came down wearing my pyjamas! Around 1–2 a.m., Lennie started getting dressed. I persuaded her to take off a large woolly vest and put on her nightie and return to bed. About two hours later it seems she'd wet the bed and needed to put on knickers with a large pad, both of which were randomly situated and had to be found."

At the Bookham Group, I led the discussion on 'Generational Changes'. The discussion "was OK but not particularly inspiring". Poor Lennie embarrassed herself by wetting herself during the drilling at the dentist. Stephen took himself off to visit an exhibition in Whitstable. "For some reason I'm occasionally getting powerful aches in my jaws; I suspect it is heart-related ... But when we both woke just before 7 a.m. we had a gentle cuddle and Lennie told me how much she loved me." We both went to Sainsbury's to do a weekend shop. Later, "I was washing up when my sister Ann phoned. Lennie answered the phone and had a warm and lively chat for about ten minutes without realising I was Ann's brother and that she is my sister. She has just said to me that she will tell Mike all about the call when he gets home." In the evening, we were visited by Richard and Will and Iris and "we spent a delightful three hours with them ... Lennie asked some strange questions, so it was quite clear even to Will that strange things were happening". The following day I wrote: "Last night had its irritations when around 2 a.m. and at two-hour intervals Lennie was getting up and dressing herself. At one stage I shouted at her quite aggressively and I wonder what our next-door neighbours must have thought."

On the first day of October, I wrote that "as usual Lennie did strange things in the middle of the night and at one stage, I had to get her to take off everyday clothes and put on her nightie again. But I didn't shout this time." Gilly came round and was very upset by the death of her dog Fellah, and they were planning to return Joey to the original kennels. "Lennie started acting strangely: she wanted to phone Maureen (who died about ten years ago) and Nana (who died around thirty-two years ago); and wanted to go home (this is our home). On Monday we went to the evening Mass and Mgr. Tony came over to ask how I was and said what a nice son Stephen was." The next day I recorded that "there are times when my jaws/ears and top arms ache and it isn't easy. Lennie still mucks around in the middle of the night and needs to be talked through fitting pads inside her knickers. Eventually, we left to take Katie to Cote for lunch. Who knows whether we will see her again when she goes off to Australia in four weeks. The conversation flowed quite easily, though I must admit Lennie's participation was quite sporadic." That evening "Lennie emptied a pile of clothes on the bed in preparation for the children going to school. When I pointed out that all our children were in their fifties it didn't make much difference. I shut my eyes for a bit until Lennie came down in my pyjamas."

Things seem to return to 'normal' in October, though this included Lennie's repeatedly distinguishng 'Mike' from me, and this house from 'our home'. After Mass on Thursday morning, it was pointed out that our Diocese of Arundel and Brighton had only five priests under the age of fifty. So, when invited to offer bidding prayers, I suggested we needed "to discern whether there is a case for women priests and married priests". When Lennie received an appointment from the Memory Clinic, she was furious, but "I was cross, too, that there was no attempt made to explain the purpose of the appointment and soften its unexpectedness. I have a big task trying to get Lennie to go to our G.P. for a consultation!" At the weekend we watched rugby and attended the monthly Family Group meal. On the Sunday Stephen walked round the estate, around three-quarters of a mile, with Lennie.

I was disappointed that Lennie didn't go for coffee with her friends after her keep-fit class. Interestingly, I recorded "I think Stephen really needs a break from the difficulties we are having with Lennie". I've had a couple of cold calls recently and regard these people as evil. I drove two men to the Men's Group lunch on the Wednesday. "It struck me that four of the ten men had wives with Alzheimer's." Lennie had been taken out for lunch by a friend. I went to probably my last Labour Party Branch meeting, just round the corner. On the Sunday afternoon, Lennie worried Stephen and me when she went off for a walk. Fortunately, she returned after shopping at Sainsbury's. On the Monday I wrote: "One of the major changes in our lives is that Lennie no longer automatically assumes it is her role to cook our meals". The monthly U3A Discussion Group was on housing policy. On Wednesday, Richard came over to watch Chelsea. "Afterwards we talked briefly about Lennie. He feels she has deteriorated badly in the past two months and is incapable of looking after herself. This poses questions for us all, especially if I die or my health deteriorates."

The following day I wrote: "We had an unusual night. Just after midnight and again later, I found Lennie fully dressed. When I suggested it was midnight and she ought to come to bed she angrily accused me of always imposing my view. I let go and she spent the rest of the night in Stephen's bed. Over and over again, she's asked what time her toes appointment is and where." I duly took her to St. John's. Andrew phoned and gave me a blow-by-blow account of his damaged relationship. On the Friday, with Stephen's help, I planted a load of tulips. "I was quite pleased with the evidence that my physical strength is showing signs of improving." Sunday's diary began with: "'You are a bossy brat. You only think of yourself', an angry comment hurled at me by Lennie around 5 a.m. when she was wandering around searching for Optrex or her glasses". Perhaps I deserved it; I'm still not on top of my irritability with her repeated going round in circles. After they'd been out for lunch, Gilly and Doug came to visit us. After Richard had driven Stephen back to Cranleigh, Stephen phoned and he and Richard had had a long discussion about Lennie and he said he didn't think he would ever be able to be a full-time carer for Mum (Lennie). They both think Lennie must be forced to go and see our G.P.

"On Monday, Andrew phoned about his coming hospital appointments. On Tuesday, Lennie and I were rowing but we decided to go to the Clandon Park Garden Centre and there we both enjoyed an excellent lunch. The following day we both attended the appointment at Farnham Road Hospital, where the nurse was gentle, understanding and encouraging, and Lennie was calm and cool and coped well with intrusive questions and my occasional corrections. At the end there was a clear memory test, which Lennie struggled with. On Thursday, we attended the Requiem Mass of Mr. Kenney, who had been two beds away from me at the Royal Surrey. Mgr. Barry mentioned me by name, noting the beautiful prayer he had said in the middle of the night in the hospital."

British Summer Time ended that Sunday. "There was a clear invitation to make love – nightie buttons undone, etc. As Lennie said afterwards, 'it was a lovely love-making'." I think that my reading this morning was probably my "last official selection as a reader. I'm withdrawing because of declining mobility though I promised to be always available as a standby." We were invited to lunch at Gilly's "to say our goodbyes to Katie before she flies off to Australia".

Later, Gillian raised with me the discussion with the memory nurse. "I'm always a little surprised that Gilly and Stephen and Richard tell me that they think I'm coping well with Lennie's dementia, as they see it." Our stair lift was finally installed on the final day of October, and I have taken it for granted ever since.

Concern about Lennie's dementia tended to dominate our everyday lives. "Lennie was angry with me for discussing her with the children and not taking her side in the exchanges." We attended Mass on both the Feasts of All Saints and All Souls. On the Thursday, I had first driven Stephen over to Teddington where he was exhibiting sculptures and paintings. Sadly, he later told us that it had been removed on health and safety grounds. I took Lennie out for lunch at Ye Olde Windsor Castle. Andrew phoned the next day and "didn't sound too good. On the Saturday, we had the first afternoon session of the Family Group on the theme of the 'Common Good'." The following day I recorded "that around 3 a.m., Lennie went downstairs for 'breakfast' i.e. cereals!" Later we were joined by Gillian and Doug and their dog, Millie. "As soon as they had gone, I drove Stephen to Teddington to pick up his sculptures and two paintings."

On the Monday morning, I drove Lennie into Guildford for her keep-fit class and then did a weekly shop at Sainsbury's. Lennie eventually returned home having got the wrong bus and been taken all around the Bushy Hill estate two miles away. In my diary for Tuesday, I wrote: "I feel I have aged a lot in the last couple of months. Lennie's strange illness doesn't help. Last night we went to bed soon after 10 p.m. At 11 p.m. she woke up and for at least half an hour looked for clothes and even proposed making a cup of tea. After half an hour I lost my cool and expressed anger at having a night's sleep interrupted ... As seems to happen frequently, as the morning progressed, Lennie got more and more agitated and angry about being bullied into going to Mt.

Alvernia Hospital and bitter at being coerced 'behind her back'. I managed to keep reasonably cool and drove her to Mt. Alvernia where she had her C.T. scan very quickly." Later that evening I was driven to the Justice and Peace meeting, where "we had some lively exchanges about the 'Write for Rights' campaign; a Peace Vigil; and the 10% collection. Pat Jones told us about the three-day conference in Rome on homelessness.

"Last night around 2 a.m., Lennie returned from having 'breakfast' downstairs but left the light on, so I walked down to switch it off. Almost every hour from then on, she was thinking of getting up. At the last time my patience gave way and I exploded about her destroying my night's sleep." Unexpectedly, she took a bus into Guildford to do some shopping. I later drove two 'oldies' to the Men's Group. I ended: "It's not been a bad day, though Lennie continues to insist that another woman has been living in this house and hasn't returned tonight as we go to bed. Be with us both, Lord, and please help me control my irascibility."

After going to Mass on the Thursday, I took Lennie out for lunch at the Horse and Groom pub in Merrow. After our afternoon snooze, "Lennie made us tea and mince pies and then nattered on and on repeatedly about the old bossy woman who lives here and occasionally drives off in the car without asking. All fantasy, but she firmly believes it as factual and that we have another home." On Friday I noted: "It seems increasingly obvious that I will have to get more seriously involved with cooking our meals". That evening we went to the Mass at St. Joseph's, where our three priests were inducted into the Catholic Parish of Guildford. "Lennie observed that she doesn't find it so easy to socialise these days. A sign of the times?"

The following Monday I had my check up at the Royal Brompton Hospital. Richard drove Stephen and me in and then we had to walk a quarter of a mile to the Outpatients

Department where the Registrar "judged I was OK for six months. My pacemaker was OK, though the third wire was still a problem. A fellow parishioner, Tony Clarke, came and kindly drove us home. Lennie was very distressed when she found none of us at home and she'd forgotten I was going to the Royal Brompton for a check-up. She was kindly looked after by our neighbours. Thank God for our caring neighbours and also for Stephen's support this morning ... I think Lennie's forgetfulness became rather public today." On the following day, when shopping in Sainsbury's, I was warned by a fellow parishioner, from his own experience, "that things would only get worse with Lennie's dementia". Later two neighbours, Norma and Ian, "drove us to Carlo's Restaurant at Newlands Corner where we had a very pleasant conversation and meal. The evening was largely spent trying to cope with Lennie's loss of memory."

On the Wednesday, I warned the Bookham Group that I might not be able to continue. In the evening there was the half-yearly meeting of the trustees. "All brought gifts: Andrew a solid chair; Gillian very much on top of finances; and Richard on top of maintenance issues. Apart from Trust concerns, Richard raised 'family' concerns about Stephen, and it was good to hear they all recognised a concern for Stephen's welfare." The next day, we took our brother-in-law, Terry, out for lunch at Cote. "We then had a very pleasant meal and conversation carried on until about 3 p.m. Terry was anxious about his family. Terry didn't feel confident enough anymore to travel across London to catch the train north. He was undergoing all sorts of investigations in connection with his memory loss and depression. Be with him, Lord." The next day I managed to go to the U3A Opera Group, but in the evening Lennie and I had another explosive exchange over the timing of a women's group meeting. At Mass on Saturday, Lennie and I were asked to bring up the offertory. In the evening "she wanted us to repeat arrangements for Monday over and over again and as she went up to bed. She kept asking where Gillian was going to sleep." Gillian was sacristan at Mass on Sunday when they sang my favourite hymn 'Here I am, Lord'. When I returned from driving Stephen to the bus station in the evening, "Lennie persisted in asking me about this house. She seemed quite unaware that we have lived in this house for over nine years now."

On the Monday, the mechanics came to take out the bath and install the walk-in shower. At lunch time I drove Lennie up to the Golf House, where there was the Women's Group lunch and, in the evening, we went to Mass at St. Pius'. Tuesday was another busy day. I was involved with preparing for the 'Write for Rights' campaign. In the afternoon I went to the U3A Discussion Group on the theme of literary fiction vs other types. On Wednesday, I drove my neighbour, Ron Sloan, to a very pleasant Men's Group lunch. "Then our superbly professional workman finished installing the walk-in shower and tidying up."

I took Lennie to a pub lunch at 'The Compasses' at Gomshall. The next day was Andrew's birthday; he was having a short break in Mallorca. Stephen kindly came over and went to Sainsbury's with Lennie. "Rather disturbingly, he told me Lennie's driving had been rather erratic and dangerous and said he hoped her driving licence wasn't renewed ... Lennie thinks her deceased sister, Maureen, is around and isn't sure which is our bedroom and what to carry upstairs for our early morning tea. Help me, Lord, to cope with love and humour." The next day started with the stair lift not working. Richard came over with Will and Iris and we watched Chelsea manage luckily to draw at Anfield. "Iris had slept in my arms for half an hour or so." Sunday passed by much as usual. "Stephen kindly took Lennie for a walk around the estate. He helped me repair a door handle, at least roughly. Some rugby was on TV, I think, and then Stephen gave vent to one of his endless discourses/rants which involved supposed MI5 attempts to corrupt the

Hornsby-Smith family from Auntie Pat, to me, to Stephen. Rather like his blogs, it didn't entirely feel coherent, so eventually I broke off, and later drove Stephen to the bus station."

Monday didn't start too well. "We exploded very angrily several times and have used the F-word more times today than ever before. Lennie has been driving me mad and she has persisted in nagging me about my birthday. I drove Lennie into Guildford for her keep fit. Fortunately, I managed to park in the bus station, but I found the 200+ yard walk to Vision Express hard going. There I had an annual check-up. I have cataract problems." Around this time we were writing loads of Christmas cards. On Tuesday morning we made our way to the Royal Surrey Hospital, where I had an appointment with the cardiologist "who was responsible for my first pacemaker twenty years ago". He had kindly arranged to switch appointments from the Royal Brompton to the Royal Surrey. That afternoon Lennie returned from a small shop. Stephen joined us at Mass at St. Pius' and the three of us went to Carlo's at Newlands Corner, "where we enjoyed a very pleasant lunch". Gilly came to wish me a 'happy birthday' and there were phone calls from Benedict, Ann and Sue.

On the first day of December, I walked to the bus stop and found the quarter of a mile hard going. In Guildford I had an eye check-up and was told I had cataracts. In the evening, Lennie and I attended a bereavement Mass organised by two parishioners. After the Saturday evening Mass, "very few of them took the trouble to come and see the information sheets (for the 'Write for Rights' campaign). Four people wrote cards there and left them for me to post!" On the following day I recorded that "we again didn't get too many people taking up the opportunity to 'Write for Rights'. I think it is time for a new approach and generation to pursue the issue." I was surprised to find the following quote on 3 December: "The thought has occurred to me that perhaps I could write a book on our experiences of old age and deteriorating memory loss. Is the Lord suggesting this?" On the Monday morning, I drove Lennie into town for her last keep-fit class before Christmas. The following day Emily drove Ann and Peter down from Royston and we took them out for lunch at Carlo's. "Ann looked lovely and had a good, long and easy chat with Lennie. Peter was very friendly as usual. I just hadn't realised how serious his stroke had been, but, fortunately, he made a miraculous recovery. He has been a great spouse for my lovely sister, Ann." Later I as driven to the Justice and Peace meeting where "there was a useful discussion about a parish response to the Refugee Crisis".

It was on the first Wednesday in December that we finally had the results of Lennie's C.T. scan. Lennie and I drove to "Farnham Road Hospital for the appointment with the Memory Consultant, which wasn't easy for Lennie to cope with". In fact, the Consultant "was a charming young Spanish lady ... who coaxed Lennie along and there were occasions where I corrected her or provided relevant information. She gently told us that the evidence, especially from the C.T. scan, indicated 'Mixed Dementia' – partly stroke-like damage to the brain, and partly Alzheimer's, allowing the possibility of medication to slow it down." For me, this was confirmation of what we had suspected for some time. However, at the time this key diagnosis was delivered, it seemed very matter of fact.

On the following day, the Handicare came to make a final check on the stair lift and walk-in shower. After Mass and in the hall, a friend led a 'happy birthday' for Lennie in anticipation of tomorrow. This evening two friends took us to a very pleasant meal in Shere.

On Lennie's 82nd Birthday, I recorded that "I woke around 1 a.m. and was surprised to find her largely undressed in my study saying she was getting dressed to go shopping. I managed to get her back to bed. We were joined at Mass on the Feast of the Immaculate Conception by Stephen. The three of us later went to Carlo's for lunch and later in the afternoon, Gilly, Doug and their dog Millie arrived with cakes. Sometime later, Richard arrived, and Will and Iris brought a lovely birthday card they had written with some beautifully exaggerated expressions of love. Then Andrew came with more cake. Thank You, Lord."

On the following day I recorded: "I am sure we made quite tender and sensuous love in the early hours. That didn't stop Lennie asking me if I was her husband and had always slept in the same bed with her. Looking out into the garden she wondered if we had always lived here." After returning from the Saturday morning Mass, I wrote, "Lennie is no longer up to taking on the task of making lunch for the three of us. Stephen went into the kitchen and started organising things while I peeled potatoes." After watching a Chelsea defeat on TV, we went to the meeting of the Family Group where we "had a rather laboured discussion on tonight's theme of how we should prepare for the coming of the Incarnation". The following day was a fairly typical Sunday. After we'd returned from Mass, Gillian and Doug came with their affectionate greyhound, Fragell, for a sherry. Lennie came with me when, in the evening, "I drove Stephen to the bus station. She then entered one of her memory loss phases. She was confused between our home and Stephen's and whether or not we'd left our pyjamas there. She started an endless search of her purse and handbag. She spent a long time looking through them when she discovered she'd lost her watch." I would have liked to have watched an interesting drama on TV. "I had a bit of a verbal exchange with Lennie and reluctantly turned the TV off. Lord, teach me to be more forgiving and just give up my TV or reading preferences."

Life continued to be busy. On the Monday, Andrew contacted me and was trying to arrange a meeting with the

Surrey Alzheimer's Society. I told Andrew that "I felt this was pushing us into this before we were ready, and I had eased Lennie into acceptance". On the Tuesday, I noted that "Lennie has decided to go for a walk, and I have (lazily?) declined because of my right knee. Life seems to be definitely changing as dear Lennie repeats herself over and over again and seems unable to grasp that this is our house and that I am Mike, her husband. Lennie repeatedly talked about Nana and Maureen being around. I managed this morning to go to Boxgrove for my winter haircut. The rest of the day was spent completing the sending of Christmas cards and other domestic chores. Wednesday was also full of coping with the uncertainties of Lennie's illness. But we did manage to go to the Clandon Garden Centre on Thursday for a very nice lunch and for Lennie to buy extra presents for Will and Iris. I seem permanently frustrated that I am being frequently interrupted by Lennie when trying to read or write."

A flavour of our lives at this stage is given in this extract from my diary of the Saturday in mid-December. "When we are in bed, Lennie often whispers, 'I do love you' and seems very happy and we seem to be at one together. Other times she puzzles because she is convinced we lived in another house yesterday and needs to be reminded over and over again that our children don't live with us anymore. She frequently confuses the names of Richard and Stephen and doesn't know how old Will and Iris are. After breakfast I phoned Richard because Lennie thought he was coming to lunch today. He confirmed that he hadn't phoned Lennie yesterday as she claimed. In a brief conversation he felt I ought to go ahead and get my knee replacement, even if this presented care challenges to all our children. This set of comments indicates just how central Lennie's dementia had become in our lives those days. Asked about lunch, she ignored my suggestion that Stephen had agreed to cook pizza and when she brought in fish, I got up, irritated, because I'd suggested pizza several times and she'd prepared salad. We had a verbal exchange, and I was accused of idleness though I had already laid the table. Over and over again, Lennie told stories about the 'dominating woman' who bullied her yesterday into going shopping and making her pay, and then into going for a facial massage. Stephen and I watched football on TV and kept being interrupted by Lennie asking about the presents we needed to get for the children. I angrily banged my wine glass on the table and it broke. Stephen and I tacitly agreed to act as peacemakers if either of us lost our temper with the repeated questioning."

On the next day, "Stephen was getting more and more agitated by Lennie's late-afternoon persistent questions, interruptions and repetitions. On Christmas Day, we went to Gilly's and Doug's for a lovely meal before being driven home by a taxi. On Boxing Day, Lennie invited two friends for coffee after Mass. Later in the day we were visited by Richard and his four children and by Andrew and his partner, Caroline. On the Wednesday after Christmas, we attended the new 10 a.m. Mass at St, Edward's "and then at Sainsbury's I lost my cool and quite publicly expressed irritation at Lennie's procrastination. Stephen helped me get over it but he, like Lennie and Andrew, made it clear that I am a grumpy old devil." The next day I took Lennie to G-Live, where we saw the St. Petersburg Ballet show of *Giselle*. That evening there was an unexpected phone call from Bishopbriggs, a former colleague from Sheffield who "admitted having dementia and when Lennie answered the phone, she said that her father wasn't in". Lennie and I started our 57th anniversary making love early in the day and later we went to the Queen's Head for lunch. Later she denied I was Mike or her husband. The following night we again made passionate love, but Lennie then got dressed and had to be persuaded to come back to bed. I sat some of the time at Mass because I had a sore bottom. By the end of the year, Lennie's dementia was obvious and fully recognised by us all.

At the end of my diary for 2017 I wrote some 'reflections on a year of significant change'. Noting observations made as early as January 2nd, "I hadn't realised I was so aware of Lennie's memory loss a year ago and had thought that the significant change had occurred <u>after </u>our summer visit to Verona for three operas at the Arena and Lennie's fall at Sainsbury's; my damaged knee and then my sudden pacemaker transplant from left to right in September. The session with the memory nurse in the autumn, and the confirmation from the consultant that Lennie had a mixture of vascular dementia and Alzheimer's was also a key change. It seems to me that the children are all unexpectedly more concerned about care for me rather than Lennie; strange."

On 1st January 2018, I added that having read John Bayley's two books about Iris Murdoch, and with a growing awareness of the possible route of Lennie's dementia, I am also aware of my ageing. I'm eighty-five and the Lord will call me sooner or later. How should I prepare for our final days? Depending on the speed of the deterioration of Lennie's memory, I might have to do more than simply order regular medications but also hand it out daily. Will I have to take the key out of the front door at night to safeguard against middle-of-the-night wanderings? Will I be fit enough to cope with all the shopping? At what stage will we need to draw on care help? Should I go ahead with a knee replacement or not? Have I put all our financial affairs in as good order as I should? Please Lord, guide me through this coming year. Help me to do Your will and, as Richard of Chichester prayed: "May I know You more clearly, love You more dearly and follow You more nearly".

CHAPTER 6
The Year 2018

The year 2018 was the first one following the definitive diagnosis of Lennie's 'mixed dementia' and the way I coped was to depict her living with me at home. I notice that in the last four months of the year, that is after my two operations, we had approached almost daily attendance at Mass at St. Pius', our original parish, on Sunday and Thursday mornings and Monday evenings: St. Joseph's on Tuesday and Saturday mornings and St. Edward's on Wednesday mornings. Over the year, we averaged Mass just over five times each week and scripture reflection just over three times each month. At our age, we were still 'making love' more than weekly.

From the beginning of the year, we continued to have pretty full and busy lives. First of all, since we no longer had work commitments, we went to Mass practically every day. Stephen came to stay with us each weekend and was a great help. I was doing regular tasks such as driving Lennie to her keep-fit class, for a surgery appointment or to and from a hair appointment, making the shopping list and sometimes going to Sainsbury's, or reading the Feed In Tariff (F.I.T.) from the solar panels. I was also still driving one or two 'oldies' to the weekly Men's Walking Group lunch, going to the six-weekly meeting of the Bookham Group and the monthly Justice and Peace Group, and preparing for the Thursday scripture reflection before Mass. After a busy morning, I (and often we) tended to have around an hour- long sleep after lunch. After supper in the evening, we tended to watch television; Lennie, in particular, watched *Eastenders* while I watched sport, especially Chelsea and football. But I had a lot of difficulty finding space to read or write as this frequently annoyed Lennie. As I wrote in my diary: "There are two different Lennies these days. At night she often says how much she loves me and asks what she would do without me. Then, quite seriously late in the day, she complains about the authoritarian behaviour of my mother, who died twenty years ago, and with my burying myself in my writing."

Lennie was "incandescent with anger at my destroying a family holiday" when I told her I planned to go to a Labour Party Branch meeting. I later wrote: "I think it is an indication that my 'caring' must approach 100% and I will have to give up contacts and meetings such as U3A, etc." Interestingly, this was reflected in my diary on the second Sunday: "Gilly had advised me that times were changing, and the demands of caring really had changed and that I ought not to go to so many meetings unless I had cover for Lennie". There were new warning signs; for example, Lennie caught the wrong bus back from town and was fortunately picked up and brought home by some fellow parishioners. I noted: "I am suddenly aware that Lennie has been with me faithfully for fifty-seven years. She deserves all I've got in our remaining years." Lennie signed off from driving in January and I took her for a pleasant lunch at Carlo's. An appropriate theme for the third Sunday was 'vocation'. What is mine?

In January I wrote that "we are going through a stage of the most passionate love-making of our lives. Lennie invites closeness and caressing both late at night and during the night." The following day I added: "To be honest, I was quite relieved that she didn't initiate another session during the night". We attended the Requiem Mass of a member of our family group. Andrew's partner, Caroline, kindly drove us to a specialist photographer in Leatherhead, who gave us a splendid set of three photos which have since hung in the lounge, possibly to indicate how we looked just before we aged badly! It was Andrew's Christmas present, bless him. We went to the Odeon to see *Darkest Hour,* which was about Churchill's early days during the war, and then *Tosca*, my second favourite opera after *Fidelio*. The attempt to celebrate Stephen's birthday seems to have failed, but he told me that our four children were planning to meet together to make plans for our future social care and deaths.

"Lennie has been disturbed to realise she's never quite sure whether I'm Mike or the woman like my mother." We changed how we managed the way Lennie returned home from her keep-fit classes. Because she had recently caught the wrong bus home, I arranged to pick her up around midday at the Friary bus station. We took our recent widow, Frances Allen, to lunch at Carlo's and bumped into two friends from earlier days. We were unimpressed by *The Importance of Being Earnest* at the Yvonne Arnaud Theatre. Interestingly, around this time I wasn't impressed by "the new tabloid form of the *Guardian*. It seems to me that their 'Comments' don't have the punch they used to have." As usual, a lot of the weekends are taken up with Six Nations rugby!

In early February I had to take our car over to Woking for its annual M.O.T. Gilly had arranged to come over and keep Lennie company while I was taken to the monthly Justice and Peace meeting, where members "have arranged a meeting with the Council and Anglican Diocese officials as our next step along the road of supporting refugees". On the Thursday evening, we were kindly invited to have a meal and spent a very pleasant evening with Pat Jones and Patrick Jordan, a very interesting couple. Pat was working on a theology PhD at Durham University. On the sixth Sunday of the year, we shifted the monthly meeting of the Family Group, which had been together for nearly fifty years, from an evening meal to an afternoon tea. The host, Tony Clarke, had been widowed twice and agreed to look after the food while I'd agreed to lead the discussion "on our attempts to do regular scriptural reflection". That evening we enjoyed watching Luke, our oldest grandson, in an episode of *Encounter* on the TV.

Having dropped off Lennie for her keep-fit class, I sat in the Friary car park reading the information documents given me by the dementia consultant. On Monday, I recorded that "I found Lennie dressing herself at 2 a.m., so had to persuade her to put on her nightie again and get into bed". On the Tuesday, we attended the Requiem Mass of a former parishioner. On Shrove Tuesday, after I'd had my nine-weekly haircut, I took Lennie to Carlo's for lunch. "There we had a very nice three-course meal and Lennie nattered almost non-stop for well over two hours, reminiscing in great detail about giving birth to Andrew – a breech birth – and about our camping holidays, especially those on the continent in the camper van. The memories brought tears to her eyes as she remembered things in great detail ... Lent is just one day away. I'll try and give up alcoholic drink for forty days and see if I can fit in some regular scriptural reading each day." When we went shopping, I did most of it and all the putting away afterwards. There were indications that parish women were discreetly organising support for Lennie. Meanwhile, I wrote: "Lennie, bless her, seems very confused at times: 'Am I Mike?' 'Is this our home?' 'Who else lives here?' 'Is Maureen taking you to hospital tomorrow?' There seems little doubt that Lennie's short-term memory is deteriorating. At the same time, she repeats stories from her young years over and over again." On the Saturday morning, Gilly kindly took us to the day ward, where I was taken to the surgery to have a wedge taken off my left ear. That night I was "worried to find my ear was bleeding. Before we went to sleep, we had a fierce row over the pillows likely to be bloodied by my ear. I even threw a pillow at Lennie before regretting my awful temper." On the Sunday Andrew and his partner kindly took Lennie to Wisley, which gave me some needed space.

Monday was a busy day. After driving Lennie to the keep-fit class I returned to Burpham for my six-monthly dental check-up, after which I did a Sainsbury's shop before driving down to the bus station to pick up Lennie. On the Tuesday, I had to park at Tesco on the way to my pacemaker check-up for problems with the third wire. On Wednesday evening we went to the Yvonne Arnaud to see Charles Dickens' *Great Expectations*. On Thursday we went to a Mass offered up for a member of our Family Group and then drove over to St. Joseph's for a Requiem Mass for the sister of another former member of the Family Group. Lennie was full of fantasies at this stage on the Friday, when we went to the lunch at the Golf Course for the wives of the Men's Walking Group. On Saturday I managed a tiny bit of gardening before the Six Nations rugby all afternoon. We started Sunday soon after 6.30 a.m., "when Lennie simply couldn't or wouldn't stop talking. I find it irritating when she insists on chat with over half an hour's potential sleep left." Gilly came over for a chat after Mass and Richard came over and watched the Manchester United vs Chelsea match.

"I struggled to apply for a Blue Badge to help with parking these days. It was quite demanding. I'm having increasing difficulty walking up and down High Street in Guildford between the NatWest bank and Nationwide Building Society. The cardiologist called to inform me that he was going to leave my dodgy third wire and keep a regular check on it. We then did a large shop at Sainsbury's because of threatened snow. On Wednesday, we managed to arrange for a friend to come and have lunch with Lennie, while I went off to the Horse and Groom with two members of the Bookham Group for a discussion on moral theology. Because of potentially dangerous roads with the snow, we didn't drive to Mass on Thursday, so I had extra time to prepare for my presentation of *Nabucco* to the U3A Opera Group. I sent apologies to the leader of the U3A Discussion Group that I felt "it was unlikely I will attend any more of her discussion groups". Our Polish neighbour asked me to stop delivering parish newsletters.

For the first time, I wrote of the need to take up shopping online. We had previously arranged cover for Lennie while I was out at the Justice and Peace Group on Tuesday and the Men's Group on Wednesday. But she was very critical about it and so I had to make three phone calls to cancel my attendance at the two meetings. Richard came over on Tuesday evening and "tried to urge Lennie that it was good for both of us to socialise regularly. But I don't think Lennie took this on board." On Wednesday, Frances came with us to Carlo's "where we had a pleasant lunch and conversation". My comments in Thursday's diary give something of the challenges of my life at this time: "For over one and a half hours this morning Lennie was 'livid', to use her expression, and raved on about my not informing her about the parish retreat day, expressing anger at me and the men's group for not properly informing her, and thinking that today we were really going to a neighbourhood celebration. All the information had been in the parish handbook for Lent. Miraculously, I kept my 'cool' at her angry tirade, and comments about my being a 'selfish bugger'. I made sandwiches for both of us to take to St. Edward's. If this is like it is only a few days after her diagnosis, what is it going to be like in the future? Lord, help me to do Your will." Stephen was with us for the weekend, but both Andrew and Gillian called with presents for Mothering Sunday. Richard came on Sunday, so we saw all our children over the weekend.

On the following Monday, I recorded that I "found Lennie dressing herself at 2 a.m. So I had to persuade her to put on her nightie again and get into bed." On the Tuesday, we attended the Requiem Mass of a former parishioner who had died of dementia. Back home I was drafting notes to 'Children Carers' and also on 'Towards Women Priests' whenever I could find some free time. Because of the overnight snow it was helpful that Gilly drove us to Mass on Sunday. Not unusually, the weekend was dominated by the last three Six Nations matches on Saturday and Chelsea getting through to the FA Cup semi-final on Sunday.

There was snow early on Monday morning and we decided not to drive Lennie to keep fit but saw that she attended her Vision Express annual eye test, where was given the 'all clear'. Afterwards, I took her to lunch at Jamie's and was "genuinely surprised by how much she raved about it ... Our unusual day on Wednesday started at 1.30 a.m. when Lennie fell out of bed and cracked her head, presumably on the corner of her bedside cabinet. Blood poured out and we had a job trying to stem it. I felt it needed a paramedical response, so I phoned 999 and had to go through their lengthy questioning to assess its seriousness. In the end, an ambulance didn't come until well after 2.30 a.m. and after preliminary care they drove Lennie to A&E. I followed in the car." She was eventually treated by a doctor, and I drove her home and later drove back to pick up a jumper she'd left in a toilet. When she took off her hat, and was looking for plasters, etc., I really lost my cool and we had a very fierce verbal and almost physical confrontation. I was the bullying bugger who always wanted my own way. Later in the day I managed to go to the Men's Group. Our close friend, Frances, recently widowed, came to join us for lunch on Thursday. The following day, I had to take a taxi to the Royal Surrey Hospital for an assessment of my cataracts. In the evening, we were impressed by the film *Pilgrimage*. On Saturday I recorded that last night "Lennie spent a good half hour bemoaning what she saw as her loss of her independence, being bossed around by her mother-in-law or the 'other Mike' at Sainsbury's and being told to pay for it with <u>her</u> Visa. And this morning she asked at least half a dozen times when and how she damaged her head." On the Sunday morning, the children all met to discuss our future care at Gillian's house, but Lennie didn't know about it. Stephen and Andrew came here for lunch. They pointed out that "Gillian expected to move to Dorset within a year so they, the four siblings, were keen for me to start getting in care workers".

On the following Wednesday I recorded that: "we didn't sleep well last night and for the first three or four hours only seemed to doze until I took the initiative and Lennie responded enthusiastically to our love-making. I used my finger as a surrogate penis – since I have no erection these days – and I pray that the Lord will forgive me as I was trying to please my Nookies and encourage an orgasm ... please help me, Lord, to be a caring husband ... On Maundy Thursday I was asked if I'd have my feet washed." I duly did and we were pleased to be joined by Gillian but sadly not by Stephen. On Good Friday we went to the start of the Good Friday Walk of Witness up the High Street to Holy Trinity but having found the walk to Nationwide hard-going, Lennie and I returned home, but Stephen completed the walk. We all went to the Easter Vigil Mass at St. Pius' and took the mother of our Portuguese neighbours with us. We had a very happy and peaceful Easter Sunday, and we joined Gilly, Doug and Douglas for a very tasty lunch. "Thank You, Lord, for Easter, for Your resurrection from the dead and for opening up for us eternal life with You."

On the Tuesday after Easter, I had a pacemaker check-up and it seemed to have deteriorated since the previous visit. On the Wednesday, I drove our neighbour to the Men's Group lunch, tore up some old financial records, and slotted in more time on 'Towards Women Priests' Thursday was a bit topsy-turvy in that Lennie's attitudes to me varied. On Friday, the young son of the Portuguese neighbours came to ask us about our experiences of World War II for a school project. Sunday was much as usual. We took the mother of our Portuguese neighbours to Mass and Gilly visited us after we'd returned home. In the evening, we watched a programme entitled *Jesus' Female Disciples* and I then drove Stephen to the bus station.

I finished drafting my twenty-one-page paper *Towards Women Priests?* and sent it by email to the Bookham Group. In the late evening, "Lennie was very confused about how long we had lived in this house, been married, or whether I was her father or husband. She admits she is finding all these uncertainties disturbing." The next day was a typical domestic day following problems with my Mastercard PIN number and the rejection of my Visa. So, the latter half of the afternoon was spent making frustrating phone calls to NatWest and, after I'd checked no movement in our Feed in Tariff reading, arranging for the solar panel maintenance people to come next week. On Wednesday, I took a neighbour to the Men's Group lunch and on Thursday evening we went to the Yvonne Arnaud. On Friday, I had confirmation that I'd been granted a Disabled Blue Badge, and it was probably the result of Gilly's appeal against an earlier dismissal. It will be a great help. On Saturday, we watched Chelsea come from losing 2–0 to winning 3–2. On Sunday we took Gilly, Doug and Douglas to Carlo's for lunch as our response to their having us on Easter Sunday.

"I am going to write a note about the extraordinary and unexpected fact of octogenarian sexual love and try and reflect on it from a faith perspective. Four times last night, once before midnight and three times this morning, Lennie and I made love. I think it was mutual, but she clearly enjoyed it more fully. But I am inclined to argue that Jesus never said anything which implied that sexual love between spouses was wrong. What I do does not give me pleasure, but it does to Lennie, and it is a helpful contribution to the development of our relationship, which was very loving. If I have offended You, Lord, please forgive me and guide me in my future behaviour and love-making."

During Monday I managed to read Pope Francis's *Gaudete et Exsultate* and at the evening Mass focused on his theme of discernment. "I tried to open myself up to the Lord to try and discern how He wants me to follow Him." On Tuesday,

I had "to sort out my four different hospital appointments: cardiac, knee, eyes, cancer growths". That evening, I took Lennie to G-Live for a concert with the Czech Symphony Orchestra. On Wednesday, I presented my paper on 'Towards Women Priests' to our Bookham Group where "the discussion was quite robust". On Thursday, the engineers came "to check our solar panel system and they said the inverters were OK and didn't need changing". We had a lovely card from Katie after her first six months in Australia "before she goes up to Queensland to do three months' farmwork". We ended the day going to the Yvonne Arnaud to watch *The Kite Runner*. On Friday I attended the Fracture Clinic at the Royal Surrey but was still uncertain about whether or not to proceed with a knee replacement. On Saturday, after Mass at St. Joseph's, Lennie and I drove over to Old Woking to stock up with salt to soften our water. Interestingly, on Sunday I wrote that "Lennie is clearly enjoying and wanting close cuddles and sexual relations these days. My traditional assumption that it was always the male that initiates sexual relations has been shown to be quite wrong." Gillian joined us at Mass and afterwards "followed us home and spent the best part of an hour talking us through our first online Sainsbury's shop".

On Monday, I emailed the Centre of Catholic Research at Durham University "expressing my concern about my archives at Heythrop". I drove Lennie to her keep-fit class and then struggled at the bottom of the town to go to Vision Express, where they managed to repair Lennie's glasses. We were then told that Jill, the parishioner we'd given a lift to Mass every Thursday, had died suddenly yesterday after having attended Mass with us. May she rest in peace. On Tuesday, I went to the appointment at the Max Factor Department at the hospital, where they said my ear was OK. I cooked our supper but will "never make 'Home Cook of the Year'!" On Wednesday, we drove to St. Edward's for Mass, which we were planning to attend regularly. On Friday, I had an operation in the Cardiac Day Ward. They were unable to solve the problem of the third wire. "They modified the contacts with the pacemaker and hope it will survive for five years before I'll need another replacement – a more serious operation." I noticed that we had made love twenty times in April, i.e., as often as in the first three months of the year and roughly the same number as in the final eight months of the previous year. Strange variations.

The month of May started with a Lennie 'walkabout', "cross because I'm not with her and seemingly unaware of my lack of energy and mobility". I drove to Sainsbury's and Aldi's to see if she'd been there, having left her purse at home, and asked neighbours to keep an eye open for her. A couple of them went round the estate looking for her. I was very appreciative of their kindness and relieved when Lennie returned. On the next day, I had to "use my puffer because of chest pains but managed to drive Lennie to her hair appointment. Later, we took our recently widowed friend, Frances, to Carlo's for lunch. On the Friday, we drove to Reading to spend a couple of hours with Andrew, who "looked as if he was recovering well from his recent bike crash injuries. Caroline has done a great job looking after him over the past nine days." We had a delightful evening when Richard, Will and Iris visited us with fish and chips. On Saturday afternoon, we went to a Family Group meeting on "the theme of the place of the Holy Spirit in our lives". On Sunday, I even managed to do a spot of gardening. Our Italian neighbours came over for a glass of wine and a chat. It seems they'd "come to this country to give their children a better chance in life".

We had a lovely May Bank Holiday. I drove the three of us down to Bowers Lane, but needed to stop as I could only walk as far as the first corner, so I returned to the car to listen to Classic FM and read The *Tablet* while Lennie and Stephen went for a walk along the river. On the Tuesday evening, Richard came down to be with Lennie while I went to the monthly Justice and Peace Group meeting. "We had a pretty lively discussion about the proposed 'Refugee

Project Francis', which was seen as possibly fitting into the parish longer-term strategy for mission." Stephen came and stayed with Lennie while I went to the Men's Group lunch on Wednesday. On Ascension Thursday, Lennie decided to go to the Yvonne Arnaud to see an interesting play, *Monogamy*, billed as a comedy but with plenty of serious elements to ponder. I took Lennie to her dental appointment on Friday, and we took home fish and chips, which we found would be enough for supper too. "Lennie was full of confusion, for example about 'Mike' and again about the 'old man' who had been dumped here by 'his wife' but who kindly helped put the Sainsbury's shopping away and was pleasant company until he phoned for a taxi to go home!"

On Monday, after driving Lennie into town for her keep-fit class, I went to Nationwide to withdraw £15k for Andrew, to buy a new car as far as I can remember. Lennie's friends kindly brought her to the car in the Friary car park. We went to St. Edward's on Iris's eighth Birthday, but found there was no Mass. Stephen came, bless him, to be with Lennie while I went to the Men's Group on Wednesday. I spent a lot of time thinning old files, tearing them up and throwing them away. On Thursday, we attended the Requiem Mass of Jill. May she rest in peace. The weather was lovely, and we ate some of our meals outside. On Friday afternoon, I presented *Nabucco* to the U3A Opera Group, but "I really thought that it would be the last public event I'd be able to participate in. Stephen came and told us the bad news that his benefits had been cut yet again so that he will now receive under half of what he was getting a year ago." On Saturday, we drove over to Cranleigh for Iris's First Holy Communion. We met several old friends there and afterwards went to Richard's house, where he, Luke and Benedict presented us with a pasta meal. In the afternoon, we played football in the garden. "I went into the goal to face Will. In saving a shot from him I tore a four-to-five-inch gash down my right shin. One suspects that my blood thinners are leaving me with very vulnerable and fragile arms and legs."

After Mass on Sunday, Gillian came over for coffee outside. "It wasn't long before the conversation focused on Lennie's mixed dementia and the coming visit on Tuesday of the Memory Nurse. Lennie became more and more angry, complaining about our intrusion into her life and quite unable to interpret the visit as a monitoring exercise rather than an intrusive interference which was not wanted. Gillian, in particular, tried to introduce an NHS perspective but Lennie was increasingly angered by what she saw as our intrusion into her life. She got so angry that several times she even spoke of preferring to commit suicide than have more lecturing about her 'mixed dementia'. In the end Gillian escaped ... Stephen, bless him, cooked us a tasty meal of bellied pork. We all helped with the washing up." Later, I drove Stephen to the bus station, and we had a phone call from Ann.

On Monday morning, I phoned "Lennie's Memory Clinic nurse to warn her that things might be difficult tomorrow and she has asked me to write down reflections on Lennie's progress to give her tomorrow". I put a load of washing on the line across the lawn, but I'm finding this increasingly difficult. Looking for a couple of handbags Lennie had mislaid "under the bed, I knocked my arm and have another blood plaster". I wrote twenty points to give to the Memory Clinic nurse tomorrow and spent an hour ordering a week's shopping from Sainsbury's on the internet. In the evening, I recommended Confession "as a means of encountering the Holy Spirit". On Tuesday, the nurse seemed mostly interested in any side effects of Lennie's medication and unexpectedly, it seemed we'd now been discharged from the memory team and passed onto the G.P. We later went to Carlo's, where we both enjoyed lunch. I was spending a lot of my time thinning files and throwing away past parish newsletters, *Tablets* and *RENEW*s accumulated over years.

On Thursday morning, our explosion ended up with my breaking a glass all over the floor. On the Friday, we had agreed with our Italian neighbours to act as surrogate grandparents to Ludvica at the Grandparents' Tea Party at St. Thomas's. "I thought it was delightful. Ludvica came over and nuzzled up for a chat and several kids came to chat. I was impressed by their discipline and togetherness in the songs they sang and their general confidence, and by the staff techniques." On Saturday morning, I used my blue badge for the first time to park outside St. Joseph's for Mass. In the afternoon, Gilly turned up with her lifelong friend, Alison and her two dogs. We had a successful communal day gardening on Sunday.

After the recent cuts in benefits, I decided to give Stephen £100 per month to enable him to buy a bus pass. Stephen took Lennie for a walk along the river towards Send while I relaxed in the car. On Tuesday, we went to the Clandon Garden Centre for lunch and to buy some top-soil. On Wednesday, engineers came "and installed equipment intended to safeguard our inverters or solar panels against excessive voltage from the grid – or whatever ... Most of the morning I spent in my study filling a wastepaper basket full of redundant records. A long, slow process but with some surprise discoveries of articles I'd written in the 70s and 80s." On Thursday, we attended yet another Requiem Mass of a fellow parishioner. On Friday, I went to the Royal Surrey but was still trying "to sort out my various hospital appointments, with four over the next eight days". The following morning, Gilly came to drive Lennie and me to the Day Ward at the Royal Surrey Hospital, "where the two surgeons cut out the presumably cancerous growths, one on my left wrist, and the other on my right forearm. Gilly drove us home and stayed for coffee and a chat." On Sunday afternoon, we attended this month's meeting of our Family Group on the theme 'Faith, Politics and Conscience'. The rest of the time always felt busy.

The Monday which followed was also a bit frenetic. I started putting a load of washing on the line. But "I was finding the strain on my back too much, so I am sitting down while Lennie is finishing it off. It struck me that the time is close when I'll need to organise what she wears every day. Helping her to wash seems a long way away. Earlier, she'd lost her Visa card. It took me quite a search to find it. She lost her front door key a week or so ago. I drove Lennie into Guildford for her keep fit." I then walked into town where I bought a new battery for Lennie's watch and three front door keys. We then drove to Oxmarket in Chichester, with wine and orange juice, but sadly there were only a handful of friends at Stephen's exhibition, which I thought was excellent. On Tuesday, I submitted the weekly shopping list to Sainsbury's on the internet. In the evening, Gilly came over to give Lennie companionship while I attended the Justice and Peace Group meeting. After we'd attended Mass at St. Edward's on Wednesday, I drove Lennie home and then had a hastily arranged meeting with our G.P., who "articulated the uncertainties about a knee replacement. On balance, I think he was in favour of proceeding." There was a meeting of the Trustees that evening which "passed smoothly". Gilly kindly drove Andrew to the station afterwards. On Thursday, the Durstons in our Family Group joined us for lunch at Carlo's where we had a very pleasant couple of hours. On Friday, I went to the Clinical Measurement Department at the hospital, where I was given the impression that my pacemaker battery had been adjusted to last on two leads for ten years and that I was coping alright. On Saturday evening, we went next door at the invitation of our neighbours for an evening of socialising. On Sunday, Stephen kindly agreed to go for a walk with Lennie. "Sadly, I feel I must give up the Men's Walking Group lunch, just as I've given up two U3A groups."

On the next week, I'll start with an extract from my Monday morning reflection on Lennie's night-time behaviour, which is not obvious to those not there. "Lennie's behaviour is getting more and more unexpected. Last night she took upstairs water glasses, a sherry glass and a cereal bowl and around midnight she was looking for a cat we don't have. This morning over breakfast, she must have asked about eight times when her mother and father died, and was I her father or mother? She is totally confused by our children and sees Gillian as her dead sister, Maureen. Help me, Lord, to cope lovingly as she deserves after being married to me for fifty-seven years. Sheila Wheeler, a friend in the keep-fit group, phoned to confirm she will keep an eye on Lennie after keep fit. The four parishioners in that group have been so loving and supportive."

At Mass this evening the priest challenged us: "Are we happy to remain disciples of Jesus or are we prepared to become apostles?" On Tuesday, I went to have my three plasters checked by the nurse at our surgery. On Wednesday at Mass, we brought up the offertory gifts and later were joined by a friend for lunch at Clandon House Garden Centre. The Thursday Mass was a Requiem for a 103- year-old. In the evening, we enjoyed a meal out in an Italian restaurant, even if our friends, Michael and Sheila Wheeler, disagreed with us on Brexit and politics generally. On Friday, we went to Mass at St. Joseph's, and I later attended another Echo check-up at the hospital. Stephen came over and cooked us supper before we watched a great game of football between Spain and Portugal. On Saturday I was concerned about the need to monitor Lennie's pills to stop her duplicating them. In the evening, we had a pleasant BBQ at Richard's home to celebrate Fathers' Day tomorrow. On Sunday, I drove Stephen to catch the train to Chichester, where Richard was going to help him remove his paintings and sculptures and take them back to Cranleigh.

The following week started off with all sorts of instances of Lennie's illness, but I drove her to her keep-fit class and she was taken to the bus station afterwards, where I picked her up. We had to go to Sainsbury's, but she'd mislaid her

Visa card yet again, and front door key. In the evening, we watched England's first game in the World Cup before I drove Stephen to the bus station. On Tuesday, I had my three plasters changed for the third time. On Wednesday, Ann's birthday, I noted: "It has occurred to me that this year's diary will chiefly be a record of Lennie's development of her Alzheimer's. There are so many different aspects that I'm unlikely to be able to record them all, from being convinced a woman has been living with us; this is not our home; I am Dad or not Mike; to putting things away in strange places, which irritates me and leads to accusations of self-importance and authoritarianism; and much more besides ... I'm not joking but Lennie spent well over an hour, possibly two, deciding what dress, jacket and sandals to wear to go to the Yvonne Arnaud this evening. We were both disappointed." On Thursday, Stephen came over to be with Lennie while I got a taxi to the hospital eye department, where they confirmed I was on the waiting list for cataract removals. I drove Stephen to the bus station after we'd watched a couple of the World Cup matches. On Friday, Patrick Jordan came over to drive us to his home with Pat Jones and we had a very pleasant evening with them. "Pat was very good at keeping the conversation going and including Lennie. I do wonder what they get from us." Stephen cooked our meals on Sunday, bless him.

Monday was "an absolutely fantastic, beautiful day". As usual I drove Lennie to her keep-fit class and picked her up afterwards at the bus station where a friend had taken her. "The evening ended with a fierce argument about what was the matter with me. Why aren't I behaving normally?" On Tuesday morning, I had two of my plasters replaced at the surgery "and returned home to find the Sky mechanic replacing our satellite dish. Then I set off for the RSCH to see the cardiologist, who was very friendly and confirmed my pacemaker battery was now expected to last at least eleven years. But he saw no reason why I should not go ahead with my knee replacement and cataract removals."

On Wednesday, the three of us went to Mass at St. Edward's and I dropped off Lennie and Stephen at Jacob's Well, so they could walk home before it got too hot. I was taken to the Bookham Group lunch, where we discussed "the recent Vatican document on the ethics of financial issues, including regulation". In the evening, we watched more of the World Cup matches before I drove Stephen down to the bus station. The good weather continued later in the week and the days passed as normal with Mass in the mornings and Lennie going to bed relatively early. After April's active love-making we only made love once in June. "Gilly was a sacristan at St. Pius' this morning. After Mass, she and Douglas came for a chat. Douglas seems to have enjoyed his first year at Gloucester University and is thinking of becoming a sports/P.E. teacher. We watched a couple of World Cup matches before I drove Stephen down to the bus station."

On Tuesday, Richard was unable to cover for me in the evening, but later Stephen offered to come. Lennie didn't feel up to driving to the coast for the day so on Tuesday we took our friend to Clandon Garden Centre for lunch. In the evening, I went to the monthly Justice and Peace meeting, "where one and a half hours of it were devoted to Project Francis, which aimed to house Syrian refugees". I gave myself a bleeding nose on Thursday when getting angry with Lennie in the kitchen. "I'm finding it more and more difficult to cope with Lennie at home." But on Friday we enjoyed having a meal out at Carlo's and I spent much of the afternoon reading Pope Francis's *Gaudete et Exsultate* in preparation for the next Family Group meeting. On Saturday Richard invited us for a BBQ. "As previously, he'd prepared a great meal for us and we enjoyed watching Will and Iris play penalty shoot-out. Then at 3 p.m. we all went into the lounge to watch a solid England performance to beat Sweden 2–0 and get to the World Cup semi-finals for the first time in twenty-five years." During the afternoon, Stephen had told me "How very difficult Lennie had been when I was in the Royal Brompton". On the Sunday afternoon we attended the annual Oak Tree Gardens Party and I proposed a thank-you for Marie for organising it.

On the second Monday in July, a fellow parishioner, Tom Daly, kindly drove me to the Optega eye hospital, where I had the cataract in my right eye removed. He waited for me and then kindly drove me home. On Tuesday I recorded: "Lennie came down to me in mid-afternoon in tears of relief to find me here, thinking I'd died". On Wednesday, I wrote that "since coming home from Mass at St. Joseph's, Lennie has been unable to prepare a meal simply for the three of us". And Croatia knocked us out of the World Cup today.

On the third Monday in July, I completed a set of notes on *Gaudete et Exsultate* in preparation for the next meeting of our Family Group, and then read *Sensus Fidei*. I wrote that "I am becoming increasingly aware that the days of 'complementary' marriage roles are virtually over. More and more I am going to have to do the cooking as well as the shopping, etc. and be prepared to respond patiently to numerous repeated questions." Tuesday was a busy day, with my trying to be a good carer as the following extracts indicate. "After sending off the Sainsbury's shopping list on the internet, we drove off to Carlo's where we had a very pleasant lunch. Later, Lennie twice answered the phone and referred to me as her father. Lennie does provoke; she doesn't know what day it is or how old she is. She no longer has an automatic domestic sense ... things get put away quite randomly, and it becomes difficult to remember all sorts of things from her schooldays." But her general anxieties and confusions were apparent over the next few days. On Friday, I went to the hospital for a check-up following recent lesion removals and started writing notes on *Sensus Fidei*. On Saturday, after we'd been to Mass at St. Joseph's, we went to Samuel's to sort out Lennie's watches. On Sunday afternoon, we were visited by Andrew and Caroline and went up to Newlands Corner for a picnic and a huge ice cream.

On Monday we phoned Benedict to wish him a happy birthday and then, urged on by Lennie and Stephen, booked a holiday in Dorset in August. We also checked Mass times in nearby Wimborne, where the priest was retiring before we went there, but said he'd known me at Wonersh in the 1970s. On Wednesday, after Stephen had walked into town, "I more or less kept my cool but did warn Lennie her repeated questions were becoming very testing. 'Who are you taking on holiday? Is Stephen really my son? How old am I? Can I show the proposals to my parents? How much did it cost? Are you my husband?' etc., etc." Unexpectedly, Richard turned up on Thursday evening and we had a pleasant chat with him. On Friday, we had the first rain since May and sent emails to Ann and Sue, whose sons Jeremy and Julian had approaching birthdays. I had to drive to the hospital for a check-up on my cataract operation and try and set up the second one. On Saturday evening, Stephen and I watched a DVD, *The Sorrow and the Pity,* about the collapse of the French army in 1942. I thanked God I never had to make choices about collaboration or resistance. On Sunday, we were a bit worried about the proposal of our neighbours on the adjacent building to build an extension and its likely impact on the shade from the sun.

The last Monday in July was busy as usual. I wrote a critical letter to Guildford Borough Council about our neighbour's plan to build an extension which I feared would reduce our sun. Then there was making the shopping list for Sainsbury's online. On Tuesday, I wrote after doing "a tiny bit of gardening, I'm shocked to find I can't do this anymore. Old age and infirmity are a reality." I then elaborated at length on Lennie's loving remarks and weird questions. On Wednesday, I managed to join the Men's Group because Stephen had come over to us. I was cross with Lennie when she put the lights on and got dressed between 1 a.m. and 2 a.m. Later, after Mass, we took our two Catholic neighbours, Norma and Ian, to Carlo's for lunch to celebrate their birthdays over the next few days. A lot of Friday was spent reading an especially interesting issue of the *Tablet*.

On the first Saturday in August, Lennie was non-stop in her anxieties and queries and fantasies about the Family Group meeting on Sunday. Thus, among my recollections was that last night: "She'd come downstairs in her nightie and found two men there but not me. Yet a couple of hours later she was saying she didn't know what she would do without me. While she juggled choices about what to wear, today she asked over and over again when we were going on holiday. This is the life I'm having to get used to and try to discern how the Lord wants me to play it. On Sunday, after Mass, I helped distribute the leaflets about Project Francis to find a home for a Syrian refugee family." In the afternoon at the Family Group meeting, "I led the discussion on 'holiness', prompted by *Gaudete et Exsultate*. The discussion was OK but nothing special."

I started Monday with chest pains, which was a bit worrying just before going on holiday. Our neighbour, John Campbell, returned from holiday and we were able to discuss with him some of our concerns about his proposed extension. We attended Mass every day this week. Lennie was full of concerns about our holiday in Dorset and her questioning was non-stop. Stephen came over on Wednesday, so I went to the Men's Group lunch. In the evening, I drove Stephen back to the bus station and then we were visited by Richard who "was showing interest in the possibility of another partner. I must confess that I don't feel a compassionate Jesus would damn him for eternity if he entered a third relationship." On Thursday, I had to go to the pharmacy twice to collect prescriptions for the two of us. We did some shopping at Sainsbury's and then watched the European Championships from Berlin. We then got ourselves ready for a two-week holiday in 'The Poppies', a few miles west of Wimborne, which turned out to be very successful.

'The Poppies' was "a lot more spacious than we had anticipated". We soon drove to Wimborne and learned where there was parking and the geography of the town. On Sunday, we attended Mass in St. Catherine's and then drove back to the Botany Bay pub for a very nice lunch. I was "a bit taken aback by the rapidity of my decline in physical ability". Throughout our holiday, Stephen would take Lennie for a walk around the countryside. On Monday, we drove to Lulworth Cove and later Durdle Door, with a picnic Stephen had prepared for us. On Tuesday, Stephen and I had a stupid exchange, so he refused to come with Lennie and me as we drove to Norden and caught the train to Swanage via Corfe Castle. Wednesday was the Feast of the Assumption, and we again went to Mass in St. Catherine's, after which Stephen did some shopping in Waitrose and returned to Almer and went to the World's End pub for a tasty lunch. There was a lot of rain on Thursday, so I tried to read more of a fascinating novel about Jewish immigrants in the U.S. It wasn't easy with Lennie, who "emptied our wardrobes and drawers onto the bed ready to pack and go home. I put everything away again, but it is difficult to explain to her that her claims are fanciful. Stephen is chatting to her. This is the reality of Alzheimer's!"

On the Friday we visited Dorchester. "My mobility was so poor that I sat on a bench skimming the *Guardian* while Stephen and Lennie wandered off and soon found a delightful restaurant where we had a very pleasant meal." In the evening, we played a couple of games of rummy and later, "I wonder if this is going to be our last holiday. On Saturday we visited Wimborne, where I am afraid that my immobility was quite a hindrance to Stephen and Lennie's shopping and visiting the Minster. On Sunday we returned to St. Catherine's for a lovely Mass and then drove to

'Botany Bay' where we again enjoyed our meals. On Monday we drove to Blandford Forum and then back via Wimborne. I enjoyed the varieties of trees and birds and regretted I'd forgotten all their names since my childhood in Ampthill and Garpel in Ayrshire. On Tuesday, we made our last big visit to Portland and then had a pleasant fish meal at 'The Lobster' before we returned to 'The Poppies' because "the afternoon turned out to be the loveliest summer afternoon of our holiday". Lennie's memory went bonkers after she woke up and she didn't realise Stephen was our son. He later took Lennie for a walk round the fields as he had done several times. "What would we have done without him?" We played more games of rummy and watched DVDs. On Thursday, we enjoyed our last day with a large lunch at 'Botany Bay' and "much to my relief, all three of us seem to have enjoyed our holiday, and I'm looking forward to going home tomorrow". The drive home was slow because we passed the Dorset Steam Fair, which seriously delayed the traffic. At home: "Stephen, bless him, brought in our cases and took them upstairs and, without being asked, mowed the lawn. We had cheese and crackers for lunch before I drove him to the bus station. Thank You, Lord."

Back home, life began to get back to normal. We went to Mass on Saturday at St. Joseph's. Then Stephen and Lennie went to do a big shop at Sainsbury's, while I skimmed the *Guardian* "which seems to have replaced the punchy Polly Toynbee with trivial feminists". Andrew phoned us and then "Gilly came to drive us to their home for a pleasant meal and evening, telling them about our holiday in Dorset" where she and Doug hope to retire. Gilly joined us at Mass on Sunday. Stephen and Lennie were very angry about the proposed extension of next door's house. On Monday, we all three helped put the washing on the line. On Tuesday, our priest "gave a thoughtful homily about hope, repentance and listening to God's call" before I was relieved not to have lost a laboured Sainsbury's online shopping order. In the afternoon, "Lennie has gone off for a walk, but she is thoroughly confused about her parents and Maureen. Be with her, Lord." The second half of the day brought out all Lennie's fantasies, anxieties and angers. "She didn't realise Stephen was her son; she expressed her horror at returning to an 'empty house' after her walk. Where had everybody gone? When was I going? What was I planning to do tomorrow? Help me, Lord." On Wednesday, Lennie was pondering whether or not to rejoin the U3A keep-fit group. I find myself doing more and more of the domestic chores. We went to Mass at St. Edward's and found Stephen there on our return home. I took our neighbour, Ron Sloan, to the Men's Group lunch. I hurried home for a dental check-up. Stephen cooked our supper before I drove him to the bus station. The Mass on Friday morning was a Requiem for a former parishioner. "To my surprise, Lennie opted to have lunch at home rather than go to Carlo's. Later, Lennie's disorientation emerged strongly ... We phoned Gilly and Doug to wish them a happy holiday tomorrow. It seems that Heythrop have arranged for my archives to be placed with the Jesuits in Mount Street." On Friday, the last day of summer, "I notice that we haven't made love for six weeks now – a sign of the times? In one sense, it is all 'as usual' as we prepared to go to Mass at St. Joseph's, where the priest reflected on 'staying awake'."

Saturday, the first day of autumn, turned out to be "a lovely summer's day" and we spent the bulk of it in the garden. Sitting outside on Sunday afternoon, I was "trying to relax but aware of the catastrophic collapse of the Church in Ireland since I co-authored an article on Irish survey findings; and aware that not all our children are 'practising' and, as far as I am aware, probably none of our grandchildren". At Mass this morning, the Polish priest reminded us that forty years ago Cardinal Ratzinger referred to "a declining Church and the need for it to grow from the bottom up. All a bit depressing." Otherwise, the day passed much as usual. Stephen walked with Lennie round the block, about three-quarters of a mile. We had a peaceful afternoon and around 7.30 p.m., I drove Stephen to the bus station. "Bless him for all he does with and for us each weekend." On Monday, we took our widowed friend, Frances, to the Clandon Garden Centre for lunch. Lennie kept confusing the coming visit of my sisters with plans for this evening.

We had by now got into the routine of attending Mass every day. On Tuesday, Lennie had a perm at Hair Partners in Boxgrove. I spent a good hour sending off the shopping list online to Sainsbury's. After lunch as usual, we had a snooze. The rest of the day Lennie tended to chat non-stop, and I found it difficult to read or write. Richard kindly came for the evening so that I could attend the monthly Justice and Peace Group meeting. Stephen came over on Wednesday morning and this allowed me to join the Bookham Group and its discussion on *Sensus Fidei*. After Mass on Thursday, I took Lennie to St. John's for her periodic nail cutting. Our fellow parishioner, Voycek, came to look at what he saw as our small garden for the first time and initiated roughly fortnightly gardening sessions; another of my jobs handed on. Andrew phoned to tell us he had resigned from his job and was looking for another.

The second Saturday in September was much the same as usual. Stephen joined us at Mass at St Joseph's and cooked our meals over the weekend. Richard, Will and Iris visited us in the afternoon, looking "very brown after their recent holiday in Greece. It was good to see the three of them. They looked happy and at ease." On Sunday, Emily picked up John from the station and Gilly and Doug came home and had a chat with Ann and Sue before we drove off to take Ann and Sue, John and Emily to Carlo's for a pleasant lunch. Andrew joined us, so it was a lovely family occasion, possibly the last such family gathering. I had a busy Monday morning responding to financial matters and so on and also submitting this week's online shopping request. I went to the Royal Surrey Hospital in the afternoon and the knee consultant agreed to go ahead with my knee replacement. We attended Mass as usual in the evening. On Tuesday, I managed to phone through our Feed In Tariff (F.I.T.) reading before setting off for Mass. Later, I added two large spoons of salts into our water softener. I was monitoring Lennie's medications but, as I recorded, "I'm not being perfect these days!" On Wednesday, we were driven to Richmond for a Family Group discussion on the child abuse scandal. Later we had a bit of a row, so Lennie went to bed in the other bedroom. When I went up to bed, I called her back to our bed. "Early this morning we came closest to making love for a couple of months. To be honest, I wasn't enjoying it and was glad when Lennie had cramp and ended our caressing." On the spur of the moment, we went to the Yvonne Arnaud to see *The Goon Show*. Lennie was terribly confused on Friday, but we survived.

My Saturday diary was full of anger at the *Tablet*'s news that Philip Booth had 'slammed' the Institute for Public Policy Research (IPPR.) report. I received a large cheque from HMRC following my call to them last week. On Sunday, Richard joined us for lunch, and we sang 'Happy Birthday' for him in anticipation of his day tomorrow and his visits to the continent. On Monday, I was worried about Lennie going off for a walk and getting lost. On Tuesday morning, I noted that "our prayers have become more general in recent months compared to the detailed listings of the living and the dead being prayed for before then". I noted that my online shopping to Sainsbury's took nearly an hour and that Lennie's friend, Norma, had taken her out for a short walk. Stephen kindly came over on Wednesday morning so that I was able to take our neighbour, Ron, who didn't look well, to the weekly Men's Group for a pub lunch. Thursday was a strange day. I recorded we had made love, but my diary suggested it didn't go far beyond caressing, but because it was so infrequent in those days, I thought it appropriate to record it. I spent a large part of the day writing notes on the IPPR report, *Prosperity and Justice*, but in the evening, we took our widow friend, Frances, to the Yvonne Arnaud. My diary for the Friday showed the ambiguities and contradictions of Lennie's and my relationship as the following extracts indicate: "When Lennie kept asking questions about what we were going to do today at 5–5.30 a.m. I rather irritatedly asked her to stop talking and let me sleep. She very angrily responded with judgments that I was a very selfish individual who only thought about myself. Yet two hours later, during our prayers, she was giving thanks for all the support I have given her and admitting she wouldn't know what to do without me and that she would have to go into a home if it wasn't for me … I managed to put out fish, chips and peas for supper ... Lennie didn't get the timing right for supper and alarm bells went off for well over a minute. We had angry exchanges as Lennie denied I'd done anything to prepare supper. Foolishly, I aggressively defended myself and we had angry exchanges which only slowly dissipated during our meal. Lennie appeared to be in cloud-cuckoo land but also, sadly, very depressed, it seems, about decisions she'd not taken in previous years. I feel I'm going to need professional advice and caring."

On Saturday we saw Richard for an hour when he visited with Luke, who didn't look too well. "Be with him, Lord, and help him to keep close to You." On Sunday, the priest's homily "did seem to resonate with the lots of anger, irritability and bad temper which I shared earlier with Lennie". Richard and Ben turned up to watch the Chelsea match. Ben seemed to be stressed with a sixty-hour week and low pay. On Monday, as I was helping Lennie put out washing on the line, my right knee suddenly 'went'. Afterwards Lennie decided she wanted to go for a walk, but later a neighbour had come along to check Lennie was OK to be out walking on her own as she told him her 'mother' was at home. A reminder that it is a sort of gamble to allow her to go out for a walk on her own. "At the moment, I'm too immobile to go with her. But I must be aware that sooner or later I'll have to achieve more control or caring help. When Lennie returned from Aldi she asked if Maureen and her father had left. When I pointed out they had died she insisted she had seen them around earlier today." I told a friend that neither of us had joined U3A for the coming year. On Tuesday at Mass, "my right knee was giving me problems so for the first time I took my stick up to Holy Communion". I spent an hour doing the Sainsbury's online shopping request. "We then had a mini-squabble – Lennie seemed to have no sense that I'd been working on our weekly shopping list rather than just 'doing my own thing'." We went to the Clandon Garden Centre, where we had a pleasant lunch with one of our Family Group couples, Bob and Maureen Durston. Wednesday's Mass at St. Edward's was the Requiem for a long-standing member of our previous parish of St. Mary's at Burpham. Chelsea beat Liverpool in the evening before I drove Stephen to the bus station. I had a terrible night that night and my knee was "so bad that I felt I needed to go and check it out at A&E. Gillian drove me there and I was taken to the Emergency Assessment Unit (E.A.U.)", where I had a series of tests taken and eventually stayed overnight. I wasn't discharged until mid-afternoon on Friday, when Stephen and Lennie picked me up in a taxi. Lennie seemed totally unaware that I had just spent thirty hours in hospital. I wasn't fit enough to go to Mass as usual on Saturday, but on Sunday Gilly drove us to St. Pius'. On our return, "Gilly led us into a fiery conversation about our need for carers. Lennie took this very personally and was full of denial of recent trends and needs. Gilly was very forceful and emphatic and angrily told Lennie she was going to insist on our need for help if I had a sudden illness because of her loss of memory and problems remembering to take and arrange her prescriptions. Lennie took it all as a personal insult from her 'daughter-in-law'!"

On Monday, I phoned "Surrey Social Care, who agreed to do an assessment of our needs once I'd been given a date for my knee replacement". On Tuesday, Lennie walked down the road to have a chat with her friend, Norma. Gilly came over in the evening to be with Lennie while I went to the Justice and Peace Group meeting. On Wednesday, Stephen came over to enable me to drive our neighbour, Ron Sloan, to the Men's Group lunch. I had a friendly chat with our G.P., Dr. Barnado, who gave me a copy of my letter of denial of Lennie's dementia of August 2014. He felt "the consideration of long-term care, especially for Lennie, should be pursued". On Thursday evening, we took our friend, Frances, to see an Alan Bennett play at the Yvonne Arnaud Theatre. Last night, I forgot to put the refuse bins out so took round a bottle of wine to our neighbour, who had kindly put them out. On Friday, I had a fall and cut my knee. Andrew visited us and told us he'd left a Lebanese company and joined an Indian company. Before going to Mass on Saturday, I'd taken Lennie to the surgery to get her flu jab. But she was feeling sick, and we had to leave the church at the Offertory. Back home we were visited by Richard, Will and Iris and we played several games of 'Uno'. Sunday completed a relatively peaceful weekend.

After washing my hair on Monday morning, I noted that "I found it tiring and it made me think that sooner or later I will need help even to wash, shower and go to the loo!" Tuesday illustrated some of my problems. After returning home from Mass and buying tickets for a concert in G-Live in a month's time, clearing emails and submitting this week's shopping list to Sainsbury's online, I suggested we go to Carlo's for lunch. While I was busy on the laptop, "Lennie took herself off and left a message on toilet paper, which read 'I am sorry not to fulfill (*sic*!) your needs for a cook, but my expectations were more normal when invited etc. to someone's house's expectations. Good luck, Lennie.' How our wires got so crossed, I don't know. There's not the space to outline the strangeness of Lennie's behaviour over the next few hours. She kept referring to her parents and sister as if she'd seen them recently. She went to bed at 7.30 p.m. and complained about being coerced into going to bed. She planned to go back to Berwick."

On Wednesday, we went to Mass at St. Edward's as usual, and Stephen came over, bless him. So, I drove Ron, our neighbour, to the Men's Group lunch. Driving Stephen to the bus station, "he warned me of unexpected anger from Lennie which might become seriously violent". On Thursday, Lennie went for a walk but ended at the end of our cul-de-sac having tea with Norma. As she often does, she persuaded me to go to bed quite early. The Surrey Care nurse came to give us an assessment after our return from Mass on Friday. "In the end she was with us for nearly two and a half hours talking to both Lennie and me. I thought she was very professional in the way she kept probing without being offensive and being sensitive to Lennie's fears of losing her freedom." As always, these days, I struggled to find any time to read with Lennie's demands, which end up with my preparing meals. On Sunday, Gilly was sacristan and after Mass I helped sign up people to attend a dinner in the parish hall to raise funds for the parish refugee project, 'Project Francis'. On Monday, I struggled to find information on 'celibacy' before the Bookham Group met. Lennie thought we were having four people for supper. My diary for Tuesday indicates that I exploded several times. After going to Carlo's for a late lunch, Lennie wouldn't stop "pushing me again and again to have something to eat".

Stephen came over just in time on Wednesday for me to be taken to Bookham for our meal and discussion on the theme of celibacy. Lennie rather pressed me to go to bed around 9 p.m. and I wondered if this was fair. I forgot to go for my hair appointment on Thursday but after I was phoned hurried over to Boxgrove for it and returned in time to put away the Sainsbury's shopping. In the evening, we went to the Yvonne Arnaud, where we waited for standby tickets at a reduced price. On Friday, we went to Majestic to stock up on wine and I managed to do some reading until I had to cook our supper, after which we watched some pretty trivial and forgettable TV before going to bed. On Saturday, Stephen joined us at Mass and came home for an early lunch so that we could watch the Chelsea vs Manchester United match in which Chelsea equalised in the 96th minute! In the evening, after I'd squeezed in three quarters of an hour's notes on 'Prosperity and Justice', we watched a DVD given to us by Gilly. On Sunday, she joined Doug at Holy Trinity before calling on us for a brief chat after they'd had lunch out. In the late afternoon, the Family Group met, and I led the discussion on the IPPR. Commission report, *Prosperity and Justice*. It was a feisty discussion with other male members of the group very much taking a free-market line. I quietly asked two female members "if they could ask Lennie out for a walk sometime". On Monday, a friend kindly drove me to the Optegra hospital, where the cataract in my left eye was removed and afterwards drove me home. On Tuesday, Lennie was taken to Squires Garden Centre by two female friends.

On the way to Mass at St. Edward's, we checked our cash balances at the Sainsbury's ATM. From there we drove to St. Luke's to pick up our prescriptions. Stephen had come and I drove to pick up Ron and take him to the Men's Group lunch in Shere. Afterwards, Stephen suggested we drive out to Newlands Corner where he took Lennie for a walk. We drove him to the bus station. On Thursday, we managed to go to the Yvonne Arnaud. Before going to Mass at St. Joseph's on Friday morning, "I emailed Anne Milton, our MP, adding a personal postscript about Stephen's benefits being halved without any question about mental health". Later, I sadly noted that in sum, "the days when Lennie used to take over the cooking of our meals are over. I can't say I like it. It frustrates me and I'm irritated to have my bits of 'free time' to read, study or write dismissed as self-indulgence." On Saturday, Stephen was a long time coming home from the library and we were beginning to worry about him. Andrew turned up. He looked pretty good and was clearly enjoying his new job with Integra (associated with Pearson's). It was the end of British Summer Time, so we switched the clocks back. On Sunday morning there was a phone call from Richard who "worryingly said his boss was unexpectedly critical of him and expected him to do things which weren't in his current remit".

On Monday, I wrote early on that "I had pains or aches in my arms, cheeks and jaws and I was aware death might not be far away". It was a busy day with Gillian's "impressive and professional reflection on the care worker's social care assessment. She noticed things on her home visits which I'd glossed over but were very helpful." Later, Lennie and I went to 'The Jolly Farmer' at Whitmore Common for lunch. I passed on Judith Champ's book to Mgr. Tony, having discovered on the internet that she was both a professor and Vatican Dame. Richard came and spent a couple of hours with us in the evening. On the last Tuesday of October, I wrote, "Love-making these days means little more than a close cuddle and caressing; sexual intercourse is long gone". I submitted a shopping list to Sainsbury's online. I sat more than I kneeled at St. Joseph's because of "cramp in my right thigh". We found that the Mass at St. Edward's was a funeral Requiem. I went to the Men's Group lunch after Stephen had come to be with Lennie. We drove him back to Cranleigh in mid-afternoon. "He had taken a lot of trouble to tidy it up. Lennie and I were both sorry for his loneliness and phobias." We ended the day watching a Chelsea win over Derby in the Cup.

There were around 100 at the Mass at St. Pius' on the Feast of All Saints. For some time, one of our parishioners, Neville Vincent, had kindly passed on his copy of The *Observer* and last Sunday's "had some powerful articles on homelessness and the decline of the welfare state, for example. It was quite depressing." Friday was a lovely day as I noted: "How lovely it was being able to sit outside without a coat for one and a half hours in early November". As usual, I spent the evening watching whatever Lennie had chosen on the TV. But my frustration came out: "that I haven't <u>done</u> anything all evening". On Saturday, I tried to give a flavour of my concerns: "Our strange life started today at 2.15 a.m., when Lennie went downstairs for 'breakfast'. In fact, I think she only had a glass of orange juice. Later, around 7 a.m., I was bombarded by questions about how old we were, how many children we had, where they were, repeated over and over again. Later, around lunchtime, Lennie asked if my husband had died recently and probed away at when her father (who had died fifty-three years earlier) moved recently. All these fantasies are only obvious if you live all the time with Lennie. To outsiders she may seem perfectly normal ... I managed to clear quite a pile of emails before we drove off to St. Joseph's for Mass. Stephen joined us there ... Back home just in time for the Concierge delivery."

On Sunday, Gillian was the sacristan, and I wore a white poppy along with my red one. In the evening, I asked Richard and Gillian if they could come over on Tuesday evening to be with Lennie. But "it seems I might have to send apologies for the Justice and Peace meeting. Not only are Gillian and Richard otherwise occupied or resistant, but also Lennie feels humiliated by the thought of being looked after even by her children." On Monday I wrote: "Yesterday night, just before midnight, Lennie and I 'made love', and Lennie even took off her nightie and we caressed each other. But that is as far as we can go these days and I always end up feeling guilty. What would Jesus have wanted an eighty-five-year-old to do?" Several things during the day made me think I ought to retire from the Justice and Peace Group. I wrote to several charities asking them to remove Lennie from their mailing list. "I also wrote to U3A saying we wouldn't be renewing our membership this year. Clearly,

I'm expected to do all the cooking these days and not just 'sit in the corner and read your bloody book!'" At Mass on Tuesday, we had a row over wearing glasses and she failed to take on board my adjustment since the removal of my cataracts. "Lennie simply doesn't appreciate that I've given up U3A Discussion and Opera Groups, Justice and Peace tonight and previously the Men's Group because of her 'demands'." On Wednesday, I drove our neighbour, Ron, to the Men's Group lunch because Stephen had come over that morning. In the evening, we took Frances to a concert with the Royal Philharmonic Orchestra at G-Live. On Thursday, I coped with broken shelves in the fridge and freezer and put away the Sainsbury's shopping delivery. Richard phoned with the news that he was likely to be made redundant next April. On Friday I noted: "Shortly after midnight, a session of cuddling led by Lennie led to caressing and then to love-making and, to my enormous surprise, to my climax and ejaculation, for the first time in many months. But was it sinful?"

After Mass at St. Joseph's on Friday, there was a peace vigil led by members of the J&P Group with a Pax Christi flag and materials. "I joined in the reflection from the pulpit, which included interesting reflections on Guildford's conscientious objectors in W.W.1. On Saturday afternoon, we watched the All Blacks beat England at Twickenham. The following day was the 100th anniversary of the ending of W.W.1. Gilly and Doug visited in the afternoon and "Lennie asked if they wanted a drink at least half a dozen times". We squabbled on and off all of Monday and I was quite impressed by the Vatican document on Sport. On Tuesday, too, I felt "this has been another wasted day". Earlier I'd written: "I more quickly than usual managed to send off the shopping list to Sainsbury's. To my surprise, Lennie hadn't done a thing to prepare lunch, though I had put everything out previously. So, I boiled two eggs and prepared lunch. I tentatively mentioned that a Community Angel was coming round this afternoon and Lennie reacted strongly", so I phoned up and cancelled it. Later, Norma came for tea and a chat. On Wednesday, we attended a tea-time meeting of the Family Group on the theme of Remembrance. On Friday I recorded "some of Lennie's memory problems: (1) Though she kindly offers us to make drinks she confuses tea with coffee and leaves the kitchen in a mess; (2) She just doesn't realise that I am Mike but rather sees me as another person; (3) She doesn't seem to realise that the Yvonne Arnaud is in Guildford and not London; (4) She confuses kitchen mugs with cups in the lounge cabinet. One could go on. It all sounds so trivial, but she has completely forgotten that I have booked her to go to our Parish Ladies' lunch and paid for it and fusses around the leaflet over and over again." In the evening, we went to the Yvonne Arnaud to see *The Salad Days* and had a brief chat afterwards with our nephew, John Worthy, who was very good in it.

I had an early appointment with the Eye Clinic, which confirmed my eyes were both fine. Gilly came with Katie, recently returned after her year in Australia. "Katie is thinking about doing a Masters in Psychology as a move into work in the NHS. Lennie is strangely unclear that Katie is Gilly's daughter and kept referring to Katie as Gilly's friend, and that the two of them had similar ages." We had a normal weekend but "Gillian brought nearly £200 worth of clothes for Lennie and checked them over for me". On Monday evening at St. Joseph's, "Bishop Richard was talking to the deanery about the new diocesan 'plan', looking forward just twelve years to 2030 when there will be far fewer priests and what this might mean for the diocese. In the end, as Pat Jones suggested next to me, it was all simply bureaucratic. In the limited question time I followed a powerful observation made by Kevin Burr, a fellow member of the Justice and Peace Group, that there were strong disagreements between the National Justice and Peace Network (NJPN) and Catholic Social Action Network (CSAN) by asking whether the plan helped to promote a unity of understanding of Catholic Social Teaching and cited Philip Booth of St. Mary's, and the Institute of Economic Affairs diverging greatly from Justice and Peace people." On Tuesday, I sent our weekly online shopping request to Sainsbury's. I started writing Christmas cards. Ann phoned and said to me: "'Learn patience!' Be with us, Lord, and help me learn the role of carer better."

Lennie was very disorientated on Wednesday. After we'd been to Mass at St. Edward's, Frances took Lennie to Clandon Park, while I drove Ron to the Men's Walking Group lunch. In the evening, Andrew, Gillian and Richard all came over for the six-monthly meeting of our trustees. "It was quite straight forward with professional financial reporting from Gilly and a helpful maintenance review by Richard." On Thursday, Norma and Ian, our neighbours, took us out to Gomshall Mill for lunch to celebrate our coming birthdays. A lot of the day I spent writing Christmas cards and clearing emails. On Friday, "I drove off to the hospital for my appointment to check on my various lesions. While I was at the hospital, Stephen took Lennie for a walk round the estate, bless him." In the evening, we went to see the film *The Darkest Hour* about Churchill's early battles with his War Cabinet in the parish hall. On Saturday, we were joined at Mass by Stephen but also Gillian, who afterwards "took Lennie out for a girlie day of shopping and lunch". Stephen was very sick later in the day. In the evening, I skimmed the *Guardian,* but "it doesn't grab me as it used to with powerful and challenging articles by people like Polly Toynbee".

After going to Mass on Sunday, I had to make the lunch because Stephen was still unwell. During the afternoon we watched sport on TV and *Strictly Come Dancing*. Lennie was still not too well on Saturday, though we did go to Mass at St. Joseph's. Lennie was going through a difficult period when she just didn't realise that we had lived in this house for ten years. "I'm afraid my temper is not great, and my patience is limited. I've not been well all day and have appealed to be allowed to doss idly as much as possible." I didn't feel well on Sunday and so didn't go to Mass, though Lennie was taken by Gillian. Stephen got down the Christmas tree from the loft and put it up in the lounge. On Monday, I put the week's washing on the radiators and later took Lennie to the dentist. In the evening, we decided not to go to the Oak Tree Gardens AGM but enjoyed an André Rieu concert from Maastricht. Each day I cleared about a score of emails. On Tuesday, Stephen came over and I took a taxi to the hospital Short Stay Ward, where "the lesion under my right eye was taken out and stitches put in". Doug kindly picked me up and drove me home. On Wednesday, we went to St. Edward's for Mass. I managed to join the Bookham Group for a discussion on the Vatican document on sport. Our relations in the evening weren't great. We exchanged some harsh words and Lennie was full of denials.

My Thursday diary records that as usual I didn't get to sleep again after a visit to the loo around 5 a.m. and that our routine usually included the day's Mass readings and a mug of tea in bed before we got up for breakfast. "My jobs today included driving Lennie to and from Hair Partners for a perm and putting away the Sainsbury's shopping delivery." On Friday, the nurse from Farnham Road Hospital came. Lennie sent me upstairs, but I came down later and "the meeting ended amicably and with an arrangement to return next month. But Lennie was furious that she hadn't been directly involved over the proposed new medication. Fortunately, Stephen arrived then and eased the tension and later made our supper." Saturday was the Feast of the Immaculate Conception and Lennie's 83rd birthday. We went to Mass as usual and afterwards were joined by Richard, Will and Iris, and later by Gilly and Katie. In the afternoon we watched Chelsea become the first team to beat Manchester City.

On Sunday after Mass, the Justice and Peace Group encouraged the annual 'Write for Rights' campaign, which used to be promoted by Amnesty International (A.I.). But the clergy insisted we used suggestions from Action of Christians Against Torture (A.C.A.T.) because of A.I.'s promotion of abortion. We were invited to Gilly's for lunch in celebration of Lennie's birthday and it was good to see Katie and Douglas there. On Monday, I had my six-monthly pacemaker check-up "and was told this time that the battery was likely to last another eight years. I was very irritable this morning. In the evening, I managed to go to confession. On Tuesday, I had my regular eight-weekly haircut and then worked my way through a large online shop at Sainsbury's. On Wednesday, my G.P. thought I had a cancerous scab on my right shin and planned to have it removed. Later, I joined the Men's Walking Group for their annual Christmas lunch. On Thursday, I drove Lennie to and from the toenail cutters at St. John's. She wandered off after lunch and was brought home by a fellow parishioner who told me discreetly that Lennie was buying flowers and cake for her Nana!" Friday would have been my brother's birthday "but I don't know whether he is alive or dead". After attending Mass at St. Joseph's, I went down to Vision Express to have my annual NHS eye test. Lennie suggested I was married to our next-door neighbour, which led me to observe that "this illness seems to be progressing fast". On Saturday, after being reminded that our children and grandchildren had been given large cash presents for Christmas, "there was a very angry exchange and Lennie went out slamming the door. We do wonder how her anger will develop and about the problem of anger."

Gillian kindly came over on Sunday and helped sort out and tidy up some of Lennie's clothes and arrange to change a jumper to extra-large for me. On Monday, Lennie went walkabout and was spotted by a close friend of Richard. Fortunately, she found her way home. "Lennie admitted she'd walked too far, almost lost her way, and we discussed the possibility of companions to go with her. But she is still rather defiant." On Tuesday, I spent an hour ordering our weekly shop online with Sainsbury's. In the evening, we had angry rows when Lennie claimed I'd not told her about various plans. On Wednesday, I noted that Lennie: "seems totally confused about children, taking them to Mass or to the pantomime, repeating the same questions over and over again. In the middle of the night, she was wandering around the bedroom and tripped up; fortunately, she was able to catch onto the bed and not fall. Later, I went to the hospital to see a consultant about the scab on my shin, only to be told it wasn't her field. Medical bureaucracy!" On Thursday we "had a vicious row which left me with a bleeding left shin following a kick ... we gradually made peace". On Friday I recorded: "I'm thinking seriously because of Lennie's memory loss, this will almost certainly be the last time we take Will and Iris to the panto". Richard drove us to and from the performance of *Cinderella* at the Yvonne Arnaud. Iris was again called up onto the stage.

On Sunday, we drove back from Mass with the mother of one of our neighbours. Monday was Christmas Eve, and we were invited to Richard's, where it was good to see Luke and Benedict for the first time for ages. In the evening, we took our neighbour's mother to the Vigil Mass for Christmas. On Christmas Day, we drove to Reading for a Christmas lunch with Andrew and Caroline and her family. Wednesday was the Feast of St. Stephen and we drove off to St. Mary's at 11a.m. before Andrew and Caroline drove over and called in on their way home from their usual visit to see Andrew's friend, Vicky from his days in Turkey "and we had a pleasant and friendly hour with them before they left". On Thursday, Stephen decided to return to Cranleigh for a few days. "Bless him, Lord, for his pleasant company and the help he gives me in limiting my irritations and anger with Lennie." On Friday, I recorded that "my back was really quite painful this morning" but I managed to drive us to Mass at St. Edward's. The following day was our 58th wedding anniversary and after Mass, we were invited by Bob and Maureen Durston, two members of our Family Group, to go to the local hotel for a coffee. On Sunday, I noted that we were still following a regular routine at the beginning of each day: "tea, Mass readings and prayers before breakfast and the drive to St. Pius' for Mass". On Monday, the last day of the year, "we went to PC World to enquire about fridge and freezer replacements. Back home, we decided to continue to cope with our existing equipment." We ended the day watching a DVD on Mary Magdalene.

At the end of my diary for 2018, I added a few reflections on the year, which had included several operations. I noted firstly, "increasing signs of the approach of my 'last lap' and my ageing, physical limitations, and awareness of the approach of death, and secondly, the increasingly obvious development of Lennie's 'mixed dementia' and my often inadequate attempts to cope with it and keep my patience". Thirdly, I noted that "our passports have now run out and I've not taken any steps to renew them. This year we didn't go abroad for a holiday for the first time in recent years."

Overall, my impression is that 2017 and 2018 were major turning points. I had major operations and we had to cope with Lennie with the introduction of Everycare staff while I was away and I was relatively immobile when I came home. I rather feel that we initiated carers to help Lennie not me and that my relative immobility was somewhat denied by Lennie and possibly the family after my various operations. Indications of change were my successive ending of previous commitments such as the regular meetings of the Justice and Peace, U3A and Bookham groups. Among the major themes which emerged were changing Catholic thinking about sexuality, but also Catholic Social Teaching. The major stages of the decade of Lennie's 'mixed dementia' seem to have been (a) Denial; especially by Lennie but for a period by me in 2013/4; (b) Lennie's continual rejection of the evidence of her illness in 2015/6 and (c) Increasing conflict because of Lennie's continuing denial and my declining mobility following my operations in 2017/8.

CHAPTER 7

The Year 2019

Before I start going into detail about the year 2019, let me try and put it into some sort of context. In this book I've shown that although there were signs of Lennie's 'mixed dementia' as early as 2013 and 2014, I was still in substantial denial about it and Lennie was angry I was even discussing it with our children and our G.P. Over the next two years, 2015 and 2016, there were steady developments, and I became more aware of Lennie's illness and the changes it was making in our lives. This became more and more obvious in the next two years, 2017 and 2018, and it was eventually officially diagnosed as 'mixed dementia'. Most people we knew now recognised this, but Lennie was in furious denial. But her behaviour at home was significantly changing and I tried to record this in my recent diaries. In 2019 I had two hospital appointments for a damaged hip in April and a knee replacement in August. While I was in hospital the children arranged for Everycare workers to give support to Lennie and that became regular from then on. The next two years, 2020 and 2021, were dominated by the global Covid pandemic and Lennie's continued deterioration, which led to her going into a care home early in 2022.

The new year started as usual. I had a lot of emails to clear before we drove off to Mass at St. Joseph's. Then, on the Wednesday after new year, Lennie was very helpful when I had a serious attack of diarrhoea, leaving a lot of cleaning up to be done. We managed to go to Mass in St. Edward's and on our return, I managed to complete an online shop at Sainsbury's before taking our neighbour, Ron Sloan, to the

Men's Group lunch. Later, we drove Stephen back to Cranleigh. Lennie and I managed to cope with our disagreements during the evening. From Thursday we agreed to stop our brief scripture reflection before Mass. After coffee in the parish hall, we returned home where I prepared lunch and then put away the Sainsbury's online shopping when it was delivered. In the evening, we watched TV, mainly *Eastenders* and football. On Friday, after we'd had a post lunch snooze, we drove to friends in the parish for a pleasant chat and tasty tea. That evening, I got out the DVD of the first thirty years of our married lives together and holidays in France, Italy and Germany.

I'm going to give two quotes from my first Saturday diary to illustrate how Lennie was coping. After Mass, "I tried to read the *Guardian*. But as often happens, Lennie kept chatting and I got cross and went into the kitchen and put out all the food from the fridge for lunch before Lennie and I had yet another of our angry exchanges. The reality is that I must get used to the fact that Lennie no longer makes easy decisions in the kitchen. She doesn't know where the fridge is and where things should be put away. I escaped upstairs, cleared emails and insisted that she didn't have to do any shopping to buy celebratory presents. I do give thanks to Stephen for being with us over the weekend because he automatically takes over the cooking, which I'm no good at and dislike. It is frustrating to have to go to bed now at 9.45 p.m. and not be able to relax together. But that is how things are at the moment, and I'm trying to learn to adapt. I have a gut feeling that problems will accelerate rapidly in the weeks ahead and that I must learn to adapt much more rapidly. Please help me, Lord."

On Sunday, Stephen very kindly took down the Christmas tree and its lights and baubles and put them all in the loft. Lennie and I seemed to have squabbles every day, usually about her repeated questions and interruptions of serious programmes. She was cross when I pointed out I was too immobile to go out for a walk with her. So, off she went, and neighbours told us she had gone towards the railway. In the end she went round Boxgrove and was spotted walking along London Road and back home. Gilly came round to be with her that evening when I went off to the monthly Justice and Peace Group meeting, which was largely concerned with the Syrian refugee project. What little time there seemed to be was generally spent clearing emails and reading and writing notes on Philip Booth's book. Then, unexpectedly, Lennie had a spell of sickness which lasted a few days and limited our attendance at Mass. We coped pretty well, though. Stephen coming for the weekend was a great help. Lennie wasn't very well but managed to go to Mass on Sunday. We had a terrible exchange in the evening but made it up later. On the Monday, I finished my notes on Philip Booth's I.E.A. book on Catholic social teaching (C.S.T.) and we also prepared for Stephen's and Katie's birthdays later in the month.

At Mass on Tuesday, "to my surprise Lennie prayed for 'William Early who had died recently' (actually fifty-four years earlier!)" That afternoon I went for my appointment at the Royal Surrey Hospital, having to park at Tesco's and finding it hard going walking up to the hospital, where the surgeon suggested my knee replacement might need to be postponed until the scab on my leg had been treated. I also had to go to our surgery to have various tests. We had a pretty awful day on Friday, when Lennie was obsessed about Will and Iris coming that evening. I became angry when I wasn't allowed to skim the *Tablet*. Then, "the pyrex plate in the microwave exploded into smithereens,and the whole afternoon just disappeared as I listened to Lennie's endless and repeated reflections on her childhood and her mother's treating Maureen (her older sister) as her favourite". While Richard went to buy us all fish and chips for supper, Lennie and I played 'Uno' with Will and Iris. I ended the day praying, "Please train me to recognise the reality of Lennie's dementia and to be patient and loving and control my temper and frustration". That night I found Lennie fully dressed around 4 a.m. and managed to persuade her to come back to bed. Stephen came to join us for the weekend. He always gives me a gin and tonic at lunch time. Richard came over in the afternoon to watch the Chelsea game. On Sunday afternoon, "Stephen defiantly said he didn't want to go for a walk. He engaged well with Lennie who seemed to distinguish our downstairs lounge and dining room from the 'hospital' upstairs." Lennie was furious when she discovered I'd arranged for Stephen to cover for me when I went to the dentist and potentially the Men's Group lunch and our friend, Frances, on the same day.

At the beginning of the fourth week of the year, Lennie and I went for lunch at Carlo's. "Lennie was very happy with the opportunity to chat with me, so it was a very pleasant and enjoyable couple of hours." That evening "Lennie told me several times how much she loves me ... Help me to show her my love and patience to her, Lord." The following morning, "five or six times she called me a liar! Stephen kindly came and calmed things down as I went off for a dental appointment. Later, our friend Frances took Lennie out for lunch and afterwards she whispered that Lennie said Gilly had died a couple of weeks ago!" In spite of earlier events, Lennie persuaded me to take her to see a film at the Odeon. When the Sainsbury's shopping was delivered on the following day, Lennie remained upstairs as I put it all away. On the Friday evening, we went to see the film *Oscar Romero,* introduced by Julian Filokowsky, who'd been heavily involved in promoting his canonisation. On Saturday, Stephen came to be with us for the weekend and we also had visits from both Gillian and Andrew. "Gillian made it clear Katie and Douglas both prefer Holy Trinity Church to St. Pius'." On Sunday, in the middle of the night, "Lennie made herself a cup of tea. A quarter of an hour later, she returned to bed."

Tuesday was the eighth anniversary of Maureen's death, so I said a bidding prayer for her at Mass. After a quick visit from Stephen, we drove to pick up Frances and take her to Carlo's, where we had a pleasant lunch. During the rest of the day, I tried to find space to read the book about Romero, which was very interesting. On Wednesday, "Lennie initiated two sessions of love-making just after midnight and again around 4 a.m. On the second occasion I actually ejaculated, probably for the last time in my life." As usual, Stephen came over to prepare lunch for Lennie while I went off to the Men's Group lunch. Later, I took Lennie to the surgery for various tests. On Thursday, I recorded that "before 6 a.m. Lennie started her questioning about today and the funeral of her former teaching colleague Barbara Hanney. She asked: Barbara Hanney's funeral – was Pa going? What time was it? Was my 'husband' going? and so on, over and over again. It was maddening and repetitive and inexplicable really. But that's the way things are. I managed to keep reasonably calm." We went by taxi to St. Mary's, where "the lovely funeral service for Barbara Hanney was led by Rev. Robert Cotton from Holy Trinity. It was very tender and sensitive." In the afternoon, I took a taxi to the Royal Surrey, where the doctor confirmed that my recent lesion removals seem to have been OK, though the one under the eye had been cancerous, so she asked me to arrange a further check-up in four months.

In spite of some overnight snow, Gillian kindly took me to the Pre-Assessment Clinic for my knee replacement at the Royal Surrey and afterwards drove me home. Stephen, who had come to be with Lennie, stayed and we watched Six Nations rugby all evening. Just after midday on Saturday, "Lennie has just told me I'm like a hole in the head. She has driven us mad over the last hour, meaning we haven't been able to read. Eventually, I exploded and called her a selfish 'bitch'. As usual we soon made up." The afternoon was again taken up with some excellent Six Nations matches. Sunday was a fairly gentle day, with Gilly visiting after

Mass and Richard phoning from Oslo in the evening. On Monday, I started my diary around 10 a.m.: "I have quite successfully managed to put up with Lennie's infuriating, repeated questions and claims since we started our day soon after 6.30 a.m. For the best part of an hour, I put up with her claims that this wasn't our house but more like a hotel and that she wanted to move to a proper home." We attended the funeral Mass of a fellow parishioner, which was gentle, sensitive and loving.

The following day we enjoyed going to Carlo's for lunch. "We drove home just in time to prevent our neighbour and his workmen breaking down the front door because the alarm was going off. Lennie had put on some chicken on the stove, in spite of my saying I'd take her out for lunch. Another worrying sign that I must take on board. Thank You, Lord, that no great harm seems to have been done." On Wednesday, I caught a taxi to Milford Crossroads surgery, where the surgeon cut out about a two-centimetre diameter lesion on my right shin after giving me a local anaesthetic. On Thursday, I had an unexpected problem with sudden diarrhoea. The afternoon wasn't helped by "Lennie's relentlessly repeated questions: 'Are my mother, father, sister dead?' 'Who is going with us if we go to the Yvonne Arnaud this evening?' 'Shall I start making supper?' etc. etc." We did in fact go and "Lennie was full of love and gratitude for my care and attentiveness towards her – bless her".

Lennie is so confused these days that I let her come with me to have my various dressings renewed by the nurse at St. Luke's. We had a huge problem sorting out our freezer which had become iced up. Later, "Lennie had one of her 'evening moments'. She thought her parents lived locally; that she was going out with Maureen, I think, this evening. She needed to be told that I am her husband and that we live together; and much more. I am now aware that these fantasies are real for her and so reasonably and patiently try and talk her out of them and lead her to the reality of our lives together; that tomorrow we will go to Mass together and pick up our son, Stephen." Saturday worked out much as usual. In the evening, Stephen and I tried to select something which might interest Lennie. "Earlier, Lennie had one of her extraordinary memory episodes, repeatedly asking where her father was, when he was coming, what about our house by the river, and so on." Sunday proceeded much as usual. Gilly came over after Mass. She and Richard were concerned about support for Lennie when I had my knee operation and Gilly was concerned that Stephen wasn't overstretched. In the afternoon we switched between the England vs France rugby match and Chelsea's awful 6–0 defeat by Manchester City.

Monday was a fairly ordinary day, though Lennie went to a women's prayer group, and I started reading Pope Benedict's *Jesus of Nazareth* and told Lennie I wanted Beethoven's *Ode to Joy* played at my funeral! On Tuesday, I had to go to the surgery to have my plasters renewed. We took Bob and Maureen Durston, who have been good friends for many years, to Carlo's for lunch. But during the rest of the day, Lennie repeated questions over and over again. The following are some of them. Before going to Carlo's: "Is my mother coming? Am I going with you? Are you my dad? What are we doing about the children? Are you my husband? – repeated over and over again for at least an hour." Then, during the evening when she was 'very disturbed': "Where do I live? Are you my dad? Where are my clothes? How long have we been married? How many children did we have? ... over and over again." I put on *Eastenders* and other programmes on the TV for her. "Then Lennie came out with her anxieties: 'Where are we? Who lives here? Have we come back here?'."

On Wednesday, when no priest turned up for Mass, several of us led a Liturgy of the Word, as we used to have years ago. In the afternoon, the British Gas engineer came to give us an annual check-up. In the evening, we took Frances to the Yvonne Arnaud Theatre. When the Farnham Road nurse came on Friday, she raised the possibility of Lennie going for a 'holiday' in a care home when I was in hospital for my knee replacement. On his way home on Sunday after his weekend with us, I raised the issue with Stephen and "he agreed because I don't think he could cope as a full-time carer".

I spent a lot of time on Monday looking up information about care homes near here. After Mass on Tuesday, Stephen came to be with Lennie while I went off to the surgery to have the bandages on my shins updated. Later that evening, after doing the Sainsbury's online shopping, I wrote: "I then had quite a strong exchange with Lennie over whether she would go into a care home or have an in-house care worker when I go for my operation". On Wednesday, Tony drove us to the Martins' in Croydon for the meeting of the Family Group. On our way home, I had quite nasty chest pains and had to use my spray to cope with it. On Thursday, we had a couple of cold calls, which I think are evil. But the evening cheered me up when Chelsea beat Malmo. Friday passed by much as usual, though Lennie had one of her 'memory loss episodes' in the evening. On Saturday after Mass, I drove "Lennie to Boxgrove where she had a hairdo, including a good colouring to hide her growing whiteness". In the afternoon we watched the rugby matches but struggled in the evening to find anything worth watching. On Sunday, Richard came round with Iris to watch the Carabao Cup Final which Chelsea lost on penalties.

Monday's diary gives an indication of the variations of Lennie's dementia: "Last night when I tried to stop Lennie's repeated questioning about times, dates, parents, and so forth, she told me that all I ever think about is myself. This morning, first thing, she told me how much she loved me and that she didn't know what she would do without me. In the late afternoon, after returning from a parish lunch at the Golf Club, she denied that she'd ever slept in the double bed with me before!" On Tuesday, I had my shin re-bandaged.

On Wednesday, I was driven to the Bookham Group lunch, where I led the discussion on the IPPC report, *Prosperity and Justice*. I noted that: "once or twice I wasn't very quick in responding to questions or comments and I'm increasingly aware that my intellectual powers, which were never very great, are noticeably declining. Into Your hands, oh Lord, I commend my spirit." On Thursday evening, Michael and Sheila Wheeler took us out for a very nice meal and chat in an Italian restaurant in East Horsley. On Friday, Lennie had one of her evening "memory losses: over the next one and a half hours Lennie quizzed me at least ten times about whether her mother or father would take her to Mass tomorrow. After an angry exchange when she threw my pyjamas out and said I must sleep elsewhere, I came down and switched off the TV."

On Saturday, "Gilly turned up to take Lennie out on a shopping trip. But Lennie complained she'd never been informed about it and was quite cross with me and Stephen, but Gilly duly took Lennie off. Strangely, Lennie seems largely unaware that Gilly is her (our) daughter." Richard came over on Sunday and watched Chelsea beat Fulham. As usual, I got hooked on a continental police drama, *Baptiste*.

When Lennie went off with Norma to go to the Women's Prayer Group on Monday, I visited two local care homes. Typically, Lennie destroyed the evening by imposing demands to find and sort out her chain and brooch. On Tuesday, Katie came over and "seems to be loving her job and is working sixty hours a week helping to save for her MSc at Edinburgh next year". I'm so pleased she seems to have found a real vocation. Richard kindly turned up to watch a DVD with Lennie. John Williams drove me to the Justice and Peace meeting where "the shocking news was that our refugee project, 'Project Francis', was seen as dead without local authority support". On Ash Wednesday, Stephen came over early, so I was able to go to the Men's Walking Group lunch at the Barley Mow in West Horsley. After making love around midnight, "I can't remember what I did to provoke Lennie, but she gave me a hefty slap across the cheek, possibly the first ever such physical assault. When she went out for a walk, I fortunately caught her and called her back, and we ate our lunch in almost total silence." When we had another row in the evening over meal preparation, "as well as telling me I only thought of my own happiness and she wanted to get rid of me, she disturbingly said she almost thought of suicide. Frightening that the thought even entered her mind ... but the signs are that life is going to get increasingly difficult and I really do need to learn how to control my frustration and irritability and learn the job of being a patient carer."

On Friday after Mass, Stephen joined us before I drove off to St. Luke's, where the nurse "soon redid my plaster and bandages on my right shin. On Saturday, we watched a Women's Rugby International and then a Six Nations match. Our Italian neighbour, Giuseppe, came round to help with laptop and printer problems. Apart from the usual visit of Gilly on Sunday morning, we spent the bulk of the day watching sport. Lennie came with me as I drove Stephen to the bus station. "He told Lennie how much he had enjoyed talking to her about her teaching experiences this weekend. Thank you, Lord, for the love and support Stephen gives us."

On Monday, Lennie knocked my mug of coffee over and I exploded as I usually do. "But finding mats in the wrong drawers and finding the Fairtrade coffee with the tea and so on, makes me increasingly aware of how things are changing. I am concerned that it is not just Lennie's dementia, but also my increasing ageing, tiredness, and, I think, depression. Please, Lord, help me respond as You would like me to." In the afternoon, Lennie went off to the Women's Prayer Group. In the evening, we watched an André Rieu concert. On Tuesday, I had my shin plasters and bandages seen to. Back home I ordered our weekly shopping online, and in the evening took Lennie to the Yvonne Arnaud Theatre to see a Tom Stoppard play. Stephen came over on Wednesday, so I was able to join the Men's Group lunch. I went to PC World and bought a new printer.

On Friday, Katie and Douglas came over for a fish and chips lunch, after which I drove Katie to Nationwide to pass onto her the savings book we'd kept for her. The evening was as difficult as usual. On Saturday, we had problems with our electricity, but the bulk of the afternoon was taken up with Six Nations rugby. On Sunday after Mass, Gillian invited us to their home for a coffee. In the afternoon, Richard came over to watch Chelsea's defeat at Everton. Andrew and Caroline also paid a brief visit. Richard "told me both he and Stephen think I'm doing a good job coping with Lennie's irritating memory loss".

The main problem on Monday was that Lennie went on 'walkabout' and missed the Women's Prayer Group. She was eventually brought back, exhausted, by one of our kind neighbours; a worrying development. On Tuesday, I had my plasters redone. Stephen cooked us lunch and after we had driven him down to the library, I did the weekly online shop at Sainsbury's. On Wednesday, Frances kindly took Lennie to the Clandon Garden Centre for lunch, so I was able to join the Men's Group for lunch. On Thursday, I added the following postscript to my diary: "Lennie's sexuality at the moment seems to be that of a very flirty twenty-year-old. This month we have made love nearly every day. This evening, she caressed me and invited me to make love. I tried to respond, in spite of the fact that I had no erection. Help me, Lord."

On Friday after Mass, I had to go to St. Luke's to have the dressing on my shin changed and we then went to Carlo's. "It was pleasant, and Lennie never stopped talking about Maureen's jealousy of her because she was only four pounds when born and seemed to have taken all her parents' attention away from her. She repeated herself over and over again." There were no parish Masses on Saturday because of first confessions; strange in Lent. On Sunday evening, "Lennie was showing a lot of her 'sundown' anxieties and was insisting she had to go to our 'previous house to get her clothes' and was so convinced by this that we thought it desirable to bring her with us to the bus station" for Stephen in the evening.

Monday was fairly normal. Lennie went to the Women's Prayer Group with Norma. Late at night, when she claimed she'd had nothing to eat since breakfast, "she persisted in accusing me of lying and I'm afraid I dangerously lost my temper. Please Lord, help me to keep calm under provocation." On Tuesday after Mass, I drove Lennie to Vision Express for an annual check-up, after which we drove off to Carlo's for lunch. "Lennie seemed to have enjoyed the lunch and was very grateful." Back home, it took me an hour to order the shopping online from Sainsbury's. Guiseppe kindly came and sorted out my problem with the printer. On Wednesday, after we'd been to Mass at St. Edward's, I went to St. Luke's to have my bandage replenished and then went off to the Men's Group lunch. In the evening, I complained about Lennie, who "just doesn't have the interest or concern to watch anything on TV seriously". On Thursday evening, I took her to the Yvonne Arnaud Theatre where we enjoyed a production of *Shrek* by the Guildford School of Acting. On Friday, Lennie refused to go for a doctor's appointment. We found the Mass at St. Joseph's was actually the Requiem for the wife of a former colleague.

It was that afternoon that I had a fall on the back lawn that eventually turned out to be more serious than I first thought. I recorded that "when the phone went, I tried to get up; my leg was numb, and I fell for the first time – fortunately on the grass and I didn't break anything. But I had to wait for Lennie to come before I could get up." After chatting to Lennie for a couple of hours, "I discovered I was a lot more in pain than I'd originally thought, and I used the zimmer frame all evening". Stephen then arrived and made me take Nurofen. By now I was pretty sore and immobile. On Saturday, I recorded my right leg was still giving me a lot of pain when I moved it and when I struggled to get up, even from the lavatory seat. My mobility was very limited, so we eventually decided not to try to go to Mass. That evening my leg really was very weak and I had difficulty just standing up and couldn't walk around clearing the table or laying it for breakfast. On Monday, Lennie went off with Norma to their women's group. I started walking with her with two sticks and was dismayed at how weak my legs were, and I simply couldn't walk safely without support such as the zimmer frame.

Just before noon on Tuesday, I wrote: "I was very aware that I'm old, meaning lacking in energy, strength, guts ... with my recent accident, which Lennie seems unaware of. I didn't think I could drive to Mass." In the afternoon meeting of the Family Group, the discussion was on the meaning of Lent. Early on Wednesday morning, Stephen and I caught a taxi to go to the Royal Surrey, where it was confirmed that my lesion was not cancerous. I needed my zimmer frame on Thursday, but managed to drive us to Mass. Otherwise, the day seemed to dribble away, and the following morning Lennie was full of strange questions: "I don't know where Mike is so I don't know when he will be here. She reminisced endlessly about her father bullying her at school. By Saturday, I was beginning to wonder if I ought to go and get some medical advice as Stephen and several friends were suggesting. At Mass the priest brought me communion to the aisle where I had the zimmer frame."

After Mass on Sunday morning, Gilly drove me to Accident and Emergency, but it was six hours later before I was discharged without having been given an X-ray. On Monday, I was pretty immobile and tired and watched TV all day. It was much the same on Tuesday, when I judged that my leg problem was getting worse. Lennie, bless her, was "very sympathetic to the realities of my lack of mobility and dependence on the zimmer frame". On Wednesday, Stephen and Lennie came with me to the surgery to have my plaster renewed for the nth. time. By a stroke of good fortune, I was seen by Dr. Barnado, who "got me on a bed and examined me and immediately made out a request for a Radiology appointment at the hospital. There, I soon had an X ray on my left hip. There was apparently evidence that I had broken a bone – something they didn't spot on Sunday. Again, to my surprise, they indicated that I needed a hip operation. The rest of the afternoon was spent undergoing various tests and measurements. Stephen, bless him, stayed to look after Lennie and promised to stay with her that night and for the days to come."

In the evening, "Gilly turned up with Lennie, who was full of love and affection. Stephen and Gilly sorted out all our problems, and informed Andrew and Richard." On Friday, my recovery physiotherapy began. Andrew came and drove my car home and Richard drove him back to pick up his car. It was quite hard going on Saturday. "It was quite painful trying to roll over – mainly my right knee rather than my hip." It was at this stage that "Gilly brought a glossy booklet about an organisation called 'Everycare'". On Sunday, Richard brought Stephen, Lennie and Ben to see me, but the talk was all about Chelsea. On Monday, the physiotherapists got me exercising again. Richard brought Lennie to see me, but she had a nasty fall at the entrance to the hospital. My progress continued, though I noted on

Tuesday that "the 102-year-old operated on yesterday seems to be making greater progress than I am!"

Eventually, on Wednesday, the "physiotherapist got me to walk with the zimmer frame to the toilet and back. Exhausting." The doctor "predicted I would be home on Monday or Tuesday; it would take me six weeks to move from frame to stick; and three months or more to be able to drive". Gilly brought Lennie and Stephen to see me. Bless Lennie, she "continues to tell me how much she misses me and loves me. Gilly brought information about the Everycare contract." On Thursday, Steve Rowden, a fellow parishioner, kindly brought Lennie to see me. She looked "older all of a sudden". On Good Friday, it was a lovely surprise to be brought Holy Communion by Sr. Theresa while I was trying to read the four Gospel accounts of the passion and death of Our Lord. Gillian brought Lennie to see me in the late afternoon, having dropped Stephen off for the Wintershall Walk of Witness in Guildford. On Saturday, Andrew brought Lennie and Stephen to see me. "Poor Lennie has deteriorated so much in the past couple of weeks, but we had a lovely cuddle." In the evening, Richard brought all his four children "which was delightful". Easter Sunday was very pleasant and both Maureen Durston and Mgr. Tony brought me Holy Communion, bless them. Gillian visited with Lennie and Stephen and her long-time friend, Alison. "So, thank You, Lord, for a happy Easter."

On Monday, Tom and Edna Daly visited me and later Gilly came with Lennie. My shin still needed bandaging and the nurses were helpful. I seemed to be very uncomfortable on Tuesday with a fair amount of pain, but also persisting problems with urinating and opening my bowels and still requiring nursing support. Steve Rowden kindly drove Lennie and Stephen to see me and Fr. Roy also came. For the first time there was evidence that I had a lesion on my bottom, which was still causing me problems three years later. On Wednesday afternoon, I was "visited by the

Occupational Therapist, who is arranging relationships with the carers for Lennie". Michael Wheeler came and visited, as did Richard and Lennie. She was "very confused and thought I was her father and said that Maureen had been a bit bossy today!"

On Thursday, my shin was re-bandaged again and I was driven home earlier than Stephen and Lennie expected. The Surrey County Council care person who turned up noted the sores on my bottom, which would need looking after. There seemed to be several different nurses who came to see us on Friday. Then a mechanic came to sort out the stair lift. Saturday was a strange day, with a nurse visiting, but "Lennie nearly drove me mad at times with endless repetitions, including assumptions that we were away on holiday and needing to know that I am her husband and have been so for fifty-eight years". On Sunday, Gilly took Lennie to Mass and Maureen Durston brought me Holy Communion. During the day, three home carers came and helped me dress and put cream on the sore on my bottom. Lennie was pretty disoriented and "I sense pressure to ensure Stephen has more free time on his own".

Monday was also a bit strange, and it was clear that Stephen "wants a life of his own". Lennie went off for a walk and was picked up by one of our carers in Boxgrove. "The district nurse then came and was very helpful to me, taking the trouble to put cream on my bum. Not long afterwards, Nigel and Jane (from Everycare) came to discuss plans for the next few weeks. We are living through a paradigm shift." Not unusually, we went to bed having had an angry argument. Tuesday morning was difficult because Lennie wandered off and was found by one of the Everycare team. Stephen took Lennie for a walk round Sutherland Gardens and then made us a tasty supper. "The District Nurse and someone from the Reablement Team came, persuading me to put the Proshield Plus disinfectant gel on the sore on my bottom. Then, of course, Lennie gave hints that she would do her own thing tomorrow! Stephen is emphasising his own need to go and live in his own home."

I was depressed and angry on Wednesday morning when Lennie rolled back all the bedclothes when I was still there. "Meanwhile, she is changing her clothes over and over again and her chest of drawers remains in a dreadful mess. How am I supposed to cope with her needs and denials?" One of the Reablement nurses took Lennie for a walk round the block. Dr. Barnado phoned and was quite supportive, "but pointed out that at my age I could expect it to be two to four months before I recovered sufficiently to be at the same stage I was at before my fall". A series of nurses came during Thursday and certainly eased things for me. Tony Doherty "delivered a pile of scripture readings for me to look at ... This is the first time I can remember failing to vote in an election."

The following morning it was good to hear that UKIP hadn't recovered in the election. Frances Allen kindly brought me a three-wheeler chair which had been her husband David's, and which could be very handy. My Saturday diary recalled that twice during the night, Lennie had got herself fully dressed before coming back to bed. Gilly and Doug turned up and Doug drilled the key box onto the wall while Gilly talked us through care arrangements. On Sunday, the Reablement nurse gave me my first shower for over a month. I was grateful to her for her support. Gilly came to take Lennie to Mass and Maureen Durston brought Stephen and me Holy Communion.

My diary for the first Monday in May records, "It is difficult to find space to think or read. On Tuesday I did the online Sainsbury's shop and Stephen went off to Cranleigh. The next hour was rather fraught with Lennie angrily saying she didn't want to be bullied by 'all these women'." Jane, one of the carers, then turned up and took Lennie out for a walk. St. Luke's pharmacy were preparing to set me up with repeat prescriptions. On Tuesday evening, the Reablement nurse arrived and put cream on my bum and put on my pyjamas. On Wednesday, Alan Hughes called for a chat. My three nurses were charming and helpful, and they all put cream on the sore on my bottom.

On Thursday, Lennie got dressed around 5–6 a.m., but next time I woke she was in her nightie! Maureen Durston came to pick up Lennie and take her to Mass and Stephen went off to Guildford just before 10 a.m. "I have much wanted peace but am more likely to fall asleep than read successfully." On Friday, Faye from Everycare and Lennie went for a walk at Newlands Corner before having lunch at Squires. I then had nearly three hours on my own. I spent a lot of time clearing emails and tearing up old files before "a physiotherapist came and very professionally worked me through exercises I needed to do to strengthen my muscles". On Saturday, the Reablement nurses did a reappraisal of what help I needed and planned a reduction from the following week. Several neighbours and fellow parishioners brought me 'get well' cards and presents. On Sunday, Gilly took me to Mass for the first time in five weeks. I seem to have irritated Stephen over much of the weekend.

On the second Monday in May, Lennie and I completed our ballot papers and voted for the Liberal Democrats because they were explicitly pro-EU. "I voted against the Labour Party I am a member of because they have been so awfully uncommitted to the EU and procrastinated, sitting on the fence during the Brexit negotiations. Two Reablement Team members came and clearly the message was, we're finishing with him asap!" The Everycare worker took Lennie out for a walk by the river. They had also put out the washing on the line and prepared lunch. When I asked Stephen to bring in the washing from the line and put it on the radiators, we had another furious row. But the following morning he helpfully "put on my socks and sandals, which I'm unable to do myself". While I did the Sainsbury's shopping online, one of the Everycare workers took Lennie to the Silent Pool and bought a replacement kettle. On Wednesday morning, I tried to "recover from the various stresses of being alive but terribly immobile. It doesn't help that my lovely wife, twice last night at around 12.00 and 2 a.m,. got fully dressed and on the second occasion made her way out of the bedroom and downstairs. I had to shout to Stephen in case she had done a walkabout. But this morning she has been lovely and has put on my socks." I paid Everycare's support last week. "It worries me that the annual cost will be over £25K."

On Thursday, Bob Durston kindly picked up Lennie to take her to Mass and afterwards to Hair Partners for a perm. It was Iris's ninth birthday. Be with her, Lord. My lovely Reablement nurse came round to put gel on my bottom and dressed me in my pyjamas. On Friday, Stephen took Lennie off to walk to the bus and go to Mass in Guildford. My response: "I feel a spell of peace without Lennie's questions and anxieties and Stephen's rapid-fire talk". At this stage it looked as if we had arranged four-hour spells with Everycare. They prepared our lunches. My Rapid Response physio came and "talked and held me through a whole series of exercises and said my mobility had clearly improved since I last saw her a week earlier. On Saturday, I think I watched the EWTN Mass from Alabama, though I did find it very traditionalist and clericalist Catholicism." On Sunday, Gilly drove us to Mass where she was the sacristan. We heard that Pat Jones had got her PhD. Bless her, Lord. As always, we spent the bulk of the afternoon and evening watching sport on the TV.

The third Monday in May was a very busy day, which may explain why my temper exploded both with Lennie and with Stephen, who "warned me of the dangers of a heart attack". Early on, Stephen took himself off to Cranleigh, while Lennie was accompanied by the Everycare worker when she went off for a walk. She prepared lunch for us and then

Lennie went off to the Women's Prayer Group. On Tuesday, I recorded that I still needed help putting on my socks. "The hour between 9 a.m. and 10 a.m. was a nightmare. Stephen and I had locked the front door and taken out the key. This infuriated Lennie, who wanted her own free choices. I argued in vain that we were concerned about her safety as she had in the past wandered off and lost her way." Later, the Everycare worker took Lennie for a walk by the river while I cleared about forty emails and then ordered the Sainsbury's online shopping. On Wednesday, "for the first time, and to my surprise, I managed to pull on my socks and sandals myself". Lennie went for a walk by the river with the Everycare assistant. She became very disoriented in the evening.

On Thursday, I asked Lennie to pull up my socks and sandals, but we had a row later and I ended up with a small cut on my wrist. A carer took Lennie off to Mass and our fellow parishioner Voytek came to do some gardening for us. The carer made us a tasty lunch. I was furious when Lennie trimmed my camelias, "but this world is short, so I'll just have to put up with it". On Friday, Faye cooled the temperature between us, read my Feed In Tariff, collected Lennie's prescriptions and went for a walk in the Chantries with her. "I somehow fell over in Stephen's bedroom. Fortunately, I didn't seem to do any serious damage and I struggled to get off the floor. It was, I suppose, a 'wake-up call' or a warning of care needed, so I told all the others afterwards." During the day I looked for information about Attendance Allowance and Carer's Allowance, "which I knew nothing about". As usual, we watched a lot of sport on Saturday. On Sunday, Bob Durston kindly gave us a lift to Mass and invited us to coffee afterwards. Today's sport was the rugby sevens from Twickenham. Douglas phoned to let us know that Gilly and Doug had arrived safely in Skiathos.

"I'm most bothered about Stephen insisting on spending more time at his own home in Cranleigh. But how do I then cope when Lennie gets fed up doing nothing, and insists on going out for a walk when I fear she will get lost and not know where she lives?" On Bank Holiday Monday, Stephen kindly pulled up my socks for me and later took Lennie out for a walk, probably around Sutherland Park. Lennie and Stephen declined an invitation from Andrew to drive down to Bournemouth, where he planned to have a swim. "I replied to a letter from our Labour M.E.P., taking the opportunity to confess I'd voted Lib. Dem because they were explicitly anti-Brexit and I regretted the fact that Labour hadn't pressed for values of internationalism, solidarity, and the common good. It took me the rest of the morning to more or less complete the fifty-page application for Attendance Allowance." On Tuesday, when Stephen went off to the library I tried "to complete my Attendance Allowance claim form, first for me, and secondly, claiming legal attorney rights, for Lennie." Later, Everycare's Faye "drove us all up to Mt. Alvernia Hospital, where I was scheduled to have a DEXA bone scan. It all went very smoothly." Back home, Faye cooked us a tasty omelette for lunch, after which I completed this week's online Sainsbury's shopping. In the evening, Lennie was totally disorientated.

My diary for the last Wednesday in May starts by quoting Lennie. " 'I'm going to go out and I'm not going to come back' ... Lennie has been driving me mad. Stephen went off to Cranleigh about 9 a.m. and Faye came an hour later and soon generated peace." When she left after her four-hour shift, an occupational therapist came to try and get me to walk with two sticks. In the evening, Chelsea beat Arsenal 4–1 in the UEFA Cup Final. On Ascension Thursday, Maureen Durston kindly drove us to Mass where I stood more and knelt for the first time since my operation. At lunch time, I found "Lennie fired up to say she didn't need Everycare's Claire anymore after they'd been for a walk along the river. Lennie was arguing she didn't need any more care and she didn't want other people's decisions forced on her." Claire made us a tasty omelette for lunch, smoothed things over and helped put away the Sainsbury's shopping delivery. On Friday, the last day of May, I had an alarm pendant delivered and tested by Guildford Care. In the evening "Lennie was in 'sundown' mode, i.e., unsure about her teaching class tomorrow, whether the house was ours or not, and so on". Eventually I "encouraged Lennie to put on her nightie and take off her skirt".

The first of June was a day of taking things easy, though the three of us did water thirsty roses and Stephen and Lennie walked to Sainsbury's. As usual on a Saturday, we watched a magnificent rugby club final and then the European Champions League Final. "At this point (sundown), Lennie drove Stephen and me mad at times with not allowing him time to complete the cooking of supper." On Sunday, Bob Durston kindly drove us to and from Mass. In the afternoon, after a snooze, "Lennie came down and insisted on going for a walk. Stephen, bless him, agreed to go with her." On Monday morning, Claire took Lennie to Squires Garden Centre, which enabled me to tidy up the numerous files and papers which have been accumulating over the past year or more. I continued with the study of the Old Testament I had been reading about for some time.

Tuesday was a fairly typical day. Claire took Lennie up to Newlands Corner. Later, Lennie was convinced there was a funeral Mass, but there was no evidence in the Parish Newsletter. "She also seemed totally unaware that Nana had died thirty-four years ago and nothing I volunteered seemed to help at all." On Wednesday, Marianne, also from Everycare, took Lennie for a walk by the river. I read a chapter on the Psalms. In the evening, "Lennie had one of her angry anxiety periods, regretting we weren't doing more to get the children ready for a game of football". I was frustrated. Then on Thursday, I regretted the apparent lack of Christian commitment on the part of any of my grandchildren and prayed about the inadequacies of my 'evangelising'.

I did the weekly online shop at Sainsbury's. On Wednesday, Claire again took Lennie out for a walk. Stephen came later and we watched an O.D.I. (One Day International) match. "Richard duly called and took Stephen with him to help clear his attic of Stephen's paintings and then take him home to Cranleigh." On Thursday, my sister Ann's eighty-fifth birthday, Lennie started getting up around 3 a.m. and spent a lot of time fiddling around in her dressing-table drawers. She "eventually went downstairs and I feared she would go on a walkabout. So I didn't really have any sound sleep from 3 a.m. onwards. I did shout in anger in the early hours with Lennie and I ought to remember that Jesus linked anger with the prohibition of murder. So repent, Mike." Bob Durston kindly drove Lennie to and from Mass and in the afternoon to and from Maureen's tea party. On Friday, the longest day, I persuaded Lennie's new carer, Jane, to take Lennie to Hair Partners and later for a walk.

Stephen and Lennie took themselves off to Mass at St. Joseph's this morning. Much of the rest of this Saturday was spent watching sport on TV. In the evening "we had to cope with one of Lennie's memory loss and anxiety episodes about Mass tomorrow; Gillian taking us; we live here permanently; etc. etc., and over and over again". Gilly drove us to and from Mass at St. Pius' on the Feast of Corpus Christi. "After Mass, Pat Jones came up to have a chat. I told her how flattered I was when she came to chat with me; bless her, Lord." In the two hours after Stephen had set off for Cranleigh, "I've had to put up with Lennie's repeated questions about this house; Maureen; where our clothes are; how long have we lived in this house – and always the questions totally ignored the fact that they'd been answered many times, most recently only a minute ago".

On Monday, I was concerned about Lennie's dementia and trying to cope with it with more limited time with Stephen. With Claire (Everycare), we took her to her dental appointment. In the evening, she came down the stairs "in tears fearing I might be dead" as she has done several times recently. On Tuesday morning, Stephen came with me to the hospital for my pre-op knee assessment. In the afternoon, Pat Jones kindly brought over her PhD thesis on 'Discovering the Common Good', which I was able to read when Faye took Lennie out for a walk. In the evening, "it was 'sundown' and Lennie kept insisting we phoned Mike to let him know where we were. 'What's happened to your other half?'" On Thursday Bob Durston again drove Lennie to and from Mass, which allowed me to read more of Pat's thesis with its criticisms of Pope Benedict's *Deus Caritas Est*. "Perhaps I ought to be more responsive to Lennie's repeated suggestions that something has happened to our relationship, and I'm too bothered with football (and TV) and reading to talk to her. Help me, Lord, to respond as You would have me do." On Friday, Jane (Everycare) took Lennie up to Newlands Corner and then the River Wey, which gave me a chance to read more of Pat's thesis. As always, sport consumed our evening.

The last Saturday of June was very hard going. First of all, I made a bit of a mess of Lennie's medications. When I showed her the arrangements for Everycare next week, "this just generated fierce and angry responses about what I had arranged without telling her". Stephen reminded us that the arrangements had been made with the three of us, "but Lennie talks as if all these arrangements have been <u>imposed</u> on her so she feels humiliated". Around 1 a.m. on Sunday, "I woke to find Lennie getting dressed. Later she left the bedroom. Around 4 a.m., I felt obligated to go and look for her. She wasn't in the other bedroom but downstairs, fully dressed and setting up breakfast. Stephen was asleep on the sofa. I returned to bed, more or less reassured that she would be looked after by Stephen." Gilly took us to Mass and back ... Stephen went back early to Cranleigh. I was worried about the hob in the evening, "and that Lennie will wander off in the early hours, although I've locked both doors".

On the first Monday of July, I recalled that "at 3 a.m., Lennie was dressed and I woke to find her going downstairs". I managed to talk her into going back to bed. My physio came and "talked me through my exercises". Claire came and took Lennie out for a walk. After lunch she "ushered Lennie up to Norma's for the Women's Group". In mid-afternoon, Ann phoned; she'd broken her wrist on her birthday. For the first time, Boots delivered Lennie's prescriptions to our door. Tuesday seemed to pass by quite easily. I prepared the Sainsbury's online shopping. Claire then took Lennie down to the river for a walk before going to Squires Garden Centre. On their return, she helped me complete a pre-op questionnaire. Two Sky mechanics came and checked our TV and changed our 'remote'. Lennie cut unnecessary flowers to add to a fourth vase and took herself off for a walk.

On Wednesday, I recorded that for the first time in three months we had a tentative session of love-making. Around this period, most of my free time was spent trying to write notes and summaries of Pat's thesis. Stephen came and made supper before returning to Cranleigh. The evening was ended by Lennie's endless and repeated questions: Where was Mass? When? How to get there? Where were her parents and sister? I was limited by the zimmer frame on Thursday but walked up for Holy Communion with it after Maureen Durston had kindly driven us there. Faye brought Leanne and they took Lennie out for a walk by the river. I tried to finish writing notes on Pat's thesis, but Lennie was always pretty angry with my "always burying myself in my books". On Friday, Lennie pressed me to cancel Faye's visit this evening. This made preparing supper difficult, but somehow we survived.

On Saturday morning, "I wondered 'what can I do about it?'" Then, with the usual bouts of uncertainty about how and whether we were going to Mass tomorrow, when and with whom, would her parents be with her and so on, Sunday was very similar. Gilly kindly drove us to Mass at St. Pius', where she was sacristan today. Mgr. Tony was very friendly after Mass and said I was looking better. Lennie gave a flavour of her irritation with 'the girls' (i.e. carers). Stephen was very helpful in guiding the conversation so that I didn't explode with Lennie's repeated questions. On Monday, Gillian's birthday, Leanne (Everycare) eased things when she came around 10 a.m. for a four-hour slot at this stage and 19½ hours this week. On Tuesday Claire came and took Lennie up to Newlands Corner for a walk. I did the weekly shop online. When there were no carers there, I often exploded in anger at Lennie's repeated questions and failure to accept replies. "Today I regret and fumed she was a 'bitch, bitch, bitch'."

Perhaps it was inevitable that on the following day I felt depressed and didn't respond to her request to make love. Stephen was helpful when he came. He almost immediately found Lennie had put out chips in the oven on a non-pyrex plate. Temperatures went down, and we all relaxed. On Thursday morning, I wanted to convey my sense of old age and the inevitable approach of death. Perhaps for this reason I asked Mgr. Tony if he would hear my confession. He was very sympathetic and understanding in confession and I was grateful to him. On Friday, our carer took a surprisingly compliant Lennie for a walk by the river (or 'sea' according to Lennie!). Wimbledon tennis seemed to preoccupy us most of the afternoon and evening.

"At one stage, Lennie skipped off on a walkabout. I didn't realise this until she rang the front doorbell to see if this was the right address. Tom Daly kindly drove us to and from St. Pius' for the evening Mass." Later in the evening I added: "Lennie is repeatedly asking if we want something to eat though we had supper not long ago". On Sunday, Lennie tested my patience in the usual ways while we watched the One Day International final and had visits from Gilly and Richard. Stephen returned to Cranleigh late in the evening and I was grateful to him for the space he gave me. On Monday morning, "I couldn't do much reading before Leanne (Everycare) came ... because Lennie needed to chat and be provided with reasons for not taking herself off for a walk before Leanne came ... I had to verbally push Lennie to get her ready to go out in time for the Women's Prayer Group." In the evening, "all hell broke out when I mentioned the carer was coming tomorrow. She shouted that all these girls were interested in was 'money, money, money' and was totally impregnable against my pointing out that they ask her what she would like to go to or to do." In these evening sessions she is bitterly angry that I have invited 'these girls' in and is offended by the idea that she is being cared for.

On Tuesday, I managed to complete the Sainsbury's shopping list online. On Wednesday, Lennie initiated love-making though I was limited with no erection. "Lord, in Your mercy hear my prayer for guidance." I was then taken to the Bookham Group (where three of the four of us were on crutches) where we were led by Chris Richardson on 'ordinary theology'. What was clear on Thursday is the role the carers have in ending or softening the rows Lennie and I have almost every day about our lives, her repeated questions and failure to take on board my responses. On Friday, too, it became obvious that I needed them to organise meals because of my limited mobility. In the evenings, "Lennie was always full of urgent questions about where we lived. 'Where have we come from?' 'Hadn't we better pack to go home?' 'Where is our home?' Such discussions always destroyed the opportunities to relax in the evenings and watch serious TV," etc.

On the third Saturday in July, Stephen kindly brought us a fan. He later "managed to calm down Lennie's obsession with what to do for lunch". I escaped into the garden "to avoid (partially) Lennie's <u>repeated</u> questions about when we are going to Mass and who was looking after the children. "It is driving me mad, but Stephen is battling on, trying to explain that we are in our eighties, our children in their fifties, and so on." On Sunday we had to cope with many of the same issues. Gilly came over after taking us to Mass and I noted: "Lennie is bitterly angry and offended because Gilly took her upstairs to help her sort out her winter from summer clothes. She won't let it go. Both Stephen and I tried to soften things by saying she was only trying to help." On Monday, I struggled to cope and tried over and over again to reassure her. She then expressed concern about what the matter with her was. I tried to say she was not at fault but had "an illness. Slowly she settled down." On Thursday, the hottest day of the year, I felt it worth noting: "Perhaps this is the time to recognise the big change in our lives this year, accelerated by my fractured hip and subsequent immobilsation, and the carers helping at mealtimes". On Tuesday, I managed to complete my Sainsbury's online shopping. Leanne had taken Lennie to Polesdon Lacey for lunch and Jane took her out briefly later.

Stephen came over and cooked our meals on Wednesday. "It was just after 7 p.m., the time of the evening when Lennie has her greatest anxieties and problems with her memory. She seemed incredibly disturbed by our plan to take the Durstons (and Frances) to Carlo's tomorrow for lunch. Over and over again, she asked for details and asked about families and children she was responsible for. At the beginning of the year, I was coping with Lennie's dementia; now my life, especially since Stephen returned substantially to Cranleigh, is quite clearly that of Lennie's chief 'carer'." Bob Durston kindly drove us to Mass and after coffee in the hall he drove us to Carlo's, where we were joined by Frances and Tony, so all the remaining Guildford members of our Family Group were there and shared the cost. Later that day the Sainsbury's shopping was delivered, and they kindly helped put it away before Jane brought Ana, her daughter-in-law, for a two-hour shift. On Friday, several of the neighbours in Oak Tree Gardens had a very pleasant evening chatting under the oak tree.

We weren't able to go to Mass on the last Saturday of July because I wasn't able to drive. When Stephen came, he brought the Saturday *Guardian* and I spent the bulk of the day skimming it and the weekend *Tablet*. On Sunday, Gilly drove us to Mass and stayed longer than usual for a chat after driving us home. "We had a brief exchange over the need for Lennie to go into a care home if I died." During the afternoon, I sat in the garden chatting to Lennie for a good hour. On Monday morning we made love and I reflected on its challenges. I responded to her invitation, "but I am completely impotent these days". I reflected briefly on sexual ethical issues: "I'm not at all sure that old concerns about masturbation are correct or appropriate. Sexual relations are about pleasing one's spouse and developing the relationship, not just a matter of 'keeping rules' which may be misconceived."

While Lennie went off to Norma's and the Women's Prayer Group after lunch, I read papers by the Bookham Group on *Lumen Gentium*. In the evening, I played our DVD of the first thirty years of our married lives together. On Tuesday evening, "Lennie went up to bed, but four times came downstairs to ask whether she should wear a nightie or pyjamas and whether she should sleep on the window side of the bed or nearer the door". I expressed uncertainty over the distinction between Attendance Allowance and Carer's Allowance. Wednesday was the last day of July, and it was rather ordinary though "Lennie has been anxious all day really" and later in the day I recorded that "Stephen and I had to cope with well over an hour of Lennie's 'sundown'".

We had an ordinary day to start August. Bob Durston kindly drove us to the Thursday morning Mass and later Jane took

Lennie for a long walk along the river. I spent much of the day watching the Test Match against Australia. Friday was a little different as Lennie didn't want to go for a long walk, and while I had the Test Match on mute, I spent much of my time reading my notes on *Gaudium et Spes*. Faye took Lennie to Majestic to buy *Sauvignon Blanc*. Saturday was much the same, though Lennie and I had a fearful row when I locked the front door to try and prevent her going walkabout before Stephen turned up. The Test Match again dominated the TV. In the evening, I hurt my finger in the door.

Early on Sunday morning, Lennie and I made love in response to her repeated invitations. Gilly drove us to Mass and came for her usual chat afterwards. Andrew visited us in the afternoon. The evening after Stephen had gone was difficult and I recorded that "Lennie has spent an hour complaining that nobody cuddled her when she was a child. She seemed totally unaware that I was not her father, and she didn't realise I was her husband and that the children we'd seen earlier were hers." This continued into Monday when I wrote: "After Stephen left us last night we coped for a while with the TV on until Lennie began to insist on another meal. When I told her that Stephen had cooked both our lunch and supper, she angrily denied it and called me a liar who only thought about 'me, me, me'!" Tuesday started with: "Lennie's sexual passions at the moment seem to be unending and emerge more than once each day – when we go to bed, during the night, in the morning and sometimes expressed during the day. She seems to enjoy caressing me and though she regrets I can't penetrate her, she doesn't seem to begrudge it. I'm coping the best I can in the light of 1 Cor. 7: 3–6 but have started to call an end each time!" The Everycare carers came twice during the day which helped, and I managed to do a bit more work on Catholic Social Thought (CST). On Wednesday, I must have pressed the wrong keys on the laptop because I ended up admitting that "my morning was a dead loss". Fortunately, it cleared up later and I managed to type in some of the notes I'd drafted during the day.

Bob Durston kindly drove us to Mass on Thursday. Afterwards, Mgr. Tony kindly gave me the anointing of the sick. We had an early supper, which meant I had to cope with Lennie for three and a half hours before we went to bed. I managed very little 'work' on Friday after doing various domestic chores. Ann phoned and Frances brought a card prior to my operation. Stephen was a great help over the weekend. I tried to do more work on my article, *Catholic Social Teaching Shift*. Gillian drove us to Mass on Sunday and stayed with us for an hour afterwards. Richard came over to watch Chelsea lose 4–0 to Manchester United. On Monday, a taxi took me with Lennie and Stephen to the Royal Surrey Elective Surgery Unit by 6.45 a.m. I had my knee replacement operation later in the day, and ended up in Bramshot Ward, where Richard brought Lennie and Stephen to visit me in the evening. On Tuesday, I knocked over a urine bottle on the bed and the nurse kindly remade the bed. Andrew also visited me.

On Wednesday I read more of Oliver James's book, *Contented Dementia,* lent to me by Gilly. The physios were keen to get me walking and discharged quickly. I was visited by Lennie and Stephen and also Tom Daly and needed bandaging. Lennie and Stephen visited me in the afternoon and Gilly in the evening. On Friday, Lennie came with Stephen in the afternoon. Sadly, "Lennie didn't participate at all in our conversation". Andrew came and stayed for an hour before going off for supper at Gilly's. I spent most of my free time reading Oliver James's book. On Saturday, I struggled with tiredness and lack of energy and my bandaged calf. Gilly, Lennie and Stephen kindly visited in the afternoon. It seems that my going home was full of uncertainties and it wasn't until late Sunday evening that Gilly and Katie drove me home. Earlier, Fr. Seb had kindly brought me Holy Communion. Two nurses had put some gel on my sore bottom. I ended my diary by praying: "Help me Lord to behave as You'd wish me to".

My first day back home wasn't bad, though "my damaged leg seeped during the night quite badly". I got used to Lennie's irritation with the Everycare carers and Stephen was there to help. "A physio and occupational therapist then came and were pleasantly helpful. Mid-afternoon, a community nurse came and changed the padding on my shin." On Tuesday, Stephen unexpectedly "said he would like time to go off to Cranleigh. I was a little taken aback and apprehensive about whether I could cope with Lennie." Later, Leanne came and took Lennie down to the river for a walk before returning to make us lunch. Stephen returned earlier than expected and we had a visit from Frances and several phone calls. On Wednesday, the community nurse redid the bandage on my leg and changed my BUTEC patch aimed at controlling pain. In the evening, I noted "as often happens these days, Lennie was completely delusional about her First Holy Communion children and the difficulties parents often were to teachers. Stephen and I found it difficult to cope because it was so unrealistic, as was her thinking that she was going to Mass tonight and her unawareness that Bob Durston had driven her to Mass on several recent Thursdays." On this Thursday, Bob drove Lennie to Mass and Maureen brought her back. Claire (Everycare) was very helpful and made us lunch and helped put away the Sainsbury's shopping delivery. The Test Match took up most of the rest of the day.

I started my day on Friday by observing that "Lennie is a different person in some respects. She doesn't automatically see me as her husband of nearly fifty-nine years and repeatedly claims to have spoken to her parents and her sister, Maureen, recently. She doesn't automatically know where the fridge or kitchen are; this morning she took dishes for washing up to the loo instead of the kitchen. Be with her, Lord, and please help me be a better carer." Later, there were two unlit gas hobs on and this made me explode with anger. Fortunately, Claire came then and took Lennie for a cooler and walk. The nurse came and redid the plaster on my leg. It looks as if it will take several weeks. When I went to bed that night, I found Lennie on my side but after "irritated exchanges she went off to the single bed in the other room" but eventually returned to the double bed. On Saturday, Stephen took Lennie into Guildford for Mass while I struggled to read Luke's Gospel. A typical Saturday with the Test match, a Rugby International from Twickenham, a Chelsea win against Norwich and then Stephen's boxing. On Sunday, Gilly drove us to Mass and came back for a weekly chat. We won the Test because Ben Stokes scored 72 of the unbroken 73 with Jack Leach – one of the great cricket memories. Quite a busy first week out of hospital.

A lovely Bank Holiday with temperatures over 30° C. Stephen cooked us a BBQ and we spent a lot of our time outside. I did go upstairs to the laptop to look through Stephen's website. I recognized that I am being allowed to lounge around in view of my recent operations and slow recovery. After breakfast on Tuesday, I spent a good hour sending off our weekly shopping request to Sainbury's. A community nurse came and took out half of the pins in my knee. Lennie was in a disturbed mood and wouldn't go out for a walk with the Everycare carer. In the afternoon, I had chest pains and used my nitrolingual puffer for the first time for months. On Wednesday, Lennie went for a walk and to the Garden Centre with the carer she had resisted the day before. A nurse came to take out the remaining eight pins around my knee and a Hospital Outreach Support Team assistant practitioner came to check my exercises and wasn't too critical. On Thursday, Stephen told me that Lennie came downstairs in the early hours and went out via the patio door, a warning about the future. Stephen took Lennie for a brief walk to the shops before he set off for Cranleigh. Maureen Durston kindly drove Lennie to and from Mass at

St. Pius'. I asked the cleaners to prioritise the cleaning of the stains on the carpets. During the day I concluded that: "It is becoming more and more apparent that my life now must revolve around coping with Lennie's dementia; sometimes she knows who I am; sometimes not".

On Friday, Stephen took Lennie for a short walk before he set off for Cranleigh. On the way he took some cheques into the bank for me. Listening to Classic FM, I reflected that it was sad that Lennie didn't share my love for classical music. A new carer took Lennie for a hair appointment at Boxgrove. A community nurse came to change my bandaging and noticed another unremoved pin which she cleverly removed. She did a good job and took a lot of trouble. Stephen came home sooner than expected but Lennie was quite disturbed, and it wasn't an easy evening. While Lennie and Stephen went to Mass at St. Joseph's on Saturday morning, I worked through accumulated mail and selected which charities to support. Lennie went walkabout and when Stephen couldn't find her, he contacted the police. "Lennie was absolutely relentless in her ongoing concerns about opening the door to and providing accommodation for all our family."

Sunday was the first day in September, but it wasn't easy with Lennie. Gilly drove us to Mass and back home did a great job sewing some buttons on Lennie's blue dress. "But when she went upstairs Lennie was absolutely furious that she had had the nerve to take such decisions for her. The fury didn't abate, and she was very angry towards Gilly, who as early as 11.20 a.m. walked back home. To be honest, I was quite glad Gilly experienced Lennie in one of her angry moods so that she realises what she is like for me sometimes when I am on my own." Lennie spent much of the evening complaining about being told what to do by the carers. She continued on Monday morning when "Richard phoned to say he'd been offered a job with ESPN on a salary near to what he earned at the BBC". As usual, Lennie went up to bed around 8.15 p.m. but I insisted I wasn't going to bed before 9.45 p.m. "I forgot to mention that early on Tuesday morning, Lennie reflected on our present lives and suggested we needed soon to go into a care home. I found this a bit startling, and my gut feeling is that it is too soon to be thinking along these lines."

On Wednesday, Faye "took Lennie to Squires Garden Centre". Lennie was very confused in the evening, but Stephen cooked us a nice supper. On Thursday, Maureen Durston took an angry Lennie off to Mass and later Claire took her for a walk. They returned just in time to put away a large Sainsbury's shopping delivery. Stephen returned and a taxi took the three of us to the Royal Surrey, where "a physiotherapist gave me a rough check-over and took me through a series of recommended exercises".

On Friday, I managed to get signed up for online banking. The Test Match was on most of the day. Stephen came and cooked us a fish and chips supper, after which we watched England beat Italy at rugby. On Saturday, Stephen and Lennie walked to catch the bus into Guildford where they went to Mass at St. Joseph's. The rest of the day passed much as most Saturdays with sport dominating the TV. I recorded that I was missing Polly Toynbee in the *Guardian*. England beat Bulgaria 4–0 and Mason Mount made his England debut.

Gillian kindly drove us to Mass on the second Sunday in September. Stephen cooked us a pleasant lunch and Lennie did the washing-up. As always, she went up to bed long before my time of 10 p.m. On Monday, early on, I cleared emails. Lennie and I put out the washing, put on earlier by Stephen, on the radiators. A physio came round and "I got the impression she wasn't impressed with my failure to exercise well". In the afternoon, Frances paid us a visit, Stephen returned home sooner than expected and cooked us supper, and Richard called and briefed us on the implications of Brexit. After Stephen had left early on Tuesday morning, Leanne came and took Lennie for a walk down by the river before she returned to cook us lunch. Voytek did a two-hour stint of gardening for us. Stephen returned late in the afternoon and cooked us supper. We ended the day watching England beat Kosovo 5–3. My diary for Wednesday 11 September shows an angry Lennie from early morning to evening. She condemned carers for only being interested in 'money, money, money'. Claire took her for a walk by the river but Lennie then became "so angered by what she saw as an alliance between Claire and me" that Claire left before the end of her shift. Frances came to take Lennie out for a walk in the afternoon. "My evening was wrecked when Lennie kept coming downstairs and was furious that she'd never been told about tomorrow (G-Live) and that she'd not been consulted."

On Thursday afternoon, Lennie "complained about being coerced into 'taking Gillian to the theatre without having been asked!'" She was full of denial that she knew Gilly, her daughter, and claimed never to have met her. Later that evening, Gilly came to pick up Lennie to take her to the G-Live for *The Pirates of Penzance*. On Friday, while Leanne took Lennie out, I had a meeting with Gilly, and Jane and Faye who came "to discuss the future care arrangements. I felt it was quite useful and as a result I've made arrangements for both of us to see our G.P. in a couple of weeks' time. I think they accepted my plea/judgement that a care home would be too soon at this stage. I don't know whether Gilly agrees. Then, unexpectedly, Richard turned up with Will and Iris, who both looked taller than when we'd last seen them." On Saturday, Stephen and Lennie went off to Mass at St. Joseph's. Much of the day was spent watching the Test Match and Chelsea's 5–3 win at Wolves.

Gilly took us to Mass this morning and afterwards told us about Katie's happy first fortnight in Edinburgh. "Andrew called and seemed a little more at ease compared to his last call." Much of the day was spent watching England win the Test but not recovering the Ashes. Stephen fed us well in the evening. "Lennie is absolutely non-stop about heating the bed, laying the table, going round in circles, driving us up the wall, and so on." On Monday, "we started the new pattern of living. Stephen left us around 9 a.m. and we won't see him now until Wednesday. Please God, help me, and us, to cope as You would have us cope." Leanne took us to a Requiem Mass at St. Pius' and then helped put the washing out. Stephen had put in the machine earlier on the radiators. She also put out our supper for us before the end of her shift. On Tuesday, we had no carer for breakfast, after which I spent an hour ordering the shopping from Sainsbury's online. Claire took Lennie for a walk along the river and then to Squires before returning to make us a simple lunch. Later, "Lennie had one of her angry outbursts about the Everycare workers, and when Jane arrived, she angrily refused to be 'bossed about' and walked off. Jane followed her, and they returned fifty minutes later. Jane made us a bacon and egg supper. In the evening, Chelsea were beaten 1–0 by Valencia."

My diary indicates that Wednesday was a difficult day. "When I went up to bed (the previous night) I found Lennie on my side and I irritatedly asked her to move over. Angrily, she got up and went into the other bedroom. Half an hour later, she joined me, and we made peace. But she was full of ideas about taking out a load of schoolkids and in the early hours I found she'd got dressed. Just after 3 a.m., I got out of bed to encourage her to come back for four hours' sleep. The negotiations took a long time but eventually she climbed into bed fully dressed. At breakfast, she asked me if I wanted toast at least ten times. Instead of making us coffee, she delivered up tea, and I eventually lost my cool when she wouldn't put back the tea in the right cupboard. One thing she does do fairly systematically is the washing-up. Her illness is real enough and I'm not very good at coping with it. Please help me, Lord." The community nurse came and changed my plaster.

On Thursday, Jane drove us to Mass at St. Pius' and later took Lennie down to the river for a walk. She then prepared a big lunch for us. After she'd gone, Liz and Howell Lewis took us out to Newlands Corner – "for me, my first venture outside apart from attending Mass, in the five months since my hip operation". They then took us to the Clandon Garden Centre for tea; very kind and supportive of them. Friday was Gilly and Doug's thirty-third wedding anniversary. We drove to the hospital where I saw the physio again. In the evening Lennie was quite taken with two episodes of *Inside the Vatican*. Saturday passed by relatively easily. Today's *Guardian* didn't interest me greatly, but to my surprise Lennie was happy to watch three episodes of a dark Scandinavian police drama. Our Italian neighbour kindly helped in trying to recharge the battery in our car, which I haven't driven for months.

Howell Lewis drove us to and from Mass on the fourth Sunday in September. Stephen cooked us a tasty beef lunch. We spent the afternoon watching the England rugby team beat Tonga, but Chelsea were beaten 2–1 by Liverpool. In the evening, we watched an intriguing DVD about the leaking of information about nuclear bombs. On Monday, Stephen returned early to Cranleigh. Leanne took Lennie for a walk down by the river and I continued my reading of the New Testament and was particularly impressed with Hebrews. Frances kindly came and drove Lennie down to the Odeon to see *Downton Abbey*. On Tuesday morning, I spent an hour doing our Sainsbury's online shopping order. Leanne came and helped Lennie "get over a bout of anxiety and tears on hearing of the death of her mother thirty-four years ago". She felt Lennie's illness had progressed recently. The Millbrook team came to recover their special mattress, which didn't fit our 5 ft. bed. A nurse came and changed my leg bandage, possibly for the last time. Voytek came to do some tidying of the garden. Lennie went to bed early and when I declined to join her then switched all the lights out. Stephen came over soon after 10 a.m. the next morning and helped a lot during the day. Chris Richardson picked me up to drive to Ye Olde Windsor Castle, where Steve Rouse led us in a discussion on 'French Catholicism and the Revolution'. Stephen took Lennie out for a short walk before supper. It upsets me that key Catholic Conservatives "are all unable to promote solidarity and the common good".

On Thursday, Stephen set off early for Cranleigh and Faye drove us to and from St. Pius' for Mass. Afterwards, we went into the hall to celebrate Frances's eightieth birthday. Faye dropped me at Hair Partners, where I had a haircut and she picked me up afterwards. Later she collected a fish and chip supper for the three of us. Early in my diary for Friday, I wrote: "Lennie has been shattered that we bought this house out of our savings and sale of our previous house, and that it is not a hotel or care home. I manage our family finances, i.e., including Lennie's. Months ago, I wrote to around fourteen charities she supported with a final cheque but also a request to take her off their mailing list. Not all have conformed!" There was plenty to watch on the TV, including the World Athletics Championships from Doha and World Cup rugby. I have been reading Tolstoy's *Resurrection* with its interesting "criticisms of the dominant culture of exploitation, inequality but also submission and counter-exploitation". Seems relevant post-Brexit. The issues covered in my diary for Saturday seemed very similar to those on Friday. Japan had beaten Ireland in the world rugby and Hassan (Netherlands) had "just won a superb Women's 10,000m race".

There were signs of autumn, so for the first time for a while I wore a long-sleeved shirt on Sunday. Tony Clarke kindly drove us to and from Mass at St. Pius'. At lunch, I noted that "my appetite is declining these days. Lennie is angry about something; she is still in active teaching mode wondering where the children are!" In the evening, "Lennie then drove me into an angry explosion with her <u>repeated</u> questions about arrangements for tomorrow". Monday was a busy day. "Lennie didn't seem sure that I was her husband and at different times referred to Stephen as a potential boyfriend ... Later, Leanne then drove us to the Royal Surrey, where the physiotherapist seems very amicable and tolerant of my seemingly slow progress." In the afternoon, "Lennie angrily refused to go to a doctor's appointment in spite of my saying it was an annual check-up. But eventually Marika from Everycare drove us to the surgery, where Dr. Barnado seemed quite pleased with my progress" but advised me to check up on DVLA guidelines. He then checked Lennie's blood pressure and took a blood sample. The rest of the day was spent watching World Athletics.

On Tuesday, 1st October, I noted that Lennie had difficulty deciding on tea or coffee. "Last night she spilled a mug of coffee on the carpet, and it has left a horrible brown stain, but this morning she is in total denial that she had anything to do with it." Later Leanne did a great job with Vanish. Later still, Ana from Everycare came and cooked us a tasty supper. As usual, Lennie went up to bed early and was angry when I didn't immediately follow but stayed to read more Tolstoy. On Wednesday, Stephen encouraged me to go to the Men's Group lunch for the first time in several months and Michael Steele kindly gave me a lift. Stephen took Lennie out for a walk and Chelsea beat Lille 2–1. On Thursday, Faye and Lennie went for a long walk along the river towards Send and the community nurse came and took off my bandage for the last time. The World Athletics dominated the rest of the day. The next three days passed fairly amicably. Gilly helped for a bit with the Fairtrade stall after Mass on Sunday. Richard, Will and Iris came to watch Chelsea beat Southampton 4–1. Lennie stayed down to watch *World on Fire*, so we went to bed around 10.15 p.m. On Monday, Leanne took Lennie for a walk down by the river. "Lennie seemed angry at having been 'pushed around' or led by Leanne all the time." In the afternoon, Lennie went off with Norma to the Women's Prayer Group and "the day ended quite reasonably".

The second Tuesday in October was very ordinary, though Leanne took Lennie to Polesden Lacey, where they enjoyed a walk and a large piece of cake. I used the free time to do some work on my *Catholic Social Teaching Shift* article and Benedict's *Caritas in Veritate*. Late in the afternoon, we had a fiery row when Lennie failed to follow my instructions about the fridge in the kitchen. On Wednesday morning, I wrote that "I do find Lennie's inability to follow instructions, such as 'it is on your right,' very irritating. I must learn to be like the carers and just cope with it. Lennie is talking about going home and seeing her parents. 'Are you my husband?' she asks." Stephen arrived too late for me to to go to the Men's Group for lunch and later I wrote, "I'm frustrated by what seems like a strange waste of a day and aim to 'do some work' while I hope Stephen takes Lennie for a walk". On Thursday, Leanne drove us to Mass at St. Pius' and in the hall afterwards I found it difficult to remember names of people I'd known for years. In the afternoon, Voytek came to rejuvenate the lawn and when Frances came to take Lennie to Clandon Park "this enabled me to do a couple of hours work on *Catholic Social Teaching Shift*, getting about one third of the way through *Laudato Si'*". In the evening, apart from watching a series of World Cup matches, I managed to read to the end of the second part of Isaiah i.e,. Ch. 55.

It was a wet Friday morning, but Leanne took Lennie into town to sort out problems with three watches. "While they were out, I managed to do another spell of typing up on the theological and scriptural analyses of *Laudato Si'*. In the evening, Lennie kept changing her clothes every time she came downstairs. On Saturday, Stephen came after he'd been to Mass at St. Joseph's, so I went upstairs and managed to finish my draft on *Laudato Si'*. Because of a tornado in Japan, there was no World Cup rugby to watch but I read as far as Ch.9 of Mark. On Sunday, Gillian "drove us to Mass on the day John Henry Newman was canonised in Rome". After being given the host, I walked round to receive the chalice for the first time since my operation. Norma came to tell us that from now on the Women's Prayer Group would be monthly. "Stephen, worryingly, said Lennie had left the gas on without burning it ... Please Lord, help me to do what needs to be done."

On Monday, I wrote: "Lennie and I have had an angry verbal exchange as the washing schedule ended and I have to learn she doesn't know where the washing machine is and how to put clothes out on radiators. Earlier, she didn't realise I am her husband and that this is our house." Claire came and took Lennie for a "pleasant walk around Squires and then Clandon Garden Centre ... So relieved to be free from Lennie's endless repetitions." I went upstairs, replaced batteries in my hearing aids, prepared the cash for the cleaners, and then spent an hour doing the Sainsbury's shop online. After an hour's break after lunch, Lennie became very disoriented. "Today, for example, she came down at 3.30 p.m. in a panic about what clothes she ought to be wearing. I decided to give her 100% attention and she wasn't sure if I was her husband of fifty-nine years or that this was our house and home, and that some of the stories about earlier today were simply rejected as lies e.g., that she had been to two garden centres this morning."

A great deal of Tuesday morning was taken up with answering Lennie's repeated questions: "I don't know where Mike is! Will we still be here next Tuesday (for my hair appointment) because I am on holiday? Are you (me) my husband?" I only had peace when Leanne turned up and took Lennie for a walk by the river. Wednesday was difficult. In the morning, I lost my cool at Lennie's repeated questions and in the afternoon, Stephen, having earlier walked 'round the block' with her, later felt obliged to follow her when she went off on her own. "But she does see this as an impingement on her freedom." On Thursday, pondering on Stephen's role, I recognized that "he is a vulnerable man with his own illness and needs". When I enquired whether Norma could take Lennie for a walk, she told me that our neighbour Ron Sloan had died this morning. May he rest in peace. Lennie's demands persisted, and when she spilt a glass of red wine on the carpet on Friday, we were lucky that Jane helped clean it up. I was being coerced to go up to bed long before my preferred time of 10 p.m. Because of my poor mobility, when Lennie insisted on doing her own thing and walked off, it was Stephen who was the only one who could help when it wasn't one of the carer's shifts. No wonder there were regular tensions and explosions of anger. In the meantime, on Saturday, England reached the semi-finals of the rugby World Cup. On Sunday Gilly drove us to Mass and coped with "a fuming Lennie, angry at other people bothering about her lost purse". Andrew phoned with worrying news about his loss of sight in one eye. On Monday morning, I completed this week's online shopping order with Sainsbury's. Claire and Lennie went to Squires and Clandon Garden Centre. From about 3 p.m., Lennie "basically stopped me working on writing up a joint first draft of my conclusions to *Catholic Social Teaching Shift*. When I tried to continue with some writing, Lennie was furious about my always 'busying myself in my books'."

I started my Tuesday diary feeling sorry for myself: "It is not easy being married to a wife with dementia. She got dressed at 4 a.m. and got undressed when I told her there were three hours to go." I proceeded to explain how difficult it was for me to push a zimmer frame with one hand and try and do domestic chores and cope with a variety of Lennie's concerns such as 'was I Mike?' Leanne drove Lennie to Hair Partners for a perm, cooked our lunch, and took Lennie out for a short walk. Confused in the evening, she kept asking where all the children were.

During and after breakfast she went on and on about whether Maureen her sister, who died eight years earlier, knew about my hospital appointment. I took a taxi to the hospital, where the physiotherapist "rather surprised me by suggesting the surgeon might suggest another knee operation if my movements didn't improve". In the evening, we were surprised when Chelsea beat Ajax 1–0. On Thursday, Bob Durston drove us to Mass and afterwards Norman Barber told me about his difficulties with Eileen before she went into a care home. The Durstons then kindly took us out for lunch in East Horsley. A sign of the times was an email I sent on Friday to "the children, saying I didn't want any 'stuff' for birthday, Christmas or anniversaries. Lennie is going on and on, wanting reproductions of photos to 'take home' because 'we only come here once a year'!" Later in the day I finished work on my *Catholic Social Teaching Shift* and sent copies to the Bookham Group and Pat Jones, asking for her comments.

My Saturday diary recorded: "Last night wasn't perfect. Lennie got dressed in the middle of the night and spent some time in the other bedroom. In the end, she returned fully dressed to bed." The TV showed England's great semi-final win against New Zealand. Later in the day, we watched Chelsea beat Burnley 4–2. The clocks went back at the end of B.S.T. On Sunday, Gilly drove us to Mass and Stephen fed us and took Lennie out for a walk. In the evening, we watched Luke suffering from shell shock in the film *Dunkirk*. On Monday, I did a large online shop at Sainsbury's. As often happens, Lennie was anxious in the late afternoon, and I recorded: "There then followed an awful three-quarters, of an hour with Lennie going on and on about 'the children' and 'the schools' and my responses just did not register at all".

On Tuesday morning, I noted that "Lennie is fine but in a memory loss mode: 'Have you seen my husband this morning?' And basic things like making tea or coffee get mixed up. She spends hours changing clothes and shoes." Leanne came and took Lennie down for a walk along the river while I started to write Christmas cards. In the late afternoon, Lennie came downstairs "in a sudden change of mood to complain that no one was taking over the First Holy Communion programme which she claims she has been involved with over the past few years". The beginning of my Wednesday diary showed how difficult Lennie can be: "Lennie got dressed around 3–4 a.m., left the bedroom for a while, returned to bed fully dressed, wanted a chat, so I had a mixed sleep. At 9 a.m., Lennie went out for a walk saying she was a big girl now and didn't need to listen to a 'cranky old man'. She wouldn't wait for Stephen. She soon returned with some Cadbury's chocs but had no idea that Stephen was her, and our, son. Lennie is driving me mad." Stephen came around 11 a.m. and while he took Lennie out for a short walk, I continued writing Christmas cards with mini letters. Stephen had earlier put away the weekly online shop from Sainsbury's. Later, we had two comments from Lennie about doing what I wanted to do, writing, and only concerned with 'me, me, me!' I was writing about a dozen or so Christmas cards and got as far as eighty-three now completed. I felt that this was a helpful contribution, but Lennie saw it as a bit of self-indulgence. We watched the TV the rest of the day, including Chelsea's 2–0 defeat of Crystal Palace.

The next day was Remembrance Sunday and Gillian took us early to St. Pius' where she was sacristan today. Back home, she kindly sewed buttons on Lennie's coat, which made it look so much smarter. In the afternoon, Richard came for over an hour and told us that his first week at ESPN had gone quite well. On Monday I recorded that Lennie had watched a DVD with Stephen into the early hours fully dressed, and I had to persuade her to come back to bed. This morning, I got the AA to install a new battery in the car. In the evening, we were told we needed a new inverter for our solar panel system.

Tuesday was another busy day. Leanne drove us to the hospital, where the physio seemed pleased with the improvement I'd made. Lennie always seemed to push for supper early, but we survived and, in the evening, I read the *Tablet*. On Wednesday, I wrote, "I find these days alone with Lennie very testing, but somehow we managed and I informed Lennie about our four children and six grandchildren, only two of whom were still at school. On Thursday, Stephen went off just before 9 a.m. and Lennie said that one of these days she'd marry him. Leanne drove us to Mass, where we unexpectedly found it to be a funeral. Stephen then turned up to join me on my first drive for seven months. I drove him back to G-Live, but to my surprise, Lennie was absolutely furious, claiming that for about four of us there had been a misunderstanding. There was an awful-looking form from HMRC for the Trust, for which I will need Gilly and possibly an accountant. We coped during the rest of the day and watched England beat Montenegro 7–0.

On Friday morning, we went to John Moore's funeral at St. Joseph's. He was at one stage the Chairman of the *Universe*. May he rest in peace. In the evening, we were rather hooked by *Children in Need*. On Saturday I noted: "Please help me, Lord, to respond as You would wish me to. 'Remind me of your name.' 'Mike.' 'And your wife's name?' 'Lennie.' 'I am your wife?' 'Yes.' 'Blimey, I hadn't realised that.' Lennie then had one of her lengthy and intrusive memory lapses when she tearfully regretted she'd never been told about her parents' or Maureen's death." Stephen was very helpful during the rest of the day. We watched England Women's rugby's last-minute win over France and the final two episodes of *The Spiral*.

On Sunday, Gilly drove us to St. Pius' for Mass and afterwards we had a pleasant chat about Katie's and Douglas's plans after graduation. I phoned Andrew, who sounded cheerful enough, but his eyes may take some months to recover. He is still struggling to find employment. In the afternoon, we watched Vera Brittain's *Testament of Youth* and later England beat Kosovo 4–0 and Mason Mount scored his first goal for England. We ended the day watching the first episode of H.G. Wells's *The War of the Worlds*. On Monday, Leanne took Lennie for a walk down by the river while I ordered the week's shopping online from Sainsbury's. At the last minute she seemed to agree to go to the Women's Prayer Group. In the evening, she had one of her difficult periods complaining about carers 'only in it for the money' and then I tried to insist that it was a form of bullying to demand that I go to bed before 10 p.m.

I started Tuesday's diary by reporting that between 3 a.m. and 5 a.m., Lennie ranted for the best part of an hour about Leanne's 'bossiness' and 'come along, dear'. It is difficult to know how best to handle these sudden and quite violent eruptions which can't easily be stopped or softened. Leanne came and took Lennie for a walk down by the river. I phoned Michael Walsh to ask for his comments on my *Catholic Social Teaching Shift* paper. We watched *Vienna Blood*, a murder mystery set in 1908, and then the political contest between Boris and Corbyn, and I read to Ch. 29 of Exodus. On Wednesday morning, when Stephen came round, I managed to read Exodus before going off to the Men's Group lunch where it was my turn to pay for the drinks. Mass on Thursday morning was Ron Sloan's funeral. May he rest in peace. In my diary I added: "Lennie oscillates between being nice to me and telling me how much she loves me and exploding angrily at what she claims is my selfish bullying and 'me, me, me'. On Friday morning, Lennie insisted on going out for a walk. Leanne brought Lennie home again, having picked her up on Boxgrove Road. But Lennie just doesn't have a sense of our concerns and simply states: 'I am a big girl, not a three-year-old.'" Saturday was a mixed and quite busy day. Everycare suggested a meeting after carers had a couple of times this week found Lennie wandering. We joined Stephen at St.

Joseph's for 10 a.m. Mass, after which Gillian took Lennie on a shopping expedition to buy birthday presents for us both. I took Stephen home and we enjoyed the respite! On their return we completed our postal votes. I voted "strategically" for the Lib. Dems.

Sunday was Andrew's fifty-eighthth birthday. He phoned on his way home from Bridport with a possible broken arm after a fall. My glasses case has disappeared this morning. "Lennie often moves things and then later denies having ever seen them. Stephen was very good with Lennie, who was at her most infuriating evening phase where she was full of demands and queries about what was going to happen to us: are we going to sell this house and move elsewhere? What are we doing tomorrow? Who else lives here? Where have they all gone? etc." On Monday morning, Lennie's endless chatter held up my Sainsbury's online shopping, but when Claire came, I was able to complete it. In the evening, we had a bit of a disaster. Lennie insisted on preparing supper much earlier than necessary, but she was unable to find the apples for stewing. After half an hour, I went to the kitchen only to find that the fridge had had everything taken out and the quiche and pork pies were all in the oven. I exploded and we had a serious row and I probably threatened with my stick, so Lennie shut the lounge door and I went to tidy things up in the kitchen and started peeling the apples. This was interrupted by a knock at the door from Laura, a neighbour, who said she'd seen Lennie wandering near George Abbot school. She'd clearly left by going out of the lounge and round the back. Laura kindly drove off and picked her up and brought her home. Bless her.

"Life is becoming very difficult" is how I started Tuesday's diary. "Last night, I found her on my side of the bed, and nothing would move her. For the first time in eleven years I slept on the other side of our double bed. In the afternoon, we watched a police drama on the TV. Then, Jane from

Everycare phoned to suggest taking Lennie to a meeting of the Alzheimer's Society. To be honest, I don't think Lennie accepts her analysis and would be fairly resistant to going ... Lennie has never stopped asking where all the children are, and the cats, and trying to envisage what our house looks like." On Wednesday, I led the discussion on my *Catholic Social Teaching Shift* paper with the Bookham Group. I introduced the discussion by referring to the collapse of *Progressio* (associated with the shift to advocacy from amelioration) with help from emails from Michael Walsh and Pat Jones. At 8 p.m., Lennie came down wondering why I was not joining her upstairs in bed. On Thursday, I drove Lennie to Mass at St. Pius', after which Frances and Lennie then went off to the Women's Christmas lunch at Clandon Golf Course. I took advantage of Lennie's being away to watch the DVD of the film *Iris,* which I saw as very much a celebration of her husband's everlasting love, but I am not sure it helped me much in discerning how to cope with Lennie.

On Friday, I had two hospital appointments and both Lennie and Stephen came with me. "The Registrar in the Fracture Clinic agreed with my request not to contemplate any additional surgery and was happy to discharge me." The physiotherapist kindly "managed to slot me in early and worked at straightening my right knee". There was worrying political discussion in the *Table*t and papers about "fears that it was going to get more difficult for Catholics to get elected to parliament". Saturday was my eighty-seventh birthday and "we went to Mass at St. Joseph's and later went out for lunch at the Queen's Head in East Clandon where we rendezvoused with Richard and Will and Iris who had invited us to celebrate my and Lennie's birthdays. We had a very pleasant meal with them with friendly chat all the time. Andrew and Gilly both phoned to wish me a happy birthday." On Sunday, "Gilly came to drive us to Mass. There was a pastoral letter from Bishop Richard, which I thought was excellent and a call to action to address the

2030 issue of climate change." Watching documentaries in the evening, I noted, "I found it difficult to pick up the details of conversations – my hearing is going." On Monday, I had an email from "my cousin Keith Harrison who, relying on Grandma's Irish background, is applying for an Irish passport because of Brexit". Claire and Paula took Lennie down to the river and on their return put out the washing on the radiators. In the afternoon, the Family Group met at the Durstons' for delicious soup and rolls and an apple cake and ice cream and a rather unfocused discussion.

On Tuesday, Claire slotted in beautifully and took Lennie for a 'cut and blow-dry' at Hair Partners. I had a very thorough check -up from the physio who came round. Voytek came to do some gardening, for probably the last time before Spring. My sister-in-law, Jean, phoned to tell us that our nephew Paul's wife has terminal cancer. Be with them, Lord. In the evening, "Lennie has come down and is rummaging for her front door key! I locked the front door as she was threatening to go out and search for the group who were planning to go teaching or something like this. When she went out from the back window, I phoned Norma but Lennie came in the front anyway. How can I cope if this gets worse?" Marika came and helped with supper. I finished reading Deuteronomy and in the late evening we both enjoyed André Rieu's *Love in Maastricht*. On Wednesday, as a result of Lennie's repeated pushing, we went to Mass at St. Edward's. After Stephen's arrival, I drove off to the Men's Group at the Barley Mow Thai restaurant in West Horsley, where I set up the arrangement to pay for the drinks since my birthday was this week. I was an active participant in the discussion. Several of them said how good it was to see me back with the group. During the rest of the day at home Stephen was the leader and led us through several episodes of the detective series *Luther*. On Thursday, Leanne drove us to Mass at St. Pius'. In the afternoon, we watched Stephen's DVD *Stan and Ollie*.

"Maureen's jealousy emerges not infrequently in Lennie's reminiscences about her childhood relations."

On Friday, Lennie and I changed the bed linen on the two beds upstairs. When Leanne came, she took Lennie off to a garden centre. In the afternoon, we watched a slightly daft police drama, and I was urged by my physio to contact the District Nurse about the sore on my bottom. Then Lennie "had one of her late-afternoon episodes. She was angry about the coming of a carer at 5.15 p.m. and that it was being considered as a regular thing, in spite of the fact that it has been regular for six or seven months since I first went into hospital." The half-yearly meeting of the Trustees was on Saturday morning and was chaired by Andrew with financial input from Gilly and maintenance issues input from Richard. During the day we watched Chelsea being beaten by Everton. Stephen was very helpful with a disoriented Lennie. Sunday was Lennie's eighty-fourth birthday. I drove us to Mass at St. Pius' where we were joined by Gilly. Stephen helped by putting on our 'Memories' DVD of 'Our First Thirty Years'. During the rest of the day, we watched a series of programmes ending with David Attenborough's *Seven Worlds; Our Planet*. Then Stephen and Lennie brought down the Christmas tree from the roof.

I started my diary for Monday 9th by noting, "Lennie seemed to agree she needed a female helper to get dressed. I doubt if she would if we set it up, but it did indicate a need. For example, she put on a blouse inside out today and needed help." Leanne came and helped put out the washing on the radiators. "I then drove the three of us to the Royal Surrey for my six-monthly check-up on my pacemaker." Everything was OK, so we returned home, and Leanne took Lennie out for a walk before lunch. I cleared emails, skimmed to the end of Joshua, and selected charities to support while Lennie went to the Women's Group meeting. In the evening, we felt too tired to go to Mass, so we watched some TV including "an election debate with an under-thirty audience".

Early in my diary for the second Tuesday, I noted: "Lennie's dementia grows ever more serious. She doesn't know Maureen died eight years ago or that her father is dead. She confuses 'dad' with 'husband'. She doesn't know where the fridge is or what the plans for the day are. She got fully dressed in the middle of the night and returned to bed fully clothed." Leanne took Lennie to Mass at St. Joseph's because I stayed at home expecting a Feed In Tariff (F.I.T.) engineer. I read about nine chapters of Judges. In the evening, "Lennie's mind was miles away with children from school who had to be fed, and also were we going to church that evening? Even after Aurelia (Everycare) left, she persisted; I'm glad I locked both doors!" Chelsea managed to get through to the last sixteen of the Champions League. On Wednesday, I read from the book of Ruth before driving us to Mass at St. Edward's. In the afternoon, Stephen put on a film, *Calvary* about an Irish priest. On Thursday, we attended the funeral of Pat Sloan on Ron's birthday. At 9.30 p.m., I wrote: "I am having to cope with an angry Lennie who has come downstairs two or three times after going up to bed shortly after 8 p.m. She accuses me of driving our children out of our home. She rejects the reality that they are all in their fifties; sees me as a selfish bully in always wanting my own way in not going to bed around 8.30 p.m.; accuses me of being a liar; brought down my pyjamas which she says she found on the stairs, totally denying that she put them there. Time to go and join her around 10 p.m."

Early Friday morning, I wrote: "Lennie, in the middle of the night and this morning, was quite different from last night; warm and affectionate ... We set off for the hospital around 8.30 a.m. and at the Maxillofacial Department, I was seen by the doctor who examined me for cancer growths." I chose the option of seeing my G.P. if I had any future problems. Frances Allen brought me her husband David's three-wheeler, which some nurses have urged me to use. The big news today was Boris's big election win. The following day, Saturday, was my brother David's birthday but I don't know if he is alive or dead. "May God give you peace, joy and love always." Stephen joined us for Mass at St. Joseph's. Afterwards, we went to Sainsbury's, where Stephen and Lennie bought presents for our carers and a very kindly man helped me fill up with petrol. After Mass on Sunday, Lennie and I gave out envelopes for the 10% collection. Stephen cooked us a nice lunch after which he took Lennie for a long walk via Briar Way to Sainsbury's. I did three-quarters of the washing up. Gilly then turned up with her two dogs. In the evening, the three of us watched a catch-up movie, *Nativity*.

On Monday I wrote: "Twice during the night, at 2 a.m. and 4 a.m., Lennie got dressed and had to be persuaded to return to the bed". Before Stephen set off for Guildford, he put the washing out on the radiators. "Lennie was furious with me that we weren't going to Mass, and she went off in tears with Leanne to go down to the river (sea)." I finished our weekly online shopping with Sainsbury's before driving down to Nationwide, where I arranged to transfer £600 from our savings account to each of our six grandchildren's savings accounts. "I definitely felt that this could easily be my last venture into central Guildford. The 2–4 p.m. party given by Everycare to its clients at St. John's Village Hall was very pleasant – unassuming, family-run and community orientated." I made a brief 'thank you' speech on behalf of the clients. Back home, we had a brief snooze "before Faye called, but by then Lennie had come down in her nightie. I phoned Norma and sent our apologies for not attending the Oak Tree Gardens AGM that night. Shortly after Faye left, Lennie came down wearing my pyjama jacket, asking when I was going to bed. In anger she threw it on the settee. I went up to bed about 9.10 p.m. In the early hours we had quite a strong session of caresses and it was the nearest to love-making for some months."

"There was no Mass at St. Joseph's, so we drove to the Clandon Garden Centre." We managed to work through the rest of the day, although Lennie had one of her evening spells when "she denied having had any supper and went off to make herself a sandwich or two. She thought that we were going off to Mass tonight instead of tomorrow. She is in total denial of things that happened recently and frequently claims to have seen her parents. Her latest worry is concerned with our taking Will and Iris to the pantomime on Saturday." On Wednesday, we drove to St. Edward's for Mass and then to the Royal Surrey County Hospital where I saw the physiotherapist "who seemed reasonably pleased with the state of my right knee and was happy enough to discharge me." I wrote my last Christmas cards, helped put away the Sainsbury's shopping delivery, and enjoyed the supper Stephen had cooked. Lennie stayed and watched *Night Train to Lisbon* until we went to bed together.

On Thursday, after an angry start to the day when "I blew up and even thought I might have a heart attack," I drove us to the Bereavement Mass for Norman's son. Afterwards, Leanne took Lennie down to the river for an hour while I booked a shopping delivery before the New Year. Faye came around supper time and we managed to see out the rest of a busy day. At this stage in our lives the laptop was still in Stephen's bedroom, so I almost invariably cleared emails before going downstairs. On Friday, I managed to put up with Lennie's anger at my having booked her a hair appointment and took her to Hair Partners where she had a 'cut and blow-dry'. The carer, Justyna, cooked our supper and somehow we managed to get through the evening without carers. On the last Saturday before Christmas, I drove us to St. Joseph's for Mass. Stephen joined Lennie while I went to confession with Fr. Roy who, as "a former married man, was aware of the difficulties of dementia and very sympathetic to its challenges". Reviews of books by Pettifor and Klein led me to order them for New Year reading and for topics for the next Bookham Group. In the evening, Richard came to drive us to the Yvonne Arnaud where we took Will and Iris to see this year's pantomime, *The Sleeping Beauty*.

Gilly joined us for Mass on Sunday, and I think she was a sacristan. Back home she and Katie visited us. Katie had enjoyed her first term at Edinburgh. Stephen cooked us a meal of roast pork with Christmas pudding to follow. Afterwards, I conked out for an hour or more while Stephen kindly took Lennie out for a walk. We then were pleased when a strong Chelsea team beat Spurs 2–0 away. Stephen helped Lennie and me to cope with the evening. On Monday, before he set off for Cranleigh, Stephen put on the washing machine and later Leanne helped put the clothes out on the radiators before taking Lennie for her favourite walk down by the river. While they were out, I managed to work through a couple of domestic chores, including sending wishes to The Lighthouse in Poole where my nephew, John Worthy, was performing. In the late evening, "my head suddenly began to swim, and I called Lennie and wrote on a piece of paper what to do if I suddenly became ill or had a stroke. At the very least this is a warning that life is coming to an end."

I felt last night's strange episode was quite a reminder, but Lennie had forgotten it on the morning of Christmas Eve. There was no 10 a.m. Mass in the parish. Faye took Lennie out for a coffee at Starbucks /Sainsbury's and a walk around the store. This gave me a chance to read Chapters 5–7 of Matthew. In the afternoon, Lennie went wandering around upstairs and in the early evening we enjoyed André Rieu's *Christmas at Home* from Maastricht before going to the Vigil Mass at St. Pius'. Pat and Patrick were very friendly afterwards. My Christmas Day diary starts: "Unexpectedly, we stayed up to watch the first episode of *A Christmas Carol* and then were hypnotised by the promise of Mozart's Credo from Croydon Minster's Midnight Mass, which was very moving with lovely choirs. I wondered why there was such a schism between us and pray for greater unity – as Gillian and her children will be doing with Doug at Holy Trinity today. Lennie's fantasy, which eventually drove us to bed by 1.30 a.m., was that she'd seen her father in the past couple of days."

We got up about 8.30 a.m. and worked through the opening and recording of presents until we drove off to Albury, where Richard and all his four children had invited us for a very nice Christmas lunch. Iris apparently wants to be an actress like Luke. Mass on Thursday morning was for the parish servers and members of the Guild of St. Stephen. "On the way home, Lennie wondered whether we were going home in a couple of days and when she was going to see her sister Maureen. This is very common at the moment. I sense that things will get more difficult in 2020 and pray that the Lord will give me the love and patience that I will need." We then drove to Gilly's for a very pleasant lunch and a game afterwards before we returned home expecting Andrew on his way home from the coast with Caroline. Lennie went up to bed at 8.30 p.m. which gave me the opportunity to read the first thirty pages of John Le Carre´s *Agent Running in the Field*. Lennie came down ready for Mass. Time to go up to bed with her around 10 p.m.

My diary for the Friday noted: "Last night, Lennie got dressed and returned to bed in the middle of the night fully dressed. Life isn't straightforward." I had driven Lennie and Leanne to Mass at St. Joseph's. In mid-afternoon I wrote: "I'm beginning to get worried. Lennie went on one of her walk-abouts an hour and twenty minutes ago and she just wouldn't accept my lack of physical ability. I could have physically prevented her but that would have caused a serious row. So, I stayed and at 3 p.m. the Sainsbury's online shopping was delivered and at 4.05 p.m. a resident in Glendale Drive dropped Lennie to our front door; *Deo Gratias* and thank You, Lord, for her safe return. She is lovely several times during the day, but at other times she is angry and in deep denial about what we have done."

On Saturday morning I dropped a full milk bottle in the kitchen. "Typically, I exploded and swore out loud but Lennie, true to form, got out the mop and gradually cleared it up without a single note of criticism. Bless her for her coolness and kindness on such occasions." I drove us to Mass at St. Joseph's. After returning home I noted: "Lennie's memory is cockeyed. She isn't aware her mother and father are both dead (thirty-four and fifty-four years earlier) or that we don't have any 'family' living with us or needing to be fed." Stephen cooked us lunch and then took Lennie out for a walk. "Gillian unexpectedly turned up with her two dogs; I think she may have brought an anniversary present which she left with Stephen." After supper we watched some films until Lennie and I went to bed around 10 p.m. On Sunday, we celebrated our fifty-ninth wedding anniversary and the Feast of the Holy Family. Gilly and Katie came home after Mass but didn't stay long because Katie was returning to Edinburgh. Andrew phoned; he seemed to be having a rough time with his Indian company. I told him that in my view he was overstretching himself. We were delighted with Chelsea's gutsy 2–1 win at Arsenal. When Leanne came on Monday morning, she took Lennie out for a walk, and I was able to catch up with domestic jobs such as booking a Vision Express eye test. I wasn't sure what I ought to do about Lennie's tendency to go on walkabouts.

Tuesday was New Year's Eve and I noted: "It's been quite a year really, the first I can remember without a holiday. For me, I had three operations on my right leg including two stays in hospital for two weeks for hip fracture and one week following my knee replacement. But possibly more significant has been Lennie's deteriorating memory and often her worrying tendency to go for walks and get lost. She frequently says she's seen and talked to her parents and sister, all long dead. I feel increasingly old and lacking in energy. I'm learning to live with Lennie's repeated questions, half a dozen or more times, this morning about our families, and so on." We went to Mass at St. Joseph's and found Stephen back home. The three of us went to the Horse and Groom for lunch and later I finished reading *Agent Running in the Field*. We watched André Rieu in the last hours of the year.

At the end of 2019 I wrote in my diary: "The future use of this diary: on 15 July I read an article I'd totally forgotten I'd written in 2002 but which tries to explain the purpose of the diaries for future researchers. The article notes: 'I have committed myself to writing a daily diary, around 4–500 words every day, to try and record for future generations of scholars, what living as a Catholic academic was like in the last quarter of the twentieth century. I hope to offer a more-or-less systematic record of the complexities of reconciling the conflicting tugs of work, family, professional and religious aspects of life. What sort of sense did he make of his life? What sort of values were expressed through his choices? How did he allocate time and reconcile often competing demands? How did he cope with ethical conflicts? What constituted religious authority for him? How did he relate to the clerical caste? I see this diary-keeping as part of my sense of the vocation of a sociologist researcher in my area of interest, a gift, hopefully, to future generations.' (p.143) in 'Researching Religion: the Vocation of the Sociologist of Religion', Int. J. *Social Research Methodology*, 2002, Vol. 5, No.2, 133–146."

CHAPTER 8

The Year 2020

Increasingly, my diary has plotted developments with Lennie's dementia and how we coped with it through thick and thin, and with patience and impatience. It may be that this might be a useful source, rather like that of Iris Murdoch's husband. I remember being surprised earlier this year when Dr. Barnado gave me a photocopy of a letter I had sent him in 2014, explaining that the children and grandchildren had drawn attention to Lennie's memory loss, but that I was in almost total denial. Things are more obvious now. But it has lasted at least six years now.

New Year's Day was a Wednesday and after Stephen had cooked us a lovely breakfast, we drove off to St. Edward's for Mass. There was a sense of peace and joy today. Bob and Maureen Durston came home for a coffee and chat. Stephen took Lennie for a walk. Gilly phoned to wish us a happy new year. Richard, Will and Iris came to watch Chelsea and afterwards Stephen put on the DVD with memories of the first thirty years of our married lives. But Richard didn't want Will and Iris to see pictures of his marriage to Anna-Lucy. I read the first three chapters of Matthew's Gospel and started reading Ann Pettifer's book *The Case for the Green New Deal*. On Thursday, Stephen returned to Cranleigh. We drove to Mass at St. Pius' and on returning home, played rummy with Faye, who then took Lennie out for a walk. Later in the afternoon, we drove over to Howell and Liz Lewis's for tea. Faye came on our return home to cook supper and I joined Lennie relatively early in bed. My diary for Friday notes Lennie's complaints about me last night. "The gist of what she said was that I was letting her down; that we weren't relating together as smoothly as we used to; that she ought to be getting ready to go teaching; and who pushed her out of teaching?" After Faye arrived, I drove the three of us to Mass at St. Joseph's.

On Saturday, we were joined by Stephen at Mass at St. Joseph's. He took Lennie for a walk and cooked our meals. Most of the day we spent watching the second Test Match in South Africa and in the evening, we watched a Scandinavian police drama. Sunday was much the same, with Lennie worrying about arrangements for the next day. I drove her to Mass at St. Pius', where we were joined by Gilly, who visited us at home for a chat afterwards. Again, the Test Match was followed until around 4 p.m. when Lennie was insisting it was time for a sandwich prepared by Stephen. The evening was difficult too, and "Lennie is now asserting we've never told her about her dental appointment tomorrow ... Lennie blew her top that food hadn't been put out for six people and a celebration. It is difficult to make sense of what she is doing. Dear Lord, help us."

On Monday, Claire took Lennie to the dentist while Stephen managed the weekly wash. Later, Faye came and took Lennie for a walk round the block. "When I told Lennie we were expecting the next carer to make supper, she was furious, angrily complaining that I was forcing her to 'make meals' for another carer. She was so angry, threatening to go out, that I locked the front door." By the time the carer left we both felt too tired to go to Mass, so we relaxed with André Rieu and *The Magic of Maastricht*. On Tuesday, we drove to St. Joseph's for Mass and afterwards Leanne coped pretty well with Lennie and cooked us a tasty lunch. Emma, the toe specialist, came after lunch and sorted out Lennie's toes. As always Lennie went to bed around 8.30 p.m. I muted the TV and spent over an hour reading Ann Pettifor's book arguing in favour of a Green New Deal.

On Wednesday, before driving to Mass at St. Edward's, I cleared emails and booked an M.O.T. with SEAT. Later, we drove off to Carlo's where the three of us had a pleasant lunch. When the Sainsbury's online shopping was delivered, Stephen put it away. Later, we drove him to the bus station because he had a dental appointment in Cranleigh the next day. Unusually, Lennie watched two episodes of *Silent Witness* "and she said afterwards how much she loved me". Thursday was, unsurprisingly, a bit different. "Lennie is anxiously changing her shoes umpteen times. Earlier, she spent a quarter of an hour searching her drawers for knickers. Her drawers are an absolute shambles." We went to Mass at St. Pius'. Around 4 p.m., Lennie was pushing for supper and at 9 p.m. she'd had enough of *Eastenders* and kept wondering about Maureen, who died nine years earlier. When I joined her later, she was wearing my pyjamas. On Friday, I was surprised that the *Tablet* had nothing on the theme of the Global Green New Deal (GND). Lennie's main problem today was "a small necklace which she couldn't clip off". On Saturday, "Lennie got herself dressed around 2 a.m., I think, and returned to bed fully dressed". Stephen joined us when we went to 10 a.m. Mass at St. Joseph's. Later, he put on the Anglo-French murder drama, *The Tunnel*. On Sunday, "I am increasingly finding it hard to stand for long spells at Mass. So, I sit as much as I can. Lennie's anxiety this morning was how to take the host; at least eight times she needed assurance about taking the host in her hand." Later, we watched two episodes of the Norwegian police drama *Wisting* and quite unusually, Lennie stayed down until 11 p.m. watching several episodes of *The Tunnel*.

On Monday, "Lennie is disorientated, annoying Stephen, not realising he is her son, repeatedly asking whether he works in London, whether he is an only child, and so on". Leanne came and took Lennie out for a walk before it rained, while I spent an hour ordering the Sainsbury's shopping online. "After lunch, Lennie was very disorientated, not realising that it was our bedroom. Then Ann, bless her, phoned for our usual post-Christmas chat. In the evening, we watched the final episode of *The Tunnel* and then André Rieu and *Love in Maastricht*." Tuesday was a difficult day because Lennie had memory problems and the SEAT driver didn't turn up. "I have been Lennie's dad, and she is furious at not being able to go to Mass this morning." I ordered a taxi to take me to Vision Express, "where I was told I had 20/20 distance vision, but my left eye might have deteriorated. Lennie and I watched *Eastenders* but then Lennie started being very critical about the carers, who 'just come here to have a meal and then go off ' and just for 'money, money, money'. I gradually eased the tension, turned off the TV and Lennie went up to bed at 8.15 p.m. I read Mt.26 and then Kleine until 9.35 p.m."

Wednesday's diary notes there was a powerful storm in the middle of the night, which severely shook the garden fence. We drove to Mass at St. Edward's and found Stephen when we returned home. He took Lennie out for a walk around the Charlock Way block. When Janani, the physio, came she "accompanied me on my first walk since my ops round the green in Burnet Avenue. Lennie came out and asked me where her dad was and then whether I would join her in bed tonight!"

Thursday was a fairly typical day. We went to Mass at St. Pius' and afterwards had a chat with Fr. Roy who, like many converts, was anti-women priests. In the evening, we went out with Michael and Sheila Wheeler for a very pleasant meal. Friday saw us both go to Mass before Leanne and then Faye took Lennie out for a walk. "After Faye left at 4 p.m., the next one and a half hours was a nightmare in that Lennie never stopped asking how many people were coming for supper, what was for supper, who was coming, when it was going to be cooked and what choices had we made. When I went up to bed Lennie told me I ought to go into my bedroom. But I resisted and said that the double bed was my bed. Then I easily fell sleep."

On Saturday, "Lennie started the day by saying how pleased she was I was taking her to Mass and how grateful she was to have me, though earlier she'd regretted she hadn't found a young man! After Mass, we picked up two boxes of wine at Majestic ... Stephen took Lennie for a walk, and then the two of them took me with the three-wheeler to the end of the road and back." In the evening, we watched three episodes of *Cobra* and then episode seven of *Wisting*. On Sunday, Stephen kindly scraped off the ice on the car and I drove us off to Mass at St. Pius'. "Later, Gilly, who'd been a sacristan, came round and we had a good old natter on Katie's 24th birthday."

Monday seemed to be a fairly ordinary day. Faye came and took Lennie "out for a walk and later helped me with a laptop problem so that I was able to send off our shopping list online to Sainsbury's. I drove to the surgery for a blood pressure test. It was apparently a bit high." In the evening, Lennie kindly agreed to come with me to the Burpham Village Hall for a meeting organised by the Guildford Environment Forum, addressed by a member of Al Gore's team. On Tuesday, I offered up Mass "in thanksgiving for all that the Lord has done for me in a pretty long life of eighty-seven years, especially with my wife, Lennie, over fifty-nine years". In the evening, "Andrew came to watch the Chelsea vs Arsenal match and experienced Lennie frenetically denying we'd had any supper and threatening to go out for a walk, which both Andrew and I prevented; I locked the door but tried to be a peacemaker. Interestingly, Andrew said he'd been impressed by the way I'd coped with Lennie's memory loss."

On the fourth Wednesday of January, we drove to Mass at St. Edward's and returned home to find Stephen already there. He surprised us by not wanting to go to Carlo's for lunch, but he took me and the three-wheeler round the green at the end of our cul-de-sac. We watched two and a half episodes of *The New Pope*. "I welcome the respite Stephen gives me. But usually, I have difficulty coping with Lennie's endless repeated questions and total ignoring of the 'This is Home' notice which Stephen put out. Lennie asks, 'Who put the children to bed?'" On Thursday, I broke the arm of my glasses but still coped with driving to St. Pius' for Mass. "On our way to Mass, Lennie wanted to know what my name is and who I am." We were introduced to a new carer, Charlotte, who took Lennie out for a walk and a chat while I drove to Hair Partners for a haircut. In the afternoon, after we'd both had a good hour's snooze, we watched episodes three and four of *The New Pope*. In the evening, Lennie's interest in *Eastenders* was minimal. "So, after the usual period of repeated questions and anxiety at having heard of the loss of her parents and sister, I managed to persuade her to watch the Wolves vs Liverpool match. Halfway through, Lennie thought it was time for supper. In spite of my saying I'd already had supper, she made enough sandwiches for both of us so half of them went into the fridge."

On Friday morning, Faye drove us to Mass at St. Joseph's and then to Vision Express, where I had a series of tests before ordering new glasses. Faye and Lennie drove me home and made us a pleasant lunch. After Faye left us, we managed to get through the afternoon watching the Test Match before Marika cooked us supper. After she'd left: "True to form, Lennie went through a fearsome phase, <u>very</u> angry when I locked the front door and prevented her getting out – from my perspective keeping her safe. But she was furious and twice banged violently on the front door. Verbally, she battered me saying I always did what I wanted and angrily objected to my not allowing her to do what she wanted. All very frightening at times, but I kept my cool and eventually eased things by getting her a Baileys."

Then it was a very ordinary Saturday. We went to Mass at St. Joseph's, where we picked up Stephen and did a brief shop at Sainsbury's. Richard, Will and Iris came over for a while. In the evening, we were invited to a Burns Night by Marie from next door. Lennie chatted to her about her teaching experiences. Sunday's diary said we "had a bit of a broken night. Lennie got dressed and then returned to bed. We gave Stephen his birthday present today since tomorrow is Holocaust Day." Much of Monday I found it difficult to find space to read or write because of Lennie's repeated questioning. Charlotte brought Lennie home after she'd had a fall in Sainsbury's. She put the washing out to dry on the radiators. In the evening, we watched an hour-long documentary, *Holocaust Memorial Day* and then André Rieu. When I went up to bed early, "Lennie was wearing my pyjama trousers. In the middle of the night, I managed to get her to take them off and put on the nightie I found." Tuesday was another difficult day. "Around 5 a.m., I woke to find Lennie fully dressed and insisting on going downstairs. Concerned about safety issues, I got up and went downstairs, where I was harangued non-stop for locking the front door and so preventing her from 'going to Mass'. When I pointed out it was three hours away, I got a non-stop verbal bashing for always wanting my own way, and so on. It worries me about how to cope. Lennie stopped me snoozing over and over again as she changed her shoes at least half a dozen times and kept asking if I was going to Mass. So off to Mass at St. Joseph's we went. To my delight Lennie thoroughly enjoyed our two-course lunch at Carlo's. I tried unsuccessfully to stop her wandering off by reminding her that we'd had carers for nine months and that by the grace of God she'd had a carer with her when she fell yesterday at Sainsbury's. Please God, keep her safe." In desperation, I phoned Everycare and Jane sent Sheena out to look for her and when she arrived, I sent off Ana. By the grace of God, Sheena soon found her and brought her home. "To my concern, Lennie showed absolutely no awareness of the problems she is causing. She can't understand where

Mike is and wants to see her parents 'at home'; she is totally dismissive that this house is our home and is searching for a bag to take spare shoes home."

"Around 2 a.m., Lennie got dressed and went downstairs. This left me worried and uncertain, and I spent two hours wondering what I ought to do to avoid accidents." Stephen came in time for me to be taken by Chris Richardson to Ye Olde Windsor Castle at Bookham for our small group of four meeting to discuss Tony Doherty's paper on theology. On our return, I was allowed to have an hour's sleep. There was a T20 match and then the Carabao Cup Final to watch and then "during the evening, Lennie had one of her normal phases, talking on and on and on about her mother and father and their house and even which country we lived in. Was I Mike? Her husband? Stephen, as always, was great, continuing to dialogue with Lennie for a couple of hours, which gave me respite."

The following day was a Thursday, so we drove to Mass at St. Pius' and had a coffee and a chat in the hall afterwards. I tried to start writing about the Green New Deal (GND). In the evening, we went to the Yvonne Arnaud for a light meal and then a performance of *Jane Eyre*. On Friday, I helped Lennie complete a women's health questionnaire.

On Saturday, Stephen joined us for Mass at St. Joseph's. During the afternoon we watched Chelsea draw at Leicester and then a couple of rugby internationals. It was much the same on Sunday. After Mass, Gilly joined us for an hour's chat and in the afternoon, we watched France beat England in a Six Nations match. I was persuaded to go to bed quite early. I missed Stephen after he set off for Cranleigh after the weekend with us. Leanne and Lennie went off for a walk while I completed our weekly online shopping with Sainsbury's. In the afternoon, I did a bit more work on my GND paper and then put on the 1948 film, *Red Shoes*. Lennie persuaded me to go to the 7.30 p.m. Mass. "Sadly, the rest of the evening was a disaster as Lennie insisted on making a second supper and I repeatedly stressed I didn't want it. 'May the Lord forgive you for what you do' she says to me, denying that we'd had an earlier supper. I'm behaving like a spoilt brat, she said to me, angry at the way I'm treating her, reminding me that we might meet her friend, Mike, and not to be nasty to him because he was a nice guy! *C'est la vie!*" We went to Carlo's for a pleasant lunch. "Lennie spent a lot of time telling me over and over again that Maureen and also her friends had warned her that I was a nice guy and if she didn't think it was going to work, she ought to break off the relationship as quickly as possible." The evening didn't get any better and Lennie "angrily asserted she wanted to go home and threatened to walk out and if I locked the door, smash it". When Ana from Everycare came round, she suggested I phoned Stephen and he had a conversation with Lennie, which cooled things down. Sadly, I also had to go to bed a good hour earlier than I would have chosen.

Wednesday was another challenging day. "Lennie got dressed around 1–2 a.m. and I later discovered she'd gone downstairs. Going to the loo, I asked if she was OK, and she replied that she was but later complained that the front door was locked and she couldn't go 'home'. She eventually returned to bed around 4 a.m. When we woke around 6.30 a.m., she was concerned about her job with children at school twenty-four years after retirement, and later asked politely if I'd drive her to Mass." Stephen stayed with Lennie while I went to the Men's Group at Send/Ripley. Later, back home, Stephen put on *Who lives here?*, *Mrs. Lowry and Her Son*, and other DVDs. On Thursday, I recorded that "last night Lennie had a fall and late this afternoon when Leanne came, she took Lennie for a walk along the river". On Friday, I emailed a 'thank you' to Sainsbury's and arranged to have a concrete support added to our garden fencing. We then drove to St. Joseph's for Mass before going to the surgery to have my bandages updated. For the rest of the day, Lennie really wasn't with us, but I kept my cool. After Lennie had gone to bed, I managed to watch a Francophile police thriller for a couple of hours. Late on Friday night, I was a 'spoilt brat' but early on Saturday morning Lennie was 'loving and caring'. Stephen joined us at Mass at St. Joseph's and cooked our meals for us. Six Nations Rugby dominated the rest of the day and we saw England beat Scotland in Edinburgh.

My diary for Sunday suggested the concrete supports for our north-side fence had been added just in time to cope with Storm Ciara. After Mass, Gilly helped on the Fairtrade stall before coming over for a coffee and a chat. We are so grateful for all she does for us. In the afternoon we watched England scrape a two-wicket win in South Africa in a one-day cricket match. Richard called in the evening and kindly agreed to drive Stephen back to Cranleigh.

I suppose Monday was a fairly normal domestic day. I put the weekly washing into the machine. When I phoned the Feed In Tariff to British Gas, they said it was the same as November so I phoned ESE to come and check our solar panels. Charlotte from Everycare came, put out the washing on the radiators, prepared lunch for us, and took Lennie up to Newlands Corner for a break. Ana came and prepared supper for us, after which I tried to write some notes on *Laudato Si*. In the late evening, we watched André Rieu in Bucharest. On Tuesday, after going to Mass at St. Joseph's and before driving to Carlo's for lunch, I asked Lennie if I could do some work upstairs, but she kept interrupting me and called me something like a 'selfish bastard'. We enjoyed our lunch, but Lennie spilled her cup of coffee all over the table. We spent a rather aimless evening but when I went up to bed, "I found Lennie in my pyjamas, so got her to change as soon as I could".

On Wednesday, I recorded that "Lennie got dressed in the middle of the night, but I woke and encouraged her to come back to bed". After I'd seen she'd swallowed her medication, she needed persuasion that she could have breakfast because the rules about fasting before Holy Communion had changed about seventy years earlier. We drove off to St. Edward's for Mass and returned home to find Stephen there. Among the emails I checked was one from Nigel, the Everycare CEO, who raised the suggestion of Lennie going into a care home. I drove off to the surgery, where I had my bandages changed. I added a bit to my draft paper on the GND, and in the evening we watched a couple of episodes of a French police drama.

On Thursday, we went to Mass at St. Pius' as usual. When Leanne came to take Lennie out for a walk, I did some useful phoning; first to Domestic and General to arrange a repair of our oven and then AEG from whom we bought three new drawers for our fridge. In the evening, we went to see the film *1917* at the Odeon, in which our grandson, Luke, had a part. Lennie and I decided to wait until the next day to open our Valentine presents with Stephen.

On Friday, we went to Mass at St. Joseph's and remained a few minutes afterwards for exposition. Back home, Leanne took Lennie for a walk along the river, and I phoned HMRC about our trusts. I phoned the authorisation codes through to Gilly afterwards. Around 1 a.m., Lennie had gone into my study and switched off all the various gadgets, including wi-fi, so I had problems that morning with emails. In the afternoon, we watched a T20 match from Durban, which in the end England won by two runs. It was much the same on Saturday. I clumsily smashed a jar of tartar sauce in the kitchen and Lennie quietly wiped it up, bless her. On our way home from Mass at St. Joseph's, we bought some wine at Majestic. After Stephen's lunch, we watched athletics from Glasgow and then Richard turned up with Ben, Will and Iris. It was nice to see them. We then watched England beat South Africa and win the series 2–1. We ended up watching the French police drama *Public Enemy*. My

Sunday diary records that Storm Dennis reached its peak during the night and, as always, I was concerned about our solar panels.

Lennie and I drove to Mass, but Gilly didn't come because she was on NHS 'call'. At St. Pius' I bought two books about Matthew's Gospel, intending them as Easter presents for Will and Iris. Stephen prepared us lunch without an oven. Lennie had one of her periods of anxiety, thinking that Maureen had died but nobody had told us. England won another T20 match in the last over. On Monday morning, Stephen put on the weekly wash before setting off for Cranleigh, When Leanne came, she took "a very flirty and frisky Lennie to Squires". While they were there, I did the online shop with Sainsbury's. "Two mechanics contracted by ESE came to look at our solar panel system. We need a new inverter as well as net covering" to keep pigeons away. I managed to spend a bit of time trying to find key themes in Naomi Klein's book to insert into my GND article.

On Tuesday, I noted that "Lennie was in a different world this morning, imagining she was going off to school to teach children". We went to an earlier Mass at St. Joseph's, after which I managed to slot in about one and a half hours on Klein's book before I gave in to Lennie's demands. We then drove off to Carlo's for an enjoyable lunch. Back home, we had a snooze until woken by a phone call. "As I feared, Lennie was miles away: 'Are you married?' 'Where do we live?' 'Where are we going?' 'Shall I go and start packing to go home?' 'Where do you live?' 'Where do I live?' 'Who lives here?' 'Am I still teaching?' 'Do we have any children?' 'I've been looking at you for I don't know how long and I don't think I've seen any improvement.' It got worse and worse until I got up. I'd thought that my lunch at Carlo's would ease things on Tuesday afternoons, but three weeks running it has failed and nearly driven me mad." Faye came and calmed things down by playing Uno cards with Lennie, who then went to bed at 7 p.m., which enabled me to finish some drafting, but I went up to bed about

237

9 p.m. I felt "a bit narked but perhaps this is the cross I must pick up".

Wednesday was also a difficult day. When I was talking to two Domestic and General oven engineers, Lennie went on a walkabout, and I didn't know what to do. Fortunately, Norma brought her back. We drove to Mass at St. Edward's and Stephen joined us back at home. This enabled me to send email birthday wishes and do a bit more work on my GND. Then I drove off to the surgery to get my latest bandage update. Dr. Barnado popped in and was very friendly. Stephen had installed the new plastic boxes in the freezer, just in time for the Sainsbury's shopping delivery.

Thursday 20th February wasn't an easy day, and I wrote: "Around 1 a.m., Lennie got herself dressed and when I failed to persuade her to get back into her nightie and then got out of bed to 'help' her, we had a very fierce and angry wrestling match which ended with her pushing me backwards over the bottom of the bed. This frightened me and I thought about the possibility of a heart attack. At one stage I angrily stopped her taking clothes off my chair." We then went to St. Pius' for Mass and coffee afterwards. Back home, "Leanne drove Lennie for a cut and blow-dry hairdo". We had other problems during the day, including a power cut, but we managed to go to the Yvonne Arnaud Theatre for an excellent production of *Oklahoma*.

On Friday, I wrote: "We didn't have a bad night, though Lennie did dress and go downstairs for an hour or so around 1–3 a.m. before returning to our bed and leaving lights on all over the house". After going to Mass and back home, I noted: "Lennie isn't 'with it' and was so angry with me as I tried to tell her where the milk in the fridge was that she even spat at me". The rest of the day passed OK after Ellie from Everycare came and took Lennie out for a walk. I was able to go upstairs and repair our broadband connections.

After Ellie's shift, we survived the evening with *Public Enemy* on TV.

On Saturday, after Mass, we spent much of the day watching Chelsea beat Spurs and France beating Wales in the Six Nations match. On Sunday morning, "I found all the clothes from my chair in Stephen's room". We had no visit from Gilly after Mass because they were visiting Katie in Edinburgh. We then watched the Twickenham match and a variety of Stephen's DVDs before going up to bed. When we took Stephen down to the bus station on Monday morning, he had already put on the clothes wash. I then completed the online shopping to be delivered on Wednesday. Leanne was very good at coping with Lennie, who was furious not to have been consulted about the carer for the supper meal. I had a good spell working on my GND paper. Gilly came round to show us pictures of Katie in Edinburgh. In the evening, we watched André Rieu for a while. On Shrove Tuesday, I wondered what I should do during Lent. After returning from Mass, I managed to slot in three-quarters of an hour on my GND paper before we drove off to Carlo's for an enjoyable lunch, where Lennie kept reminiscing about "Maureen's warning to her not to mess me about 'because I was a nice guy!'" But later, her anxieties took over and "she expressed denial that we'd ever slept together in the double bed. Her illness is real. She has no idea that I took her out for lunch today and has been pestering me since 3 p.m."

On Ash Wednesday, we were anointed with ash at St. Edward's Mass. I prayed: "Help me be a more understanding carer this Lent, Lord. I need to be; Lennie's memory loss is becoming more and more challenging." Back home, we waited for Stephen to turn up before I drove off to St. Luke's, where a fellow parishioner, Carole, "cleaned and tidied my two leg sores". Oven repairers were expected on Thursday morning, so we were unable to go to Mass, but instead I managed to read Mk. 12–16. The mechanics came and quickly replaced the oven heating coil. Leanne came and took Lennie down to the river for a brief walk. I had a couple of sessions working on my GND paper. In the evening, we went to the Yvonne Arnaud Theatre, where we had a light meal before a performance of *The Last Temptation of Boris Johnson*. Lennie seemed to enjoy our evening out.

On Friday morning, we went to Mass at St. Joseph's and on our return helped put out washing on the radiators and did some domestic chores before Leanne came to help us at lunchtime and, later, Faye at suppertime. In the evening, Lennie seemed surprisingly cool in watching news channels. The main news of the day was a big hit on the stock markets as a result of the coronavirus pandemic and my concern for our Fidelity savings.

On Saturday, we watched an interesting DVD documentary about MI5's attempts to mislead the Germans about the plans for the invasion of Europe. On Sunday, "I drove Lennie to St. Pius' for Mass, where we were told there would be no chalice today because of fears about the coronavirus. Afterwards, Gilly called for her hour-long session, and we exchanged family news about the past week." Stephen cooked us a nice lunch, and in the evening, we watched a fascinating documentary about the GCHQ leak about the Iraq war. On the first Monday in March, I wrote that the previous night, when I went up to bed and found Lennie on my side, I went to the bed in the other bedroom. Later, when I went to the loo, I found Lennie had gone downstairs to Stephen, so I returned to sleep in my side of the double bed. Later, Lennie joined me but remained fully dressed.

Today's Mass at St. Joseph's was a funeral Mass attended by Faye and Jane from Everycare. Leanne made us lunch, but also put out the washed clothes on the radiators. In the afternoon, we went to see Dr. Barnado. "Rather to my surprise, he invited us both in together. He took Lennie's blood pressure and a sample and chatted away with her a bit and Lennie seemed quite robust in her responses. But in his subsequent session with me, he expressed no doubt that Tuesday was another mixed day and that Lennie's illness had deteriorated, and to my surprise seemed to think I was doing very well in the circumstances." We drove to St. Joseph's for Mass, where I kissed Lennie at the kiss of peace, although advised not to due to coronavirus precautions. I managed to slot in some work on GND before going off to Carlo's for lunch. I felt very sleepy during the afternoon. In the evening, Richard came over to watch the Chelsea win over Liverpool. "Lennie came down a couple of times angrily asking where all the children were."

My Wednesday diary reflected a bit on Lennie's anger, which Richard had commented on. It shows the 'ups and downs' of life with someone with dementia. "After half-time last night, Lennie went up to bed but during the second half, two or three times she came down agitated that we hadn't seen or looked after 'the children'. She was so angry that we were mainly concerned with <u>our</u> desires that Richard went off home quickly. So, I went up to bed about 10 p.m., a bit surprised to find <u>my</u> side of the bed free. But Lennie was pretty hostile about my only being concerned with 'me, me, me'. I tried arguing at first, mentioning Carlo's and Yvonne Arnaud visits, but they were disregarded; she wasn't being informed about things happening in her life and so forth. So, I kept quiet, and I suppose we dozed off for a couple of hours. Then right out of the blue, around 12–1 a.m., she started cuddling me and caressing me intimately, taking off her nightie and encouraging lovemaking for the first time in months. I responded quite keenly but prayed to Jesus, asking Him how he would respond. After half an hour we'd had enough and tried to sleep. During the rest of the night, I struggled with sleep as Lennie got dressed, went downstairs, came back, undressed into her nightie and returned to bed. A mixed night, typical of Lennie's ups and downs with her dementia."

We drove to St. Edward's for Mass, then back home to await Stephen. I then drove off to St. Luke's where a nurse, Carole "undid my plasters on my leg but anticipated the need for two more weeks' redressing". Andrew phoned and told us he had lost his job; be with him, Lord. Stephen fed us and, in the evening, put on *Public Enemy*. I wasn't very well early on Thursday, but we managed to go to Mass as usual. In the hall afterwards, I sensed that a couple of the ladies were keeping an eye on Lennie before I took her to her hairdresser at Boxgrove. Later, I picked her up and Leanne was helpful in keeping conversation going. I skimmed papers including the diocesan *A&B News*, which included an outline of Pat Jones's marvellous talk at the annual Justice and Peace Assembly.

On Friday, I recorded that "Lennie was quite incapable of helping me to get a simple breakfast of cereals and milk and orange juice. I find it frustrating because I am so physically limited." Mass was at St. Mary's and the homily was given by Deacon John Lamb, a former university colleague. Back home, Leanne took Lennie for a brief walk and cooked our lunch. Lennie also took me for a brief walk along the cul-de-sac and I managed to write a small amount for my GND paper. At suppertime, Lennie appeared to be very disturbed. She "kept on referring to her parents and Maureen. 'Where do I find Mike?'" When her angry outbursts prevented my watching any TV in the evening, I joined her upstairs and wrote: "I began to think that there really is no point in my wanting to watch a TV series, and that I simply need to give in to the reality of my cross; Lennie's developing dementia". On Saturday, as usual, we were joined by Stephen at the Mass at St. Joseph's and back home watched interesting episodes of *Babylon Berlin*. During the day there were a couple of rugby internationals. When I went up to bed, Lennie took off my pyjamas and put on her nightie!

Sunday's diary was rather mixed: "Lennie said, 'I do love you, darling', but then complained that she didn't like living in our house, she didn't feel free and regretted her loss of freedom". Gillian joined us at Mass at St. Pius' and afterwards helped on the Fairtrade stall. When she joined us at home we had an interesting debate about politics. "I shared Gilly's concern for integrity vs Stephen's for realism." We watched Chelsea beat Everton 4–0. Andrew came about 7 p.m. and we had "a lively discussion about our faith and rules about divorce and pastoral responses". Before we went to bed, Lennie came down with my pyjama top on. "It was good to have seen three of our children today." Monday was much as usual. When Leanne took Lennie for a walk by the river, I did the online shopping with Sainsbury's. She said she expected to see her mother or sister at Mass this evening. It was a prayerful and pastoral Mass. Later, I enjoyed Berlioz's *Symphonie Fantastique* and another episode of *Babylon Berlin*. On Tuesday, after we'd been to Mass at St. Joseph's, I was allowed time to type in more summaries to my GND file. I told Lennie I thought it was a form of bullying to expect me to go up to bed at 8.30 p.m.

The second Wednesday of March indicated Lennie's memory problems: "I came down to breakfast this morning and Lennie had put out a lunchtime salad. She's just said she hopes this is our last day here, i.e., on holiday, and wants to go back to Berwick. Her parents are alive, etc. Last night was one of those when she got up around 1–2 a.m., dressed ready to go out with her overcoat and hat on. After one and a half hours she returned to bed for a while but then, around 6 a.m., got up and dressed again. This is the reality of my/our life these days. Last night Lennie thought she was going to school as a teacher; this morning she thinks we are here on holiday. We drove to St. Edward's where Mass is always peaceful and friendly. Just after Stephen came, I drove off to St. Luke's where Carole changed the plaster on my left shin for probably the penultimate time. When

Lennie came down in the middle of the evening and wondered where all the children were and Stephen, I told her they were all in their fifties and had left home in their twenties, rather as she had done when she left Berwick for Charlbury. It got us nowhere."

The coronavirus pandemic panic hit St. Pius' after Mass on Thursday, when there was no coffee afterwards. Later Leanne took Lennie for a walk down by the river, which gave me precious space. In the evening, we went to the Yvonne Arnaud, but early in the second half Lennie was in a lot of pain and I had to ask the lady in front of us to help me get her out. She kindly brought her as far as the car. On Friday, we drove to St. Mary's for Mass. Andrew phoned us, saying Sue had contacted him, as she was worried about our vulnerability to coronavirus at Mass. Rugby and Premier League matches were also cancelled. I managed to do a few more drafting notes on Pettifor's book before going to bed. On Saturday, we attended Mass at St. Joseph's. I spent much of my time typing up summaries of Pettifor's chapters while Lennie "spent most of the afternoon worrying, mainly about the children, or school, but also the coronavirus panic which dominates the news".

We went to Mass on Sunday morning, after which Andrew called, anticipating a lockdown for the over-seventies to counter the coronavirus pandemic. "Stephen later agreed to come and look after us. Gilly came to have a long discussion about the anticipated shutdown with Stephen and me. To our astonishment, there was no Sainsbury's delivery slot for about three weeks! Andrew phoned and drove over to give us some shopping in case we were isolated. Bless him." Richard phoned on his return from New York, "where attitudes to the pandemic had reversed in a few days. Stephen let me watch two episodes of *Babylon Berlin*. Lennie came down and found me dozing. I never do anything for her, she accused me."

Early on Monday, there were emails from Sue, who was recovering from a fortnight's isolation in Italy, and from Gilly about Everycare cover for us if/and when we would become isolated. I managed to do some more work on the GND paper before driving to St. Luke's, where Carole discharged me after a final change of bandages. I noted that: "Lennie seems totally unaware of the present situation". In anticipation of lockdown, we went to Mass at St. Joseph's on Tuesday 17th March, recognising that it could be the last time for weeks. From there we drove to Cranleigh to pick up Stephen, who had a large amount of food purchases. "Lennie had one of her awkward patches. Astonishingly, she still has absolutely no sense that we might be confined to our house because of the global pandemic. If she wants to go for a walk, she will go." Faye turned up and kindly went to Sainsbury's, where she found many of the shelves empty because of panic-buying.

On the Wednesday, following suggestions from Liz Lewis, I think we viewed Mass on livestream for the first time; I think it was EWTN from Alabama. Otherwise, the day proceeded much as usual with Stephen organising our meals. On Thursday I followed Mass on livestream from an abbey in Belfast and found a church in North London later for Lennie and Stephen. Later, it emerged that the Bishops in England and Wales had agreed on a total shutdown of churches. In other words, the isolation policy has now filled all our lives together. Claire agreed to go to an ATM for me. "Schools will be shut tomorrow and all across Europe there is total shutdown – a global war." Gilly came to the door with loads of loo rolls she'd kindly bought for us. On Friday, we watched Mass on livestream from St. Mary's in Hampstead. "Lennie was very much in need of constant attention and was in denial." News from Italy warned us that the situation might become desperate in a couple of weeks. We spent the day watching several episodes of *COBRA*. On Saturday, we watched Mass from Glasgow. We spent most of the lovely afternoon outside on the patio. "Stephen was a great conversationalist with Lennie, who was miles away from the present reality and kept interrupting Stephen and me."

On Sunday, we watched Mass from Bishop Stortford and only later found a livestream from St. Joseph's. Gilly and Katie brought round a delicious lunch for Mothering Sunday. We coped in the evening, watching several episodes of *The Big Bang Theory*. On Monday, I recorded that "Lennie is white-hot angry with me for having 'humiliated' her by having asked Leanne when she arrived at 3 p.m. to do a shopping run for us. We've had a vitriolic phase as she insists I should have consulted with her beforehand. She seems totally unaware that I've been shopping online for us for nine months and also that we are facing an increasing level of shutdown." Later the three of us attended Mass 'spiritually' from St. Joseph's. On Tuesday, we watched the livestream Mass from St. Joseph's after I'd done some editorial work on my GND paper. Leanne came and chatted with Lennie before taking her for a walk. Lennie "was incredibly anxious, unaware of the realities of the coronavirus pandemic, where she was, where her home was, and so on". When I went up to bed, I found my pyjamas had gone so I went to bed with my pants on.

On Wednesday, we attended Mass on livestream from St. Joseph's and I emailed them afterwards to ask them to turn up the volume. During the day I managed to do some more work on the GND paper. Stephen cooked all our meals, and we spent a lot of time outside in the sun. "Richard phoned to check on us ... Lennie didn't know she'd been a wife to me." I went up to bed hoping to find my pyjamas.

On Thursday, I noted that we were still regularly reading the Mass readings and praying for the living and the dead before we got up for breakfast. We attended Mass from St. Joseph's on livestream. The news was dominated by increasing death rates from COVID-19. Stephen put on a

DVD, but we joined neighbours at 8 p.m. with applause outside for NHS workers. Before going to bed, I read some Isaiah and John. It was much the same on Friday, though I had more trouble with my laptop. Leanne came and took Lennie for a walk round the estate. I managed to get a one-and-a-half-hour slot, which was quite fruitful. Leanne made us lunch, after which I had a usual doze outside in the sun. I walked up and down the garden a dozen times to try and improve my mobility. Gilly phoned to check we were OK. My Saturday diary noted that I'd had a terrible night. Outside, the garden looked lovely, from snowdrops and primulas to camellias. We attended Mass from St. Joseph's on livestream. Michael Wheeler phoned. I then unexpectedly had a bout of diarrhoea and had some clearing up to do. In the evening, we followed Stephen's DVDs.

I had a better night at the beginning of British Summer Time. After livestream Mass, Stephen cooked us a splendid lunch. We then had phone calls from Andrew and Richard. Stephen cooked our supper and decided what DVDs to play during the evening. On Monday, I noted: "Lennie just doesn't seem to get the reality of the pandemic and the consequences, such as watching Mass on the laptop each day. Today, the three of us decided to take a small piece of bread to share and participate in the Holy Communion, 'take and eat'. Faye came in time to take Lennie for a walk and then went to Sainsbury's, where she had to queue for half an hour. She observed how much cleaner the air seemed to be with the big reductions of transport." Stephen presented us with a pizza and salad supper. We ended the day with a couple of episodes of *Spooks*.

On Tuesday, I had a fair range of problems with my laptop; I'm just not on top of the differences between pdfs and whatever. "I'm just not keeping up with technological developments and am feeling helpless." When Faye arrived, she took Lennie for a walk and then "very helpfully helped me contact NatWest to set up online banking; signed up for

Sainsbury's shopping but only finding no delivery slots for three weeks! Also, I ordered some printer ink from Amazon."

On Wednesday 1st April, around 4 a.m., Lennie had a fall and damaged the blind on the adjacent window. After breakfast, I cleared emails before we attended Mass from St. Joseph's on livestream. Lennie "just doesn't accept the fact that she can't go out for a walk whenever she feels like it; after all she's not a three-year-old!" I regretted that I hadn't kept photo albums since 2015. On Thursday, I noted that we were still starting our days with the Mass readings and prayers. As usual now we watched online the Mass at St. Joseph's. Leanne came and took Lennie out for a walk. "Around 7 o'clock Lennie had one of her fantasy spells. She wanted to put sandals into a bag and take them to put in the car. She is totally unconcerned about the pandemic taking up nearly all the news and the reported instructions to remain indoors." At 8 p.m., I joined the national clap for NHS workers.

On Friday around 3 a.m., Lennie was fully dressed and angrily refused to come back to bed. Stephen must have heard us and gently eased Lennie into the other bedroom. "Two hours later she rejoined me, and we slept pretty well until about 7 a.m." Then, suddenly, I had another episode of diarrhoea which I couldn't control. We watched Mass on livestream but had to struggle with sleep. Leanne came and took Lennie for a walk while Stephen and I walked up and down the garden. Leanne made us lunch and Stephen supper and put on DVDs in the evening. Lennie twice came downstairs wearing my pyjamas, obsessed with her sister Maureen. Stephen persuaded her to go to bed in the other bedroom. She came and joined me at 4 a.m. on Saturday morning. There was a friendly email from Pat Jones with attachments about her research with sex workers, asking for comments. Marie looked over the garden fence and told us she and John had probably had the virus, which was worrying. On Palm Sunday, we managed to follow Mass from St. Joseph's on livestream in spite of computer hiccups and then Pope Francis in an empty St. Peter's Square, followed by a Franciscan from Walsingham.

Later, I worked on my GND article. "I'm trying, not very successfully, to be a companionable husband to Lennie but she doesn't seem to be registered with current reality – seemingly totally unaware of COVID-19 and its consequences and demands, and also quite frequently unaware that I am her husband of nearly sixty years and that we have lived in this house for twelve years." Late in the evening, "Lennie came down angry that I'd paid her no attention all day! Oh wow!"

On Monday, I started my diary: "During the night we had a disturbed Lennie who angrily wanted to go out to 'her own home', dressed and going downstairs, where Stephen was very good. When she came up, she angrily said she didn't want 'sex, sex, sex'. That was a new one and I defensively said I was eighty-seven and she was eighty-four. After a while, she took over 'her' bed and I moved to the other bedroom. Two hours later she came, woke me up and suggested I joined her in our bed. I slept in until 7.30 a.m. Later, an anxious Lennie was looking for her purse and her parents. So, we watched Mass together on the laptop." My Italian neighbour, Giuseppe, kindly came to sort out some of the mess on my laptop. Leanne made our lunch, after which "Lennie and I spent over an hour sitting in the garden enjoying the occasional sunshine. Her memory really has gone, and she needs reminding that I am her husband of nearly sixty years and that we live here, in our home." Faye came and took her for a walk and made us supper. "After she'd gone, Lennie started fuming because we didn't seem to take seriously her concern for her coming 'wedding'. Stephen and I showed her wedding photos, but they just didn't register. One expression of anger was frightening: 'I might kill myself'. Please Lord, guide me; I'm asking, seeking and knocking at Your door pleading for guidance and the grace to follow You."

On Tuesday, I recorded that several times last night I had to stop Lennie getting dressed and encourage her to get back into our bed. I finished my article on the GND and sent a copy to the *Tablet*. We attended Mass online, after which I started reading one of Pat Jones's documents on her research with sex workers. After lunch, we sat in the garden on a very pleasant day. Marika took Lennie out for a walk and on their return made us supper. In the evening, we watched the fascinating Zeffirelli film, *Jesus of Nazareth*.

My diary for the second Wednesday of April notes that Lennie got dressed in the early hours and after going downstairs, returned to be with me. Around 6.30 a.m., she cuddled me and told me how much she loved me. After breakfast, I spent nearly an hour reading Pat Jones's *Women at the Well* before we switched over to Mass from the Catholic Parish of Guildford (CPG). The volume wasn't great, so I read the Gospel and the three of us shared bread and a mug of water and wine at Holy Communion, a sort of symbolic reception of Holy Communion. In the afternoon, we both went out into the garden and for a full hour Lennie told me over and over again about how roughly Maureen used to treat her in their childhood. Afterwards, I was able to finish reading Pat Jones's draft letter to the bishops. In the evening, Lennie was angry about going 'home' and quite unable to take on board the realities of the present 'shutdown'.

On Maundy Thursday, I wrote, "Lennie got dressed in the early hours and at one stage went downstairs, probably for a couple of hours. She returned and, as always, was very loving early on though she didn't appreciate my trying to stop her talking in order that I might sleep. I wasn't very successful. As usual, we read today's Mass readings and prayed for our family and friends, living and dead." I managed to finish reading Pat Jones's *Appendix to the Bishops*. Stephen put out sheets on the radiators and made our bed all by himself. Andrew phoned; he planned to drive over with a leg of lamb for Easter; he came over but distanced himself at the door because of the lockdown restrictions. Richard, Will and Iris phoned for a chat. We applauded the NHS and care staff outside before following Mass from St. Joseph's. The evening was seen out with an interesting film, *The Pilgrimage*. On Good Friday, I noted that "my feeling is that my energy levels have declined a lot in recent weeks. I even felt that I was entering my final days."

I suggested watching Part IV of *Jesus of Nazareth* as it was appropriate for Good Friday. Sadly, I dozed off and missed some of the key discussions in the Sanhedrin. When Leanne came, she took Lennie for a 'walk round the block'. In mid-afternoon, we watched "Deacon Tom lead the Good Friday Passion with Liturgy of the Word, the Passion, then adoration of the cross, and then Holy Communion. It was strange without a single other person." Later, Faye came and took Lennie for a walk before preparing supper for us. Afterwards, we sat out in the garden on the hottest Good Friday I can remember. Gilly phoned to make contact and to check on us. "In the evening, Lennie carried on her strange lack of memory about the purchase of this, our house, twelve years earlier. Over and over again, she repeats the same questions, totally ignoring all our previous explanations. She was still unaware that we have been married for nearly sixty years, that I am her husband, and this is our home."

Saturday's diary noted that: "We had a loving caress and cuddle early in the night. This morning, as she often does, she told me how much she loves me and how she couldn't manage without me. Thank You, Lord, for giving me such a loving wife, even these days when she is not at all sure I am her husband and that we have four children." Lennie gave me a little space to read some of Pat Jones's letter to supporters. We went into the garden together and Gillian brought a small box of Easter eggs. In the evening the three of us watched a long Easter Vigil.

My diary for Easter Sunday is rather ambiguous. It suggests Lennie must have gone downstairs fully dressed at some stage. It then refers to a phone call picked up by Stephen around 4 a.m., apparently from Gillian, who must have had a call from Social Care, whom Lennie had apparently phoned. Lennie then returned to bed with her nightie on. We watched Mass from St. Joseph's, after which we enjoyed a sherry before Stephen's lunch of Andrew's roast lamb. I finished off a letter to Pat Jones. Stephen gave us a supper of cheese on toast. On Easter Monday, Stephen put out our washing on the radiators. "At 10 a.m., all three of us gathered round the laptop to finish skimming the *Tablet*. True to form, Lennie became restless after 8 p.m. and eventually went up to bed and brought my pyjamas down, telling me not to wake her up when I went up to bed. At one stage, Stephen pointed out that seven-year-olds were allowed to stay up until 9 p.m. but she was treating me like a three-year-old. She was pretty angry at that."

On Wednesday around 6 a.m. after a difficult night, "I blew my top when Lennie asked half a dozen or more times what time Mass was and whether she needed to take any food, and so on. Stephen kindly came up, took her away and I probably dozed for an hour. "Lennie was asking when we are going to watch Mass from St. Joseph's and I struggled to keep awake. Again, we simulated the eucharist with a piece of bread and mug of water and wine. Afterwards, Lennie was in memory-loss mode; she didn't know this was our house, that we'd bought it twelve years earlier and have lived in it ever since. She repeatedly asked about this. Her memory loss is difficult to cope with, asking, for example, 'Are my parents and sister alive?' over and over again ... Richard phoned to make contact."

On Thursday, I received an email from Pat Jones, who had suggested to Brendan Walsh that I was a potential contributor for a forty-year reflection on the 1980 National Pastoral Congress. The livestream Mass was difficult to follow because there was a mismatch between the visual and audio elements. Leanne bought our shopping and then took Lennie for a walk. Stephen asked me to type his *Force Majeure* blog. Claire took Lennie out for a walk before cooking supper. In the evening, we watched the film *Brassed Off*. "When I tried to write this diary, Lennie wouldn't stop talking but, bless her, she was full of love for me, even though there are times when she doesn't know we've been married for over fifty-nine years."

On Friday, I cleared emails before Mass. "As before, I offered up a piece of bread and a glass of water for the three of us to try to follow the guidance of the Last Supper." Leanne came and took Lennie for a walk round the estate. On their return, they cooked our lunch. Meanwhile, I tried to type more of Stephen's text. Richard phoned and we had a chat with Will and Iris. The evening dribbled away, though Lennie did stay down for the DVD of *Coppelia*. Saturday was much as usual. We all three watched Mass on livestream. When Lennie had one of her memory-loss sessions, I took her outside and we coped with the deaths of her parents and sister. We watched Part II of *Giselle* and then some of Hilary Mantel's *Wolf Hall*.

Mass on Sunday from St. Joseph's was said by Fr. Roy on the anniversary of his wife's death. We watched *The Bourne Ultimatum* during the day. I made out my cheques for the charities I was supporting that month. In a spot of anger, I slammed the door of the fridge and broke off some plastic. On Monday, Stephen was helpful with the weekly washing. I continued thinning old financial records. Mgr. Tony said Mass today and reflected on the Easter to Pentecost liturgies and the response of the early Christians. Leanne came and took Lennie out for a walk and to post some letters. After an afternoon in the garden, I did some more typing for Stephen, and then Faye came and took Lennie out for a walk. During the evening, we watched *The Bourne Legacy*. Much the same on Tuesday. "Lennie was talking about going to school etc.; she still seems quite unaware of the reality of the pandemic. I'm afraid my irritability gets the better of me, even when she comes over to flirt." I spent an hour thinning old insurance records. After Mass, "Lennie was full of the need to go to 'her' house and she'd brought down three or four pairs of shoes to take home". When Leanne came, she took Lennie for a walk. After lunch prepared by Leanne, I spent some time in the garden with Lennie. I was also trying to read the Bible a bit more regularly. That day, I managed Luke 11–12 and Jeremiah 12–17. At the end of the afternoon, Claire came and took an anxious Lennie out for a walk before she cooked our supper. During the evening, we watched Episodes 2 and 3 of *Wolf Hall*. I felt sorry for Tyndale, burned at the stake for having promoted an English version of the Bible.

On Wednesday, we prayed for Peter Worthy on his ninetieth birthday. I spent three-quarters of an hour thinning Nationwide files before we attended Mass on livestream. Afterwards, Nigel from Everycare delivered our shopping. Stephen made us lunch, after which I joined Lennie, who never stopped talking, in the garden. Dr. Barnado gave us a call and seemed quite happy with how we had been coping over the previous five weeks. An episode of *Spooks* helped cope with the evening. Thursday, the Feast of St. George, was another glorious, cloudless day. I had another unexpected 'loosening of my bowels'. The three of us participated as best we could in the Mass from St. Joseph's "with a piece of bread and glass of water but also reading the prayer about participating spiritually in the consecration and sharing of the bread and wine". During the day I printed a document on 'The Preferential Option for the Poor' by Chris Richardson. Faye came and took Lennie for a walk before she helped prepare supper. While they were out, I struggled to type more of Stephen's *Force Majeure*. At 8 p.m. we joined neighbours in clapping for NHS and care workers. During the evening, we watched Episode 4 of *Wolf Hall* with More's execution.

On Friday, we found Mgr. Tony more audible at Mass. Afterwards, while Leanne took Lennie for a walk, I did some more typing for Stephen. In the afternoon, I joined Lennie in the garden and read the *Tablet* whenever I could. Faye arrived and took Lennie for a walk 'round the block'. She helped Stephen and me cope with Lennie's obsession with an early supper. Stephen put on *Last Tango in Halifax,* but I had to go up to bed at 9.35 p.m. On Saturday, after clearing emails and thinning out old records, we attended Mass online from St. Joseph's. Afterwards, we had coffee in the garden. "Lennie was delighted that this was 'our' house and has gone upstairs to explore it." Stephen cooked supper for us. To cope with the evening, he put on another episode of Last *Tango in Halifax*, "but, as usual, an anxious Lennie got up and wanted a meal, denying she'd had anything since breakfast". Richard, Will and Iris phoned after having a great day with a BBQ. Andrew also phoned and had a long chat with Lennie. On Sunday, Bishop Richard gave a brief podcast homily at Mass based on today's meeting at Emmaus, which was quite thought-provoking. "Lennie was very affectionate, but needed reminding that I was her husband." After lunch, Stephen took Lennie for a walk. Frances phoned to ask how we were. Stephen cooked us a tasty three-course supper. "Lennie was very difficult, going on and on about a supposed marriage we were going to and had to prepare for."

The last Monday of April was busy but fairly normal. After breakfast, I checked emails and didn't manage much thinning of files before it was time for Mass, which focused on the ministry of Stephen. Steve and Norah Smith phoned to ask how we were. I was trying to thin my dementia files. Leanne came and took Lennie for a walk. "After lunch, we went out into the garden to try to ease Lennie's anxieties." Marika came and took Lennie for a walk. We put on the final episode of *Wolf Hall*. During the day, I had managed to read a couple of chapters from the Old and New Testaments. On Tuesday, I pointed out to Lennie the potential dangers to the water system of putting sanitary towels in the toilet but, unsurprisingly, "she denied any responsibility and was furious I'd even suggested it as a hypothesis". After breakfast, I spent three-quarters of an hour tidying a large collection of files related to social care and dementia. We all three watched the daily Mass from St. Joseph's. After breakfast, I cleared emails and "we then participated in today's livestream Mass with our slice of bread and jug of water". Downstairs, we watched TV and awaited the delivery of the shopping. Stephen put away the shopping and then cooked a very tasty omelette for lunch. Later, we watched one more episode of Last *Tango in Halifax* and when Lennie went up to bed, Stephen put on *Utopia,* which was very interesting. "I'm feeling critical about the way I'm living with all my physical limitations. Do I have to watch so much TV in order to be a good carer? Am I living as the Lord wants me to live?"

"This morning, after some early jobs, the three of us attended Mass and at appropriate times offered up our bread and glass of wine and water. We also read the prayer about 'spiritual communion' but there is a bit of me which quietly thinks Jesus at the Last Supper said 'This is my body ... this is my blood' without specifying only priests could say it. Today, Leanne was wearing a face mask for the first time." She joined us for lunch, after which we spent much of the afternoon watching *Cats*. I spent a long time typing more of Stephen's blog. He then put on the TV, hoping it would hook Lennie. It did for a while but then she went up to bed. I said that having seen half the film I wanted to see the ending. But at least four times Lennie came down for her father, "then her husband, in her nightie. It is now 10.30 p.m. What should I do? Or have done? Is it unreasonable not to be bullied into going to bed early? Jesus, what should I have done? Forgive me for my limitations."

I seem to have been fairly irritable on the Friday morning. After breakfast, I managed to clear emails and tidy some medical records before the three of us joined the Mass from St. Joseph's. I had a different perspective from the *Tablet*: Jesus at the last supper told us what to do. Why can't we do it? Leanne arrived and took Lennie out for a second walk after Stephen had. The *Tablet* also had an interesting article by Pat Jones on the National Pastoral Congress of forty years ago. I finished typing Stephen's blog. Marika came and took Lennie for a walk before she helped cook our supper. The evening wasn't very satisfactory, but we managed.

On Saturday, Lennie was driving me mad with questions about where we lived and which was our church after we'd celebrated Mass, so I went out into the garden. Andrew, and later Richard, Will and Iris phoned. During *Last Tango in Halifax,* Lennie came down wearing my pyjamas. *C'est la vie*! Sunday was my mother's anniversary; may she rest in peace. Before Mass, I managed to clear emails. Stephen prepared a pleasant lunch for us. In the evening, I wasn't very successful arranging a Zoom meeting with Andrew and Richard. Monday was a Bank Holiday, but I'm not sure it made any difference to us during lockdown. Mass was a bit of a disaster in that I failed to get any sound. Earlier, I'd cleared emails and made slow progress with thinning files. Leanne followed an angry Lennie on walkabout. The three of us attended Mass on livestream, after which Leanne took Lennie out for a walk. Claire came and made us supper before taking Lennie out for a walk.

On the first Wednesday in May, I recorded that Lennie's "memory loss is incredible, but I keep repeating answers to her about this home, from which we have no plans to move. Yesterday, Stephen helped with her tidying her drawers.

Last night, at one stage, she put on my pyjama trousers and for the past couple of days has been wearing one of my short-sleeved shirts. Occasionally I find my pants in her drawers, and vests, and this morning I found a dirty pair of knickers in the refuse pan in 'my' loo." Mass was very clear that morning. Stephen prepared our lunch, after which I'd hoped to have a snooze. "You must be joking! Lennie went on and on and on about who was feeding the children, just not taking on board Stephen's and my repeated references to our family, this is our house, we live here, and there are no schools open, and on and on. I got cross and whacked the settee with my stick and Stephen gradually calmed things down." During the day, I managed to finish reading Acts and Jeremiah. Stephen and Lennie walked to the post box, having left me on the Green, where a very kind lady brought me a glass of lemonade. Back home, most of the time I spent listening to Lennie's recollections of her teaching days. I ended the day spending over an hour typing for Stephen.

On Thursday, I noted that Lennie was "totally unaware of lockdown and our confinement to our homes". Ben phoned us and I had to reply to our young neighbour Ludovica, who wanted to know about my experience of V.E. Day. Faye was very helpful in helping me set up online banking, so I made my first online banking payment to Everycare. She later posted a birthday card for Will. Friday was the 75th anniversary of V.E. Day and unexpectedly all our neighbours came out after the 11 a.m. silence to celebrate. There was also a lot on TV, and I had tears flowing down my face. Richard, Will and Iris phoned. Faye took Lennie for a walk round the block. Gilly then brought some flowers for Lennie, the first time we've seen her for quite a while. For unclear reasons, we couldn't get St. Joseph's on livestream, so we watched Mass from Merton on Saturday. We phoned Ann and then Will on his birthday. "Around 4.30 p.m. Lennie became obsessed with the need to prepare a meal, sometimes for up to ten. It is infuriating when she will not recognise that Stephen has it in hand. Bless him; he calmed Lennie more than I did."

On Sunday, "as usual, Lennie was fully dressed in the early hours but came back to bed". We again celebrated Mass from Merton. We had an unexpected phone call from Katie in Edinburgh and then Gilly. In the afternoon, some rugby, and in the evening the first episode of *Informer* in which our grandson Luke had a small part. Monday was much as usual, with Lennie in place but today we celebrated Mass from St. Joseph's. Marika took Lennie out for a walk while Stephen and I watched cricket on TV. Stephen brought down Lennie's nightie to try and get her to wear the right clothes. Tuesday also seemed to be a similarly ordinary day. I was trying to read Ezekiel and Romans when I could find time, while telling Lennie when Maureen's birthday was before she died. That day's Mass from St. Joseph's was a Requiem for a long-standing parishioner. I continued to try and do a bit of gardening while avoiding falling.

Wednesday would have been Mummy's birthday; may she rest in peace. Before Mass at St. Joseph's on livestream, I did some more thinning of files and throwing away old copies of the *Tablet*. Stephen cooked our meals and put on DVDs of *Star Wars* and the *Big Bang Theory*. Thursday was a little different in that "early on we made love, as far as we can go these days, i.e., caressing". Practically the whole hour after breakfast was taken up with clearing emails, including a long one with several photos from my sister Sue in Italy. Mass was from St. Joseph's. When Leanne came at lunchtime and Faye at teatime, they both took Lennie out for a short walk. Luke, our oldest grandson, kindly phoned and was able to find my article on the GND on the local Labour Party website. Faye helped me finish off paying Everycare online. On Friday, "Lennie and I had a sensual caress and some 'naughty, naughty'. I wondered what Jesus would expect of me. We watched the Mass at St. Joseph's, and I was taken up by an excellent issue of the *Tablet* last week. Lennie and Stephen managed to change the sheets on our bed and put the old ones in the washing machine. Andrew phoned, having just had his eye operation. Stephen spent most of the afternoon watching *Star Wars* films; not my cup of tea."

Saturday was Iris's tenth birthday, but we couldn't get through by phone. Before the three of us watched Mass from St. Joseph's online, I tried but failed to solve problems with both British Gas and HMRC. I wondered whether to respond to the advert in the *Tablet* from Villanova University to submit a paper on the GND. Sunday was a pleasant and gentle day. I sent off my GND article to Villanova to see if it might interest them. "The three of us watched Mass this morning and I struggled with sleep. These days, I like to have a snooze after lunch and watch a film in the evening, but Lennie always interrupts with non-stop questions, so both of them are typically disappointing."

On Monday, Lennie and I were still reading the Mass scripture readings and saying some prayers before getting up for breakfast. The three of us attended the livestream Mass from St. Joseph's, after which I managed to complete an HMRC. tax return. After lunch, I was lucky to get a full hour's sleep. Outside, the builders seem to have returned to the extension in Fennel Close, signs of easings after the coronavirus lockdown. On Tuesday, I got a warm reply from a Villanova welcomer. We three attended Mass at St. Joseph's online. The British Gas engineer came and seemed to have solved the heating problem. The ESE engineers came later and installed a new inverter. I finished reading 1 Corinthians and got as far as Ezekiel 27. As always, Stephen tried to find some sort of film that might interest Lennie and see us through the evening.

On the third Wednesday in May of 2020, the Mass was a Requiem for a fellow parishioner. May he rest in peace. The garden was in need of some water, but we had little in the butt. We sat outside in the garden most of the day and I managed to get to 2 Corinthians 3 and Ezekiel 31 before Lennie came to chat. Stephen prepared our meals. A neighbour came to help me on the laptop, and I suppose I battled on. The following day was Ascension Thursday and again I was having problems with my laptop and beginning to think I needed a new one. But after Mass on livestream from St. Joseph's, Leanne came to make us lunch and Stephen put away the Sainsbury's shopping after it had been delivered. I joined our neighbours in the 8 p.m. 'clap' for NHS and care workers. Faye took Lennie for a walk, but I failed in my attempt to send our shopping list for next week. All in all, it was a frustrating day. Things didn't change much on the Friday. The three of us followed Mass said by Mgr. Tony, who'd challenged the lockdown restrictions by going for a cycle ride over Newlands Corner and then back via Chilworth beforehand.

Whenever I could, I chased up relevant articles for my GND paper on the internet. Leanne took Lennie for a walk before lunch. "This afternoon I tried to please Lennie by sitting with her in the garden for a couple of spells, but she was unmovedly obsessed by the needs of the 'children' for supper and being driven back home." Faye came and took Lennie out for a walk before supper. Faye and Stephen had quite a dialogue about politics before she left. On Saturday, "Lennie started by saying how much she loved me and then wondered when she would meet a nice young man!" Later, she protested that the Mass hadn't been appropriate for young children. I typed out Stephen's latest blog. In the evening, Lennie came down four times over the next hour with different sets of clothing. After attending Mass, Lennie was at her worst. We came down to watch the cricket test and she asked, "Why isn't the front door unlocked for the children?" At one stage I feared physical engagement with Lennie and the police getting involved.

On Monday, I had a painful neck and was grateful that Lennie put on my socks and sandals for me. My neck was very painful and when Lennie didn't follow my guidance, "I exploded, and she threatened me. I am frightfully explosive." Most of the day we watched the Test from Trent Bridge. My neck was so painful that I went to bed early. "Yet Lennie was lovely, very understanding and sympathetic." Things got a little easier on Tuesday. Faye took Lennie out for a walk before lunch and Claire did so before supper. In the afternoon, we all three chilled out and I even had time to read the *Tablet*. "The evening dribbled away pretty aimlessly."

Wednesday was the Feast of St. Augustine of Canterbury. After Mass and coffee, "Lennie immediately went into one of her anxiety moods. She thinks we ought to be preparing for the 'children'; the lockdown is not comprehended. When are we going to our house/home?" Stephen greatly helped by talking with her endlessly about the coronavirus. In the afternoon, Stephen "agreed to take Lennie out for a walk as she was insisting on going on her own otherwise, and for months we have not allowed that because of the danger of her falling or getting lost".

I wondered how to put in the work necessary to upgrade my GND paper for Villanova. In reality, Lennie doesn't allow such study space. Thursday was apparently the fifth anniversary of Bishop Richard's ordination. Be with him, Lord. The mechanic came today and will hopefully protect our solar panels. Marika came and took Lennie for a short walk before cooking our lunch. I had an awful time trying to follow up a letter from NatWest with three or four failed phone calls.

For the first time in over two months, the cleaners came. Claire came and took Lennie for a walk before she served us supper. "Lennie was worried sick about the children's needs at Mass tonight. A fantasy!" Part 1 of the Zeffirelli film

Jesus of Nazareth captured the attention of all three of us. For reasons I'm not sure about, Stephen asked me on Friday to postpone the next visit of the cleaners for four weeks. I was a 'bit rusty' driving Stephen to the ATM machine at Sainsbury's to withdraw some cash. After lunch I must have fallen asleep for two hours. In the evening Stephen put on the DVD *When Harry met Sally,* which kept Lennie interested until 9 p.m. Then "an angry and concerned Lennie came down and kept pressing us about the wedding which was supposed to be happening here tomorrow. Had we done all the preparations? She was totally resistant to our repeatedly saying there was no wedding."

On Saturday, I noted: "Lennie had one of her difficult nights – got dressed, angrily left all the lights on as she went off downstairs in the early hours; later, she returned and slept on the bed fully dressed". I managed to send off next week's shopping list before we attended Mass on livestream. Mgr. Tony gave a very good homily today and urged us all to spend the day preparing for Pentecost and phoning family and friends. So, I phoned Ann and Andrew and emailed Sue. Richard came round for a couple of hours, distancing himself in the garden. Pentecost Sunday was the last day of May. For a while I lost my alarm until Stephen found it in one of Lennie's drawers. The Mass was pleasant and full of the fire of Pentecost. The papers disappointed me; there was no Polly Toynbee in the *Guardian* and the *Times* seemed preoccupied with celebrities. Stephen cooked our lunch and the bulk of the afternoon we spent in the garden. In the evening, we watched TV.

On Monday, I managed to do a couple of hours work on the Villanova paper. When Claire came and took Lennie for a walk, it gave me time to read a couple of chapters of Daniel. In the evening, Lennie was bored with the TV Stephen had put on and she went up to bed but kept coming down to get me. But I resisted it as a form of bullying. On Tuesday, I didn't manage to do much work on the Villanova paper. In the afternoon I spent most of the time reading 1 Thessalonians and the first six chapters of Daniel. When Claire came at 4 p.m., she took Lennie out for a walk. Stephen put on Part 3 of *Jesus of Nazareth,* but Lennie wouldn't stop interrupting and insisting that others were coming for a meal.

On the first Wednesday of June, I couldn't get Google on the laptop and hence livestream Mass, though I do believe we watched it later from EWTN, Alabama. After lunch, Andrew and Caroline turned up "and kept their distance assiduously". We sat outside well apart and chatted for a couple of hours. It was good to see them after a couple of months. When they left, Stephen set us up with the last hour of Part IV of *Jesus of Nazareth*. "But Lennie's fantasies are not halted by us, and the result is that our watching of serious programmes is destroyed practically every night by Lennie."

On Thursday, our neighbour, Giuseppe, managed to get me Google Chrome just in time for me to find Mass at St. Joseph's on livestream. Leanne took Lennie for a brief walk before preparing lunch. This gave me an opportunity to do some more drafting. Faye later took Lennie for a walk before cooking our supper. Gillian phoned for a chat and I put Lennie in touch with her cousin, Peter Dooley. Friday was another fairly typical day. I cleared emails before Mass. Leanne came and took Lennie for a walk before lunch. I managed to add a paragraph or two to my Villanova paper. After lunch, I conked out for a good hour. After Claire had made our supper, we watched an episode of *Spooks*. I was surprised to find Lennie fully dressed when I went up and got into bed first.

On Saturday I wrote: "Last night Lennie took all my clothes on 'my' chair, and it was only early this morning that I found them all in the wash basket!" After breakfast, I managed to clear emails and complete the weekly shopping list before switching to the online Mass from St. Joseph's, which the three of us watched. In the afternoon, we watched a couple of rugby and football internationals. Andrew called on a visit. When he left, we watched two or three episodes of *True Detective* before going up to bed. Early in the morning, we read the liturgical readings for Trinity Sunday. Lennie asked me what my name was and later what were we doing about the children for a picnic or whatever. Gillian turned up unexpectedly with her two dogs and confirmed that Doug had been made redundant and was awaiting serious surgery on his legs. Katie had just got a full-time job in Edinburgh and Douglas had completed his dissertation. We watched the film *1917* which Luke appears in, and then two episodes of *Cardinal*. "It's been a mixed day; on the whole not bad. But it is difficult to cope with Lennie's anxiety episodes and anger."

On Monday, I recorded that on the previous evening, Stephen had been worried that my anger with Lennie might lead to a heart attack and that "Lennie's dementia was leading to her death. He has a point, so I am again praying for patience and love ... Mgr Tony said the Mass and reflected interestingly on the Beatitudes." Stephen and Lennie put out the washing on the line and when Leanne came, she took Lennie out for a walk. This enabled me to put in a good stint on my Villanova paper. I failed to make connections with British Gas and then "finding it impossible to get help on the internet, I wonder if it is only oldies like me that fail to cope with the multiple choices both on the phone and with internet connections". In the evening, Stephen put on episodes of *The Cardinal*. Lennie didn't interrupt badly, "but insisted she'd seen 'Dad' recently, even though he'd died fifty-five years earlier".

On Tuesday, I managed to clear emails and do a little work on my paper before the three of us followed Mass on livestream. After Leanne had taken Lennie for a walk and to post letters, I slotted in another hour on my paper. When

Claire came, I wrote a birthday card for Doug's Mum and sent donations to several charities. "Lennie had one of her difficult evenings in tears at being told Maureen and her parents had all died." It was unusual in that Lennie stayed down with Stephen and me all evening to watch some rugby on the TV.

On Wednesday our rather mixed-up lives seemed to carry on as usual. For example, it took me three- quarters of an hour to pay Everycare on online banking. The three of us then attended Mass on livestream. Then there was a problem with the TV. I'm just not competent enough. After working on my Villanova paper, I felt I'd lost some text. But Stephen and Lennie allowed me to work on it for a couple of hours in the afternoon and in the evening, Stephen put on a DVD film, *Official Secrets* about the GCHQ leak. At 10 p.m. I took Lennie up to bed.

On Thursday, I opened my diary by writing, "Lennie is not the wife of a few months ago". Interestingly, Mgr. Tony said the Mass on the Feast of St. Barnabas and spent most of his homily talking about 'vocation'. The prayer about spiritual communion was inserted in the right-hand side of today's screen. I managed about an hour's work on my paper. After lunch, the Sainsbury's shopping was delivered and then the Domestic and General men arrived and seemed to do a superb job adding protective netting around our solar panels. After Faye left in the evening, Lennie started to insist on going 'home', getting more and more angry. Eventually, she left by the back door and escaped along the path. Stephen set off to catch up with her. "How do we cope with this? At some stage, she may smash the door down because she has no key. We tried to cope with watching three episodes of the CIA drama, *Condor.*"

Early on Friday, I noted that Lennie "angrily said if she'd enough money she'd go and live somewhere else. A minute later she was saying how much she loved me! The three of us attended the Mass from St. Joseph's. Again, I felt a little uncomfortable and even bullied by the prayer on the screen and felt that we were only receiving 'spiritual communion'." In mid-afternoon, Stephen took Lennie out for a short walk and later Claire came and took her for a walk round the block. I managed to do some work on my paper. In the evening, Stephen put on a documentary with Ross Kemp about dementia. "What did come out was that the lives of carers were completely changed; relationships with spouses were never the same – those with dementia often didn't know their spouse. I can vouch for that." We were prevented by our laptop from getting Mass from St. Joseph's, so we attended Mass from Merton. Gilly came and kept social distancing outside in the garden for nearly an hour. In the afternoon, we had a phone call from Richard, Will and Iris. In the evening, we put on two episodes of *Condor*. On Sunday, I noted: "Around 1–2 a.m. we 'made love', i.e. caressed each other intimately for a while before recognising that it was time to go to sleep". Before Mass, I cleared emails and did some work on my Villanova paper. The three of us then attended Mass, followed by Benediction. Afterwards, I managed to send off our weekly Sainsbury's shopping online. In the garden that afternoon, I noted Lennie said: "'I'd like to meet a nice young man' and 'Where is Mike?' and 'He's always doing his own thing.'" Before going to bed, I managed to read a few chapters of Hosea and 1 Timothy.

Monday was a busy day, starting with putting on the weekly wash. After Mass from St. Joseph's, Claire took Lennie for a drive down to the river. Andrew came later with Father's Day presents. Faye came and made supper and took Lennie out for a walk. I didn't manage to do much work on my Villanova paper. "A lot more work is necessary because I feel out of touch." On Tuesday, Mgr. Tony said the Mass, which the three of us followed. Leanne took Lennie out for a walk while I did some more work on the contribution of Catholic Social Teaching. In the afternoon, Frances came for a chat in the garden and lent me a book about her former parish priest. I had a row with Stephen in the evening. Lennie and I watched the last episode of *Condor*.

On Wednesday, Stephen surprised us by saying that because he had a sore throat, he was going to Cranleigh for a week or so. After attending Mass on livestream, we drove Stephen to Cranleigh. On our journey home, "Lennie accused me of never telling her about Stephen's schizophrenia and our buying, in Trusts, his apartment in Cranleigh. Lennie is in a different world and I've no idea how I will cope with having to make meals three days a week." In the end, Lennie helped me unexpectedly and we watched the final two episodes of the film, *Cardinal*. On Thursday, unexpectedly, the cleaners came but we managed to attend Mass on livestream. I got a scam phone call from 'the police' but I managed to contact the fraud squad to inform them. In the afternoon, the Sainsbury's shopping was delivered and without Stephen it was a big job putting it all away. Later, Faye arrived and took Lennie for a walk round the block. Gillian and Stephen both phoned. "It is obvious how much I've relied on Stephen sharing the coping with Lennie over the past three months. Please Lord, help me do the right thing."

On Friday, the Feast of the Sacred Heart, Lennie was "again furious when I said Leanne was coming, repeatedly claiming all she said was 'come along dear, come along dear'. She then said she'd go out for a walk before Leanne came. So, again, I'm not sure how to cope; I'm frightened of her breaking a door or window. Please help me, Lord." After we'd been to Mass, two police officers came to investigate my possible scam for about an hour. Leanne duly came and took Lennie for a walk before preparing us a fish and chips lunch. But when Lennie came downstairs after a rest, she wanted to go for a walk. I opened the door to the garden, but she went out by the front gate. I struggled with two sticks to Bryony Road and was wondering what to do when a young woman brought her to our cul-de-sac. "I returned home and accused her of destroying my trust in her." Faye came and took Lennie out for a walk before she prepared our supper. I hadn't been able to do much 'work' that day.

Saturday was 'quite a day'. Around midday, I pushed Lennie back in the kitchen and she kicked me and gave me an inch-long tear on my right knee. Before Mass on the Feast of the Immaculate Heart of Mary, I managed to slot in some reading for my paper, but afterwards Lennie "exploded when I mentioned that Richard and his children were coming, seeing it as making last-minute demands to make them a meal. In fact, Richard planned to bring a picnic. The visit of Richard, Ben, Will and Iris was lovely though Lennie was very quiet and uninvolved in much of the conversation, particularly with Will and Iris, which was a pity. I cooked lasagne for supper, but Lennie insisted on going for a walk. I walked to the end of the cul-de-sac with her, and she carried on. After some time, our neighbour Laura came to the door with Lennie, and it was clear she'd had difficulty in finding the way back and had asked several people."

On Sunday, after breakfast, I managed to clear emails and do nearly an hour's work on my paper before Lennie and I attended Mass on livestream. After Mass, Gilly came with Father's Day presents and we had a pleasant hour with her. She also kindly prepared our lunch for us. In the afternoon, Andrew came just in time for the Chelsea vs Villa game in which Chelsea scraped a 2–1 win. Andrew took Lennie for a drive up to Newlands Corner. "Thank You, Lord, for the love and kindness shown to me over the weekend." On Monday, I cleared emails and did half an hour or more's work on my paper before Lennie and I went to Mass on livestream. I managed eventually to book next week's shopping online with Sainsbury's. Leanne cooked us a tasty lunch, after which I went out into the garden with Lennie until it was too hot, and I came in and did some more work on my paper. Faye came later and took Lennie for a walk.

On Tuesday, I recorded that "the reality is that Lennie no longer automatically follows or understands directions in the kitchen or is clear about coffee, tea and sugar tins, or thoroughly washes up. So, for example, she doesn't clean the insides of mugs. Lennie frequently expresses anger that both the front and back doors are locked and she hasn't the freedom to go out." The Mass today was a Requiem for a St. Joseph's parishioner. Claire took Lennie for a walk before lunch. After Claire had gone, "Lennie had a crazy spell, hanging out knickers on the line and suggesting they belonged to the children. When Faye came, she took Lennie off for a walk on the Downs. When Faye left at 6 p.m. Lennie started her panic evening: the need to lay the table and prepare food for ten people. She seems totally resistant to my view that nobody is expected this evening. Both Luke and Richard phoned."

Wednesday was a very hot midsummer's day. We were unable to get St. Joseph's, so we followed Mass from Merton. I'd managed to do some work beforehand. When Leanne took Lennie out for a walk, I had chest pains and had to use my puffer for the first time in months. After lunch, I had a deep sleep and "after struggling there, I was surprised that Lennie had apparently slipped out of the garden door and gone for a walk. Disturbing. How do I cope with her?" Later, Faye and Marie took her for a brief walk and then made us a pleasant omelette for supper. I told Gilly that Lennie and I were no longer able to do much more as trustees. We dossed during much of the day until Marie came and took Lennie for a walk round a pond near Stoughton. I managed to watch Chelsea beat Man. City 2–1. On Friday, I was tired after being woken early by Lennie, but managed to insert several references in Matthew's Gospel to Jesus's stress on doing something into my current writing. When Leanne left, we drove to Cranleigh to pick up Stephen for the weekend. "I wondered if it would be the last time I ever go there."

Stephen cleaned the freezer and watched a repeat of Chelsea's win yesterday, which guaranteed Liverpool as champions for the first time in thirty years. When there appeared to be a gas leak in our freezer, our next-door neighbours offered us an old freezer and we duly added it in our hall. On Saturday, I managed to do our Sainsbury's shopping online before we followed Mass on livestream. Sunday was "back to normal, with Lennie getting up and dressed around 2 a.m." Before going to Mass, I managed to add some more to my paper. I persuaded Stephen to mow the lawn. Gilly came round just as Lennie was walking out and took her for a walk by the river. Chelsea beat Leicester 1–0 to get to the semi-finals. "At times today, Lennie wanted to go and see her parents and she wasn't sure if I was her husband."

At breakfast on Monday, Lennie "didn't realise Stephen was her son or that her parents were dead. Stephen put on the week's washing but so far none of us have found the bags with the clothes pegs. When Lennie puts things away, it often takes ages to find them. The other day, bowls of cabbage and other vegetables were found in the washing machine. She has since brought in the washing from the line, while angrily asserting that she's finished with her teaching job!" After driving Stephen to the bus station, we attended Mass. At 11 a.m., "while Lennie and I were having a row, Claire came and immediately helped ease things". When she took Lennie for a walk down by the river, I managed to do three-quarters of an hour's work on my paper. Our next problems included a clogged-up loo and then another scam confirmed by the police and BT. On Tuesday, the last day of June, I managed to add more to my paper before we attended Mass. Claire pushed me into getting a replacement fridge. Because it was raining steadily, Lennie didn't go out for her usual walk. An hour after Claire left, Lennie was driving me mad, going on and on about Maureen, etc. I locked the front door. The afternoon was a nightmare, and it substantially consumed all my time, energy and patience. Marika was very helpful and took Lennie out for a couple of walks. Stephen came and after watching some football with him, I read some Hebrews before going to bed.

Wednesday 1st July was a bit of a mixture. I managed to get some writing done but felt Lennie should only go for a walk with a companion, so I locked the doors. Fortunately, Marika turned up shortly after the Sainsbury's shopping had been delivered. Richard came to watch the football and have a chat with Lennie. Chelsea lost 3–2 to West Ham. It was good to hear that Richard had got a good appraisal from his boss, so will now go ahead looking for a house in Guildford. On Thursday, I tried to do some work before Mass, but it wasn't easy with Lennie fussing around. The nail-cutter didn't turn up but after Marie left in the evening, "Lennie seems to have assumed we were leaving tomorrow 'to return home' or 'go to the sea'. When she came down, she was very angry to find both doors locked, and I feared she was going to smash them. Our exchanges got more and more angry and I'm afraid I lost my cool. I claimed it was my responsibility according to our marriage vows to look after her and see she didn't get into any danger, so I thought she needed a companion every time she went out and was in danger of getting lost. Lennie calmed down and was even apologetic."

Life wasn't easy on Friday. "Before Mass was difficult because Lennie defiantly wanted to go for a walk. She vigorously rattled both locked doors, front and back, and I fear she will soon break them." We couldn't get St. Joseph's on livestream, though I tried for half an hour. When Faye took Lennie out for a walk, I peeled potatoes and carrots as a contribution for lunch and edited about half of my paper. Marie from Everycare cooked us supper and was rather surprised by Lennie's anger and refusal to eat it. Saturday morning was infuriating, and Currys brought a wrong sized fridge/freezer. Stephen came and made lunch. Lennie wouldn't let go of the idea that she was teaching on Monday. Stephen and I were able to watch Chelsea beat Watford 3–0. "On Sunday the three of us went up to Mass, the first with a mini congregation for three and a half months." Gilly visited us with Fraggle and told us Douglas had got a 2:2 for his dissertation. Like Ben, he wants to be a teacher. On Monday, we drove Stephen to the bus station before putting washing on the line outside. The rest of the day dribbled away. On Tuesday, Richard came over to watch the Crystal Palace vs Chelsea match, which we eventually won 2–3, ending up in third place.

Wednesday was Gilly's 57th birthday. Lennie had knee problems today, which made it difficult to go for a walk. In the evening, Andrew and Richard called briefly before Richard drove Stephen back to Cranleigh. I watched a bit of football on TV, but when Lennie went up to bed, around 9 p.m., I switched it off and read some scripture. On Thursday, I wrote: "Life is certainly changing. Very early in the night I found Lennie fully dressed. Yet she slept most of the night in our bed. This morning, she was obsessed with what to wear and after breakfast she was changing shoes/sandals over and over again. In the kitchen, she no longer selects the right place to put different types of cutlery. Today, the cleaners came, and I seemed to have problems with scammers and cold calls." Mgr. Tony forgot to light the candles at Mass today and his main theme was the need for priestly vocations. Leanne and Faye both took Lennie out for a short walk and made our lunch and supper. Our neighbour, Imogen, kindly put our bins out. Lennie wanted to go home and see her parents down the road. She was very aggressive about it and for a while seemed totally immune to my insistence that I was telling her the truth that her parents were dead and that this was our home. Then, suddenly, she quietened down and went upstairs and later "came down fully dressed and ready to go out. I switched off the TV and closed Duffy's book, *Saints and Sinners*, that I was reading, and she eventually went back to bed. Before going up to bed, I read three chapters of Zephaniah."

On Friday, I started my diary: "Lennie remained in her nightie all night for a change and was very amicable as we read today's Mass readings and said our prayers for the living and the dead. Yet, later, I blew my top when, having found a spare comb for Lennie, she couldn't respond to my suggestion that she put the comb on the top of the dressing table. Soon we were grappling with each other's arms and shouting. In frustration I banged my hand on the top of the dressing table. I've tried to record this in my diary because it illustrates the fact that I have a short fuse which is easily sparked by Lennie's dementia. She ends up as I cool down by lambasting me as only concerned about 'me, me, me' and so on. Help me, Lord, to remember that love is patient and never let us harm each other physically." Leanne came and took Lennie for a walk before cooking our lunch. "Lennie has a shorter snooze after lunch than I have."

"Then Lennie came down quite soon and we had a very difficult half hour or more in which her time frame took over and I was very provoked and probably went over the top briefly. At least six times she told the story of the Revd. Mother at the convent saying, 'Didn't you do well?' after a hockey match. Eventually, by keeping quiet for a while instead of clarifying realities, things calmed down." Marie came and took Lennie for a walk round the block before cooking our fish supper. Lennie went up to bed early at 7.15 p.m. "Lennie went up and down the stairs in her nightie two or three times; then came down fully dressed." I switched off everything and went to bed at 9.45 p.m. On Saturday morning, Gilly brought Fraggle with her in the middle of the online Mass. She brought the laptop downstairs where we watched the Mass. Stephen came and took Lennie for a walk before his G&T and lunch. Richard and Will turned up to watch Chelsea play Sheffield United; a disastrous 3–0 defeat with poor defence.

On Sunday it was Fr. Tom's first Mass, I understand, but it was a warm and pleasant occasion. Stephen made our lunch, after which he helpfully took Lennie out for a walk. "Just as well because she is driving me nuts with her repeated questions, which fail to take note of previous replies which have emphasised how long ago her parents died and that this is our home." The rest of the day rather drizzled away and left me no time to continue reading Duffy. A difficult start on Monday with a dead car battery, which meant I couldn't drive Stephen to the bus station. The AA responded quickly. We watched Mass online. Frances phoned to tell us Andrew Martin, one of our Family Group, had died the previous night. May he rest in peace. Leanne came and took Lennie down to the river before she made us lunch. Lennie's right knee was giving her a lot of pain and I cut my right leg badly. We spent much of the afternoon chatting in the garden. Marie came and brought in the washing off the line before driving Lennie to Holmbury St. Mary's and making us supper. Chelsea managed to remain in third position, and I read a bit more of *Saints and Sinners*.

On Tuesday, we attended Mass online before Marika came and served us lunch. I informed the parish office about Andrew Martin's death. There were concerns today about a huge surge in the coronavirus pandemic. I read Duffy most of the day. Lennie's knee was hurting her and prevented her going out for a walk. Richard visited in the evening, and we watched Chelsea win 1–0 to remain comfortably in third position.

On the third Wednesday in July, Domestic and General installed the new fridge/freezer. Faye found out when it was going to be delivered on her mobile phone. It's time I got a modern mobile; I'm totally out of touch with contemporary needs and IT in general. Earlier, we had 'attended' Mass on livestream, during which Lennie was anxious about the children and whether we'd told them whatever. Stephen came for a while and watched a repeat of Chelsea's win yesterday before we took him down to the bus station. The evening dribbled away after a brief visit from Andrew and Caroline, who were both struggling to get work. I managed to read some Duffy and some scripture before joining Lennie, who was upstairs, still messing about with what to wear.

Thursday was unusual these days in that we started the night making love with my usual absence of an erection. The rest of the night was broken up by Lennie's getting fully dressed, going downstairs and then on a couple of occasions returning to bed. Lennie seemed quite unable to do basic domestic things such as putting water in every glass and dish and was full of denials. After Mass on livestream, I drove to Boxgrove for my first haircut in several months, after which I put on the Test Match. Leanne cooked us lunch, after which, as is fairly usual these days, Lennie had one of her angry spells when I didn't let her go for a walk on her own. Faye was helpful and took her for a brief walk before preparing our supper. "The Everycare workers are technically supporting Lennie, as I'm so wobbly these days that I couldn't do without them. Lennie seems totally unaware of her illness and needs, and from my perspective she contributes very little to our domestic needs." She was very demanding about going out for a walk both this afternoon and before this evening, after Faye had gone. I tried to say it was my job to look after her and see that she was safe and that she had already been on two walks with Everycare workers that day, and that she ought to be prepared to compromise. It fell on deaf ears, and she claimed that I was just a bully and "she would bash the doors down and had even on a couple of occasions threatened suicide".

On Friday I added: "Last night, probably around 2–3 a.m., she got out of her nightie and got dressed and went downstairs without waking me. I have concerns over things such as not turning off the gas on the hob and I don't know what she does when downstairs." Most of the day I spent out in the garden reading the *Tablet* and Duffy's book. On Saturday morning, I managed to order the weekly shopping from Sainsbury's before we 'attended' Mass from St. Joseph's. On Sunday, our next-door neighbour handed over to us his redundant freezer, which we parked in the hall. Gillian paid her weekly visit in the morning and Richard and Ben came to watch Chelsea beat Manchester United 3–1. Monday, as usual, was a bit frenetic. We drove Stephen to Merrow, where he wanted to visit charity shops, before going home. Leanne helped calm things down this morning, as did Marie in the afternoon. Both had taken Lennie out for a short walk. Tuesday morning was a bit different. As I wrote in my diary: "Lennie started getting up at about 5.30 a.m. and she banged away with the sliding doors on the wardrobes for the next hour, looking at the blue dress she has worn all week and putting it away because it was 'too long', then taking it out and considering it over and over again for an hour, when I finally exploded". Lennie seems incapable of making even a simple breakfast, though she does do the washing up. I phoned in my Feed In Tariff for our solar panels. Leanne drove Lennie to Boxgrove for a hair appointment.

On the fourth Wednesday of July, Lennie broke another glass while I was washing-up. I managed to prepare breakfast, which was difficult with a stick. I then paid Everycare by online banking and phoned NatWest Fraud as requested and Voytek, our gardener, came for the first time that year. Andrew came and next-door, Marie witnessed a legal document he then took up to our solicitor. Richard came and we watched a gutsy 5–3 defeat at Anfield which exposed Chelsea's porous defence. Afterwards, he drove Stephen home to Cranleigh. On Thursday, we were invited to Andrew Martin's funeral at the cathedral. Frances kindly offered to drive us. In the evening, we watched three episodes of *Outnumbered* until "I suggested it was time to go to bed. Lennie said she was waiting for Mike to come home. *C'est la vie!*" On Friday, I noted: "Lennie got dressed not long after midnight and reacted quite aggressively when I complained about her taking clothes from my chair. She went out for a while but returned fully dressed to go to sleep next to me ... I basically managed breakfast ... When it came to coffee Lennie put salad cream instead of milk into it; I drew attention to it and she said I was 'the most selfish person she had ever known'." Lennie was difficult all day and walked out of the garden gate at one stage, though both carers took her for brief walks.

On Saturday, the Mass at St. Joseph's was said by the newly ordained priest, Fr. Tom Kent. On Sunday after Mass, we went to Gilly's for coffee and to see Katie and Douglas. In the afternoon Richard and Ben came to watch Chelsea's home win over Wolves and took Lennie for a walk round the block. Andrew and Caroline also visited. On Monday, Lennie and I were still reading the Mass readings with the help of *Bible Alive* every day before breakfast. We drove Stephen to the bus station before watching Mass on livestream. It was too wet for Faye to take Lennie out for a walk. The mechanic from ESE came to give our solar panels an annual check. After a doze in the afternoon, "Lennie came downstairs wanting to go to her home. I made us mugs of tea but nothing I said about this being 'our' home worked and eventually I phoned Stephen, whose safety she was concerned about, and he had a ten-minute conversation with her which calmed her down." During the evening, I read some scriptures.

On Tuesday, I wrote: "Lennie has asked me half a dozen times whether I live locally and how long I have lived here. Last night she got dressed and went into the other bedroom or downstairs before eventually returning. I said a quiet prayer asking the Lord what I should do. In the end we put on the lights in the loft, and it worked quite well." Before Mass I cleared emails. Marie came and was very sociable to Lennie. She took her for a walk in spite of her painful knee and then cooked our lunch. The British Gas engineer came round in the afternoon for our annual boiler check-up. I watched the Test Match with the West Indies. Gilly phoned to say Everycare had emailed her "to say they were concerned about potential physical damage resulting from anger between Lennie and me". *Our Yorkshire Farm* gripped me in the evening.

On the last Wednesday of July, Frances Allen kindly drove us to Andrew Martin's funeral Mass in Arundel Cathedral and we had to sit two metres apart. It was the first time in over four months I was able to go to Holy Communion. Back home, I was surprised Frances didn't have sandwiches with us in the garden. It was good to see Stephen, who looked after us before I drove him back to the bus station. On Thursday, our Brazilian cleaners came unexpectedly early, so we ate our breakfast outside on the patio. Faye came and took Lennie for a walk down by the 'sea' (i.e. river!). Richard came and I told him that following Everycare's email, Gilly had urged me to increase our Everycare cover and that this would mean digging into our savings. "Then, Lennie came down, angrily saying she didn't know where her dad and sister were and that she'd seen her sister a couple of days ago. She was wearing my pyjama trousers, but of course hadn't taken them from under my pillow. The more she came down the angrier she got about my supposed errors, and she eventually took off my pyjama trousers and threw them in my face. Fortunately, I kept my cool, at least partly because it wasn't obvious to me what she was angry about. But I fear this sort of dementia anger is probably likely to get worse and I'm going to need Your help, Lord, to know how to cope with it."

Friday was a difficult day as I recorded: "I was awakened around 5.30 a.m. by Lennie complaining that our bedroom was like a junk shop. I first, rather gently, said I thought it was unkind of her to wake me early and pointed out that all the 'junk', i.e. jackets, skirts, nightie, etc. on the end of our bed, had been put there by her during the night. This angered her and she asserted that I was a liar and smacked me across my feet. This created a criticism about what I was doing in her bedroom. At my age I'm aware that we both may have only a short time to live. I wish I felt I could prepare for it as God would wish me to. Upstairs, I cleared emails and we then 'attended' the livestream Mass on the Lewis's 49th wedding anniversary. Afterwards, Lennie went up in tears about her sister Maureen. Later, she craftily went out of the garden and walked up the cul-de-sac. I hastily let myself out of the front door and asked young Flavio if she was walking up there. It seems he phoned his mother, Laura, who, bless her, walked up the street and brought her back. telling me not to get cross with her! But it shows the limit of trust and my need to be careful. In the evening, I lost my cool and called her a 'killing bitch'! *Mea maxima culpa.* Today's diary gives a faint idea of what life is like with a wife with dementia."

Saturday's diary reported that "last night a nearly naked Lennie invited me to make love to her, which I did using my finger to replace my failed erection. Later, Lennie didn't realise that Stephen was her son. She fancies him and can't face up to the fact that he is twenty-nine years younger. At breakfast time she poured coffee into our cereal dishes rather than mugs ... Richard turned up with Will and Iris, as did Andrew to watch Arsenal beat Chelsea 2–1 in the Cup Final. Before Mass, I'd done our week's shopping with Sainsbury's online. When I went upstairs Lennie was wearing my pyjamas."

On Sunday morning, Lennie was very disoriented and wanted to discuss/argue about what she ought to be wearing over and over again. For Mass, Stephen brought up a piece of bread and a glass of wine and water. We tried to simulate the realities of Mass and participate in the words Jesus said at the last supper, sensing that the prayer about spiritual communion doesn't speak to the 'reality' as we experience it. "There are times each day when it is hard to cope with Lennie's shifts of time frames. At 9.35 p.m., it is time to go up and join Lennie, even if she has nicked my pyjamas." Monday's diary suggests it wasn't an easy day. "We drove Stephen to the bus station, and I was full of grateful thanks for all he had done for us over the weekend. I was obviously irritated a lot by Lennie's failure to follow suggestions and was worried we were making a lot of noise for our neighbours. Both Faye and Marika took Lennie out for a walk before preparing our meals. When Lennie put my pyjamas under the pillow on the other side of the bed, I felt relegated and took myself to the other bedroom." My Tuesday's diary reports that "when Lennie got dressed and went downstairs, I returned to 'my' side of the double bed. After about 7 a.m., she began to rattle the doors, demanding the car key, and generally being potentially dangerous." The evening was quite pleasant, and we watched Ireland beating England in an ODI and a championship match play off won by Brentford.

Wednesday was an ordinary sort of day. I managed to do some file-thinning and clearing before we watched Mass on livestream. When Marie came and took Lennie down for a walk by the river, Stephen came and put away the washing. Voytek came to do a splendid job on the garden. Thursday was much the same. Leanne took Lennie for a short walk before preparing our lunch. The cleaners came and made the bed and Marie came and calmed us down before taking Lennie for a walk and making us supper. She and Lennie also took the sheets and pillowcases off the line and put them away.

On the first Friday of August, we attended Mass at St. Joseph's on livestream, and I was worried that the pandemic lockdown might have inhibited us contacting our G.P. about Lennie's knee problems. Marika came for the two shifts and took Lennie out for a walk before making our meals. We watched a range of programmes on TV. "Lennie keeps asking where the children and her parents and sister are, seemingly not knowing that I am her husband and we've been married nearly sixty years."

Saturday was fairly busy, and I recorded concerns about my archives at Farm Street and then Curry's charging for our fridge/freezer. We then attended Mass on livestream. Stephen came and made us lunch. We watched the tense Test Match with Pakistan, which England won. In the evening, we watched Chelsea lose 4–1 to Bayern Munich. On Sunday, we attended Mass on livestream and all signed cards for Ann and Peter's wedding anniversary the next Thursday. "Lennie didn't realise this was our house." In the evening, we watched two episodes of *Harlot,* but Luke wasn't in them!

My Monday diary notes that I had badly lost my temper. "The row exploded so much Lennie even said she'd kill me." Stephen intervened and I spent the next hour completing the weekly online shopping with Sainsbury's before we drove Stephen to the bus station and returned to attend the online Mass from St. Joseph's. Claire came and calmed things down and made our lunch. Later, Faye took Lennie for a walk before making our supper. In the evening, we watched an interesting film about the S.O.E. agent *Charlotte Gray* and then an hour with André Rieu. Tuesday was another day where Lennie's time frame and concern for the children were always not far away.

The second Wednesday of August turned out to be very ordinary. The laptop played games, so we tried *What's On* and followed Mass in our cathedral at Arundel. Voytek came to look after the garden and when Claire arrived, I drove to Sainsbury's to get cash from the cashpoint and fill up with petrol. Claire took Lennie out for a brief walk. As usual these days, I had a lengthy doze after Claire's shift. Stephen came and watched TV. But I drove him to the bus station as soon as Marie came and prepared our supper and helped put away the Sainsbury's online shopping. I spent the evening listening to Mozart and Brahms on Classic FM. In many ways, Thursday was much the same. The cleaners came for their weekly shift before we followed the livestream Mass from St. Joseph's. When Faye came with some welcome tonic water, I persuaded her to take Lennie down to the river. I switched on the Test Match and then bashed my arm against the door and had another bleeding cut. It was a relief when Marie came to chat to Lennie and take her for a walk. During the afternoon, I had the Test Match on but Lennie's interruptions were so non-stop that I missed two or three wickets! Shortly after the end of Marie's shift at 7 p.m., Lennie decided to go to bed, and I switched on Classic FM. "Then Richard turned up for a pre-holiday visit and chatted to Lennie a bit, but his main concern was to persuade me to increase carers' times in order to benefit my mental health and ease relationships between us. I am vaguely considering the possibilities."

On Friday, there was no Mass from St. Joseph's, so again we followed it from the cathedral. When Marie came, she took Lennie for a walk down by the river. This gave me the chance to tidy up the past week's correspondence, put away bank statements and send BT my annual payment for a TV Licence. In the afternoon, "Lennie was quite stuck in a time frame of thirty odd years ago: 'where are my father, mother, sister? Or 'where is the other chap who was here?'" The evening wasted away as usual. Saturday was the 75th Anniversary of V.J. Day and the end of WWII, not mentioned at the livestream Mass. After Mass on TV, there was a very moving tribute to the Burma Army which had me in tears. Stephen came in time to make us lunch and afterwards we watched sport on TV. I sent off our shopping request online to Sainsbury's. I had to sleep that night in my underwear since Lennie was wearing my pyjamas. The three of us attended Mass on livestream on Sunday, after which we all came down for coffee outside, where we were joined by Gilly, who came for our weekly chat. Stephen cooked us a roast chicken meal, after which all three of us watched *Jane Eyre* on TV.

On Monday, I struggled to have my shower before we drove Stephen to the library. Before then he'd done the week's wash and helped put it on the line. "Back home we 'attended' Mass on livestream, though Lennie was quite unaware that we have been doing so for five months daily." When Claire came, she and Lennie wisely brought in the washing from the line because it soon began to rain. She later made our lunch. I had to cope with a scam on the phone. The rest of the day I had to cope with Lennie's memory loss and failure to realise I was Mike, her husband and father of her children. Marie came and cooked our supper, after which Lennie remained down with me and we watched an André Rieu documentary.

Tuesday was much the same sort of day with Lennie's 'time warp'. After Mass on livestream, she wanted to go shopping so it was a relief when Leanne came, took her down to the river for a brief walk, and made us lunch. When Faye took Lennie out for a walk in the late afternoon, I did some watering of plants, but I was shaking and worried about another fall. But the evening was long and drawn-out, as Lennie planned to pack some clothes in order to go 'home' tomorrow and didn't realise that I was her husband.

The third Wednesday of the month was much the same, with Lennie in her strange time frame. She couldn't find her purse. Claire found a full dose of Lennie's breakfast pills in her bag. Just before the end of Marie's shift, she found Lennie pouring coffee into a shoe! Lennie joined me for livestream Mass from St. Joseph's. Stephen came for about three hours in the afternoon before Marie came and I drove him down to the bus station. Sadly, Lennie went to bed largely dressed.

On Thursday, as on most days, my first big job was to manage Lennie's breakfast pills and see that she swallowed them. "Before Mass on livestream I managed to pay Everycare and clear that day's emails." Marie came and took Lennie down to the river for a walk before lunch. Andrew came in the afternoon, and we had a very pleasant chat, though there were signs of a breakdown with Caroline. He took Lennie for a walk along the Downs and "it seems to have been a great success and Lennie really enjoyed it and seemingly 'fell' for the young man, her son, who'd taken her". In the evening, we both enjoyed the film *Quartet.*

After Mass on Friday, the Feast of St. Pius X, Jane took Lennie for a brief walk and cooked us a fish lunch before I drove Lennie to Hair Partners, where she had a cut and blow-dry. Most of the afternoon, we watched the Test Match, with Crawley scoring his maiden Test century. It was the Championship Final later and I decided, "I'd better go upstairs and cope with a verbally violent wife in my pyjamas". On Saturday, I cleared emails before Mass. Stephen came and cooked our lunch. During the afternoon, I socialised outside with Lennie in the garden. In the evening, we phoned Lennie's cousin, Peter Dooley, on the second anniversary of his wife Daphne's death. On Sunday morning, I managed to do our weekly online shopping at Sainsbury's before we 'attended' Mass at St. Joseph's. Gilly then came for her weekly chat. It emerged that Doug has now retired, and they were planning to move to Dorset. Stephen has given me a lot of space this weekend. "I'm going to miss him but am still uncertain how, and if, to increase my Everycare help."

On Monday, Stephen helped put the washing on the line before we drove him down to G-Live and then returned for Mass on livestream. Claire helped bring in the washing before preparing lunch and then ironed it and put it away in drawers upstairs. When Claire left at 6 p.m., "Lennie and I had to cope with the next four hours. It wasn't easy. She needed to be informed about the death of our parents and Maureen, the purchase of our house and our relationship as husband and wife. Not easy, over and over again. 'What do I do now?' 'You are a retired teacher, etc.' 'Am I married? Who to? Is it you?'" On Tuesday, I wrote: "It is more and more clear that Lennie's memory is deteriorating. So much so that she can't even make a cup of coffee ... Lennie and I attended today's Mass from St. Joseph's on our laptop." Claire was helpful during her shift. Amanda and four-year-old Clemmie on their Yorkshire Farm made the evening acceptable.

On Wednesday, my diary suggested a non-stop day of arguing with Lennie. It helped when Claire came and took Lennie down for a walk by the river before serving up lunch. Stephen came and put away the Sainsbury's shopping delivery. When Claire came later in the afternoon, she again took Lennie out for a walk and later cooked supper. When they returned, I drove Stephen to the bus station. Before going to bed, I watched an episode of *Harlot,* but didn't spot our grandson Luke. On Thursday, we had problems with our internet connection and so instead of watching Mass on livestream we said five decades of the joyful mysteries of the rosary. In the afternoon, we looked through several years of photographs from 1989–1992. "I was surprised at how frequently Stephen was with us and glad to feel we'd 'looked after' him for quite a long time."

Friday was the second day without Mass, so we said the five sorrowful mysteries of the rosary. Marika came to cook supper and also take Lennie out for a walk. I managed to phone BT to get a new hub. I enjoyed the Beethoven at the

Proms that evening. On Saturday, Chelsea Women won the Community Shield 2–0 in an empty Wembley. "Lennie has been very much in another time frame all day. She doesn't clearly always know that I am her husband, though she often addresses me as if I were her 'dad'. She strongly asserted she'd seen her mother and sister upstairs much of the time. Stephen came early and made us a tuna pasta lunch and has just taken Lennie out for a walk. She doesn't realise how immobile and unable I am." We said the five decades of the glorious mysteries of the rosary and we watched Mass on EWTN.

On Sunday, we again followed Mass on EWTN, though I dozed off a bit at times. Stephen showed signs of paranoia about the removal of his passport. Gilly came round for a pleasant chat, with a phone call from Katie. Richard came round and we watched England beat Pakistan in a T20 test. We also watched PSG win the Women's Championship final. Monday was the August Bank Holiday and by my reckoning the last day of summer. With Lennie's incessant wandering, I didn't have a very good night's sleep. Stephen kindly took Lennie out for a walk. He also guided us through a game of scrabble for the first time in years. He cooked us an early lunch so that we could follow Mass on livestream from EWTN. The large amount of Latin in the Mass annoyed me and I wondered if they'd heard of Vatican II. Stephen took over control of the TV.

"So, we've come to the end of summer 2020, the second summer we haven't had a holiday. It seems that the last lap of our lives came up on us suddenly and we are having to cope unexpectedly. The coronavirus has been an additional reality this year and we are all adjusting to it. I've not minded being 'locked down' all that much though Lennie has." Tuesday was another mixed day and I had to cope the best I could ... We drove Stephen to G-Live as he requested. Claire took Lennie down to the river, which they enjoyed, and then, because Lennie's knees were giving her trouble, went for a brief drive before preparing our lunch. Then Lennie watched the Mass from EWTN and afterwards said how moving it had been. At least today they said the 'Our Father' in the vernacular. When we phoned the pharmacy, they told us nobody had answered the door when they'd rung the bells three times ... Soon after Claire had gone, Lennie subjected me to about the worst verbal bashing yet, with frequent physical threats. "At first, she demanded to go for a walk and denied having just gone with Claire. Secondly, she expressed a concern for all the 'children' I was supposed to have been looking after and totally rejected my claim that we weren't looking after any children, that this was our home, and we weren't on holiday. Suddenly, after a spell when I shut up, she calmed down and even came over to apologise for her nastiness to me earlier ... Lennie's last comment included, 'I expect Mike will be here tomorrow morning'!! So, who am I?"

The first Wednesday of September was as mixed, and difficult as usual. Early on, Lennie "was angered to find both doors locked, and this led to well over an hour's angry verbiage about my selfishness: 'you only think about yourself: me, me, me, and you've never done anything for other people; you behave like a god, etc." The Boots man delivered my prescriptions but not Lennie's, which had to be chased up and delivered later. Voytek turned up to do some gardening. Faye came and took Lennie for a walk down by the river. Lennie claimed "that we were doing nothing and all I was doing was sitting in my chair. This became quite fierce, and she kicked the wastepaper basket across the room." Faye came and took Lennie for a walk and the Sky mechanic came to sort out our broadband problems. "After supper, Lennie had one of her time shifts and was only concerned about how many people we had to cater for, in spite of my protests that there were no such arrangements. To escape, I went upstairs to clear over ninety emails. I heard the front door and went downstairs to find Lennie had gone walkabouts. Fortunately, one of our neighbours, Norma, kindly brought her back. Give me strength and patience, Lord." On Thursday before Mass, I managed to do the weekly Sainsbury's shop online and paid the weekly Everycare bill. When Faye came, I drove Stephen to the bus station after withdrawing cash from our two joint accounts. Classic FM played Beethoven's ninth symphony for a change.

Friday was a busy and, at times, fraught day. In the morning, I tried to make bookings for the Family Group at Carlo's, for a place at Mass at St. Pius', and a visit from Andrew and Caroline's family. After chatting to Lennie for an hour after lunch and making us tea, "the Lord tested me. Lennie won't stop talking and is in the earlier time frame, needing to be reminded that her parents and Maureen are all dead and that no children are coming to be fed. It is incredible how many times I have to repeat the story of her mother being knocked down by a lorry thirty-five years earlier and Maureen's stroke in Cumbria over ten years ago and eventual move down to East Surrey Hospital and then discharged into the care home in Reigate. She now wants the key to open the front door." Fortunately, Marie came and took Lennie out for a walk and on their return made us supper. The Shortlands phoned to chat and socialise. Lennie allowed Stephen and me to watch the T20 match with Australia all evening, which we won by just two runs.

On Saturday, I wrote: "What a strange life it is trying to cope with a wife with dementia. She looks lovely this morning and 'with it' but she is going on and on about 'going shopping' and meeting up with her friends and going to school, and so on, all of which she used to do over twenty years ago." We attended Mass online in a still empty St. Joseph's. In the afternoon, Richard turned up with Will and Iris and we watched England beat Iceland 1–0. After Stephen had cooked us supper, we watched the Athletics Championships. On Sunday, for the first time in six months, we attended Mass at St. Pius', though Lennie refused to wear a mask. Gilly joined us and later came home with us. She was pleased that Douglas had been offered a teaching assistant's job at St. Peter's next year. Andrew called with Caroline and all her family. Lennie's anxieties peaked and Stephen chatted to her for a couple of hours while I watched a film about Berlusconi.

On Monday, Stephen put on the weekly wash, which he managed to put on the line outside before Lennie and I drove him to the bus station. Lennie and I then 'attended' Mass on livestream. When Leanne came, she took Lennie for a walk and then made us lunch. I found a spare key for the back door, so Lennie managed to bring in the washing off the line. Faye took Lennie for a walk 'round the block' before preparing our supper and, at her suggestion, watched a couple of episodes of *Strike* during a quiet and peaceful evening.

On Tuesday, I noted that Lennie had gone to bed fully dressed. As usual, she left all the preparations for breakfast to me. After we'd watched Mass on livestream, Katie unexpectedly called round. It was lovely to see her, but we weren't allowed to cuddle because of COVID-19 restrictions. Leanne took Lennie out for a short walk and then cooked our lunch. In the afternoon, we dozed off outside, made ourselves tea and cake, and when Marika came, she took Lennie out for a short walk.

On Wednesday, Lennie had had a good night's sleep and enjoyed Mass and we then put out the washing on the line. We cancelled a proposed visit to Carlo's because of anticipated COVID-19 restrictions. Stephen put away the Sainsbury's shopping. Faye prepared supper while I drove Stephen to the bus station. "The four hours after Faye left us are always difficult but we just about managed today with a variety of programmes on TV. Lennie repeatedly came downstairs with different clothes on. She was full of love and thanks, but at other times is weeping at hearing her parents and sister are no longer here."

Thursday was a mixed day with problems with my laptop. Leanne took Lennie down to the river but had a struggle cooking us lunch. During the afternoon, I tried to read *RENEW*, which was difficult with Lennie's non-stop chatter. Faye took Lennie for a short walk before preparing supper. We then had angry exchanges over plans for Christmas presents but ended up watching a programme about Beethoven's 7th Symphony.

Friday was another mixed day, starting with the slow movement of Beethoven's 9th Symphony on Classic FM. As always, we 'attended' livestream Mass before Leanne came. Leanne took Lennie for a walk and then cooked us a fish and chip lunch. We dozed a bit in the garden in the afternoon until Marie came, took Lennie up to Newlands Corner and then made our supper. England lost the O.D.I. "Lennie came down to ask me what to do to go to bed. I suggested she take off her cardigan, blouse and skirt and put on her nightie. It didn't work, so I had to go up to bed before 9.30 p.m. But when a woman can't dress or undress herself there are real problems. I helped her find her nightie and we had lights out around 9.40 p.m.; earlier than usual." On Saturday, we celebrated "a lovely Mass on the Feast of 'the Name of Mary.' Stephen made us lunch and I spent most of the afternoon outside skimming the *Guardian* and *Tablet*. In the evening, we watched the last night of the proms."

On Sunday, I noted that: "Lennie wasn't easy last night. She was fully dressed and at least once went downstairs, and Stephen told me she could have gone walkies through the lounge door because I hadn't locked it and taken out the key as I usually do." The three of us followed Mass on my dodgy laptop. I had a session typing some of Stephen's blog before he cooked us roast lamb for lunch. "For much of the afternoon I sat out in the garden with Lennie, just to be with her, trying to keep her calm and at ease. Then, in the evening, we had a very difficult hour or more with Lennie going on and on about looking after 'the children' and totally ignoring our responses about how old they were, where they are, and so forth. I tried to keep the peace when Stephen was reacting angrily to Lennie's explosive criticisms of him. I'm dreading five nights without Stephen to share the difficulties with Lennie."

Monday was much the same, though in the afternoon we were invited to a Family Group picnic at the Durstons'. Richard came to watch Chelsea win 3–1 at Brighton. Tuesday, again, was much the same and in the afternoon, "I took us both outside and devoted the bulk of the afternoon chatting to Lennie and answering her repeated questions about this house, where it is, who owns it, do we know any of the neighbours, how long have we been here, etc." I phoned the Church Bookshop and ordered two Bibles for Will and Iris and while Natalie took Lennie for a walk by the river, I managed to do some scripture reading myself and ended the day watching a mix of things on the TV, including the 80th anniversary of the end of the Battle of Britain.

My diary for the third Wednesday in September contains evidence of difficulties resulting from Lennie's illness. For example, Stephen found his wallet in Lennie's bag, and I found Lennie's cards in my drawer and my pullover in her drawer. She seems quite unaware that we have been watching livestreamed Mass every day for about six months. We spent much of the day watching the T20 match with Australia and an episode of *Harlot,* looking for Luke, our grandson.

Thursday started with a mini disaster; we had no internet, so we watched Mass on TV from Alabama. Much of the afternoon was taken up with Lennie's numerous confusions: 'Was this our house or not? Was it Berwick or Burpham?

Did her parents live here or not? Was her sister here or not?' Natasha took her out for a walk before serving us supper. I had the same sort of problems on Friday. Again, with no internet, we had to watch Mass from Alabama and "I miss our Mass from St. Joseph's, which is closer to our sensitivities, not so clericalist or traditional". A BT man was very helpful and talked me through my internet problems. I struggled to water the garden in the afternoon and did spells of typing for Stephen and printing for Richard. When Marie came to take Lennie for a short walk before serving supper, I managed to pay Everycare with online banking and prepared half of next week's online shopping with Sainsbury's. I also managed to read a few chapters of Acts and Isaiah.

On Saturday, we had difficulty getting livestream from St. Joseph's at first, so I tried several alternatives until we returned quite late in the Mass. But we tried. The next hour was a nightmare with Lennie's time warp until Stephen turned up. After lunch, Gilly came and had a very pleasant chat with us outside in the garden. I tried to find time to read the *Guardian* and the *Tablet,* but it wasn't easy with Lennie's persistent demands to chat. It was much the same on Sunday, with Lennie confused and getting up early. Before breakfast I managed to finish editing and typing Stephen's latest blog. Lennie was strangely quiet during the afternoon, so I managed to skim the *Tablet*. We watched Chelsea losing 2–0 at Anfield before going to bed after a reasonably quiet day.

On Monday, concerns were growing about another wave of the coronavirus pandemic. "To be honest, I haven't so far objected to the 'lockdown'." Earlier, the three of us had put the washing on the line before driving Stephen down to the bus station. After Mass, Leanne took Lennie down to the river. In the afternoon, Lennie was unaware that I was physically unable to take clothes down from the line because I needed to use a stick to stop me falling. In the evening, Richard came to watch the football. We had a lovely hour and a half with Richard, reminiscing about Lennie's hockey ... Lennie responded beautifully to Richard's flirting.

On Tuesday, I kept dozing off during the livestream Mass from St. Joseph's. Afterwards, I nudged Leanne to go with Lennie down to the river. Lennie and I had a good, chatty afternoon. Later in the afternoon, Marika took Lennie for a walk before serving us supper. "Then, suddenly, Lennie entered a thirty-year time warp. She wanted to go to the school she was teaching in. When I suggested she'd retired twenty-five years ago, she accused me of trying to take her job."

My diary of Wednesday 23rd September is full of details of Lennie's shift of time warp in detail, particularly during the morning when she expected to be going to school and get instructions from her mother and sister. After our livestream Mass, she was searching for a lost £50. When Claire arrived, she took her for a walk around Whitmore Common. Voytek came to look after our garden. Stephen came, but Lennie wasn't interested in an international hockey match which he'd thought would appeal to her. In the evening, we put on a DVD about Mary Magdalene. Lennie's demands also dominated Thursday's diary, when she complained that nobody had told her about her mother's death thirty-five years earlier. Otherwise, the day proceeded as usual. In the evening, I put on the fifty-five-year-old film, *Dr. Zhivago,* which we both watched for over an hour. Friday was another day dominated by the need to cope with Lennie, who spent the early hours searching for her lipstick. As usual, both carers took Lennie out for a walk before serving up meals for lunch and supper. During the evening, Lennie came downstairs several times wearing my pyjamas.

Wednesday was Sue and Mario's 48th wedding anniversary. "Bless them, Lord." Our day was fairly typical. In the early hours Lennie "had an obsession with a woman or women who were trying to exploit me. Such obsessions go on and on and over and over again." I managed to do a bit of work before we watched livestream Mass on the laptop. Because it was raining when Faye came, she and Lennie played Backgammon while I did an hour's work on my paper. Stephen put away the Sainsbury's shopping before I drove him down to the bus station. Faye took Lennie out for a brief walk before cooking supper. Shortly after Faye left, Lennie started to be awkward, wondering "whether Pa was back and what confirmation there was that the meeting with the schoolchildren was going ahead the next day. Please, Lord, help me to do Your will with Lennie."

My Thursday diary noted that Lennie got dressed before midnight but joined me in bed throughout the night. Vicky came early and watched Mass on livestream with us. Voytek did a great job in the garden. "The rest of the afternoon dribbled away without a war, but Lennie became very disoriented, endlessly and repeatedly wondering about 'the children', despite being told that they were all in their fifties living in their own homes." Naomi came and took Lennie out for a short walk before making us supper. Andrew came for around two-and-a-half hours and talked mainly about his work with 'A Call to Action' (ACTA).

On Friday, we had difficulties trying to arrange an eye test for Lennie, who was full of denial and memory-loss issues, so that I was unable to do any work on my paper. The two of us watched Mass on livestream. Claire came and took Lennie for a walk around the lake at Whitmore Common. Later, Natasha took her for a walk round the block, but she wouldn't stop talking and I recorded that it was a dreadful evening. But, unexpectedly, Lennie suddenly became very apologetic. After a difficult evening, we caressed and made love as best as eighty-year-olds can manage.

Saturday was fairly straightforward, with Lennie still in a time frame of thirty years ago, anxious about where "'the children' were and whether we'd got food for them". After lunch, I went upstairs to the laptop and ordered next week's Sainsbury's shopping online. Richard came over in the evening and the three of us were mightily relieved when Chelsea managed to get a 0–0 draw at Old Trafford. On Sunday, we celebrated the 50th anniversary of the canonisation of the forty English martyrs, including Philip Howard. Bishop Richard gave a lovely homily. Gilly came over for an hour-and-a-half's chat about family matters.

On Monday, we all helped put out the washing on the line before we drove Stephen to the bus station. After lunch, "Lennie brought in all the washing. Earlier Faye had discovered a ruined kettle which had been put on a hob and burned! The clothesline rod had disappeared, but Lennie says she doesn't know anything about it." Faye got out the draughts board and played a game with Lennie. We watched Spurs score a late winner at Burnley. On Tuesday, I managed to do a bit of work on my paper before the two of us attended livestream Mass. Faye took Lennie out for a drive to Newlands Corner and later Natasha took her for a walk round the block. I spent all the time I could working away at my GND paper. In the evening, Lennie joined me in watching Manchester City beat Marseilles 3–0.

"Our long-standing prayer session at the start of each day seems to be slowly slipping today, with Lennie falling asleep." We attended Mass together on livestream before going downstairs for coffee. Faye came and took Lennie for a walk round the pond at Whitmore Common. After Faye had left, "Lennie was a bit disoriented and criticised Faye 'for treating her like a three-year-old'. Stephen came and took Lennie out for a short walk and when Faye came in the late afternoon, I drove Stephen to the bus station." We watched an episode of *Harlot* in which Luke appeared, but we decided it was not for us.

On Thursday, the two of us attended Mass on livestream. "It was a pleasantly peaceful Mass, and Mgr. Tony gave a simple but relevant homily suggesting that we respond to the fact that the Wonersh Seminary has just closed as an indication perhaps that we are not responding to the news about Christ; instead, we are ignoring it, rather like many did when Jesus was in Galilee." Marie came and took Lennie for a ride around the countryside and central Guildford before preparing our lunch. "Everything was interrupted by an increasingly angry Lennie, who didn't believe that this was our house where we lived." I put on a T20 match and made us a mug of tea with a blackcurrant tart. "I am becoming increasingly aware that even such basic tasks are beyond Lennie now. She doesn't automatically know where the fridge is and though she is very good at washing up, she puts things away any-old-where." In between all this I tried to conclude the revising of my Villanova paper. Friday was a very similar type of day. Lennie "was full of ideas that there were four of us and she was totally unreceptive when I stressed there were just the two of us, and that we had been married for nearly sixty years and so on". We attended Mass together on livestream and Natasha took Lennie round the block. I found it difficult to do any work on my paper and we got through the afternoon watching an Indian Premier League (IPL) cricket match. In the evening, I put on the Northumberland detective drama, *Vera*, but Lennie was only mildly interested for half an hour. So, I ended my evening checking emails and then paying Everycare with online banking.

On Saturday, we learned that there will be another 'lockdown' to cope with the COVID-19 pandemic, for four weeks from Thursday. I managed to do some work before we followed the livestream Mass, and we then watched another IPL match until Stephen came and looked after us. In the afternoon, we watched Chelsea work together as a team and win 3–0 at Burnley. Later, we watched the England vs Italy game "and coped with a combative Lennie coping with a combative and angry Stephen". Sunday's diary for 1st November records that in the early hours Lennie dressed herself and went downstairs. "Sometime around 4 a.m., Stephen gently brought her up to me to go to bed. And she did sleep until 7.30 a.m." The three of us then attended Mass on livestream and shortly after Gilly came with some flowers for Lennie and some pearls for me to give her on her birthday. In the evening, we watched Arsenal beat Manchester United at Old Trafford.

Monday was much the same sort of day, with Lennie threatening to go walkabout when I was physically not able to go with her. I had to vote for the N.E.C. of the Labour Party and decided to vote for those who mentioned a Green New Deal. After Stephen had put the week's washing on the machine, we drove him to the bus station and got back in time for the readings at the livestream Mass. Both Leanne and Faye took Lennie for a walk before preparing our meals. Andrew called with some presents in the evening and "told me I ought to start planning for the time when both of us ought to go into a care home". Fears that Lennie might leave the gas on were among our concerns about her on the Tuesday as we drove over to Cranleigh to pick up Stephen and a huge amount of art material for the second lockdown. Before lunch, Claire took Lennie for a walk. Ann phoned us and we had a pleasant chat. Richard phoned and aimed to come and watch the Chelsea match the next day. Naomi came and took Lennie for a brief walk before cooking supper.

On Wednesday, I managed to do the online Sainsbury's shopping before we attended Mass, with Stephen bringing bread and wine to offer. We watched Chelsea win 3–0 and were a bit worried about the American election, where Trump has called postal votes a 'fraud'. On Thursday, we watched Mass on livestream from an empty St. Joseph's, but Stephen made it feel more like the Last Supper by bringing to the laptop a piece of bread and a glass of wine.

Both Leanne and Faye took Lennie out for a short walk before preparing our meals. In the evening, after she'd gone up to bed, she came back down and wouldn't stop talking. So, we turned off an interesting French film. From my perspective it had been a wasted evening. On Friday, I managed to do some thinning of files before we watched Mass on livestream. I then started planning to send around seventy-five cards for Christmas. Stephen took Lennie out for a walk and after supper Marie played a couple of games of draughts with her. It was another mixed night. Lennie went up and put on her nightie and then came downstairs three or four times to complain and kiss me 'good night'. On Saturday morning, I cleared emails and tried to sort out accumulations of charity cards before we attended Mass on livestream. We then drove to Sainsbury's, where I withdrew £410 from the ATM. Stephen made us a tasty tuna pasta. We watched a Women's T20 match which went down to the last ball, and then Chelsea's defeat of Sheffield United 4–1.

On Sunday, after breakfast, I cleared emails before we attended Mass on livestream from St. Joseph's. At 11 a.m., at Mgr. Tony's suggestion, the three of us went to the front door to observe two minutes' silence on Remembrance Sunday. Gilly, in lockdown, phoned us and we had a good half-hour's chat. It was good to hear that Katie had achieved a very good MSc in Edinburgh. As usual, Lennie mucked up the evening with her time gap. On Monday, I had problems with the laptop, and we didn't get the livestream Mass until Fr. Tom's homily. Leanne took Lennie out for a brief walk and later we noticed that Lennie's mobility has declined noticeably in the last couple of weeks. I arranged for Dr. Barnado to phone us on Friday about Lennie's problems and also made her an appointment with Vision Express. Faye took Lennie for a short walk before cooking our supper. On Tuesday, I cleared emails and paid a charity subscription by phone but was again late in getting through to the livestream Mass. Faye took Lennie for a walk around Whitmore Common and then made us a tasty lunch.

"Stephen and I then watched the T20 Final while trying to cope with Lennie driving us mad. Faye cooked us a nice supper." We were worried about a potential civil war situation in the U.S.

On the second Wednesday in November, I recorded a modest day. I was having problems with the laptop, but we managed to get to the livestream Mass on time and "the three of us watched it in peaceful harmony". Accidentally, we discovered that "the BBC were showing the service in Westminster Abbey to commemorate the 100th anniversary of the service for the 'Unknown Soldier'. It was beautifully choreographed and very moving." Leanne came and took Lennie out for a very short walk. "She is in increasing pain with her legs." In the afternoon, the week's shopping was delivered, and I ordered next week's online. In the evening, we watched a couple of episodes of *Harlot* because my grandson Luke had a small part in it, but we decided not to watch it anymore.

On Thursday, I forwarded the Ed Miliband and A. Dodds Green Plan to members of the Justice and Peace Group. Two cleaners "brought up bread and wine to 'concelebrate'". After lunch, Stephen put on a DVD about the Battle of Britain. Lennie refused to watch it and slipped out of the back door. Stephen, bless him, went after her. Before she made our supper, Faye took Lennie out for a short walk. In the evening, we watched England vs Ireland. Three Chelsea youngsters were in the England team.

On Friday 13th, Dr. Barnado phoned and judged Lennie's knee problem was osteoarthritis and recommended a paracetamol before going for a walk. "A little to my surprise, he was a bit concerned about how I was coping and seemed to imagine a future when it may be necessary to find some other way of caring for Lennie." After this, the three of us "attended livestream Mass. When Leanne came, she drove Lennie up to Newlands Corner before preparing our lunch. Stephen took her out for a short walk with a paracetamol as Dr. Barnado had suggested. Lennie's restlessness continued and she just doesn't realise my limited mobility." As usual, an angry Lennie destroyed our evening. On Saturday, I cleared emails before we attended livestream Mass. Afterwards, we drove to Sainsbury's where Stephen did a forty-minute shop. Back home we watched an interesting Women's rugby match between England and France, which we won. Lennie now has a forty-year memory loss and is wondering where the children are. All three of us enjoyed Mozart's Requiem from the Coliseum, where we used to go years ago. On Sunday, around 1 a.m., Lennie got dressed but returned to bed. I had problems with my laptop, but we managed to follow Mass on livestream. Soon afterwards, Gilly phoned, as did Richard in the evening. We then watched Belgium, with four ex-Chelsea players, beat England 2–0.

On Monday morning, Stephen and Lennie put out all the washing on the radiators. We then participated in the livestream Mass with our piece of bread and mug of wine and water. Faye took Lennie out for a short walk before she gave us a tasty lunch. During the rest of the day, I tried to read more of Richard Gaillardetz's book on Vatican II. We gave Lennie an Ibuprofen and it seemed to work, so that when Vicky took her out for a walk later, she managed to go round the block. It was much the same on Tuesday. After breakfast, I managed to clear emails before the three of us attended Mass with our bread and wine. Leanne played draughts with Lennie before preparing our lunch. In the afternoon, we watched Australia's women beat India's women in a T20 match in Melbourne. In the evening, we watched a couple of episodes of *Utopia*. Andrew phoned and talked non-stop for half an hour. He was expecting his eye operation shortly.

Wednesday was a fairly typical day. "Lennie came to bed fully dressed. The three of us attended Mass online with our slice of bread and mug of wine. Have faith! Leanne came and took Lennie for a short walk. When the Sainsbury's shopping was delivered, Stephen kindly put it all away." I went upstairs to pay Everycare on online banking and then order next week's Sainsbury's delivery. Ann kindly phoned and we had a pleasant chat. Then Terry Dobson phoned, and he sounded OK with his Parkinsons. In the afternoon, I watched the England vs Ireland match, which we won 4–0. On Thursday, Lennie wasn't too well but after paracetamols she did get up and "I caught her trying to put on a bra as a pair of knickers". Later, Leanne took her for a walk round the block by the police station. In the afternoon, Stephen coped well with Lennie's interruptions while he watched a film and I tried to read more of the book on Vatican II. When Faye came, she took Lennie for a walk before preparing a salmon meal for us. When Faye left, Lennie changed her time frame and was concerned about the 'children'. Gilly phoned and chatted to her for a while until she calmed down.

On Friday, after breakfast, I cleared emails and thinned some charity requests until the three of us attended Mass on livestream from St. Joseph's. Leanne took Lennie out for a short walk before cooking us fish and chips. All the time I was trying to read Gaillardetz's book on Vatican II. Stephen was great at keeping the temperature down and he prepared supper. When Marie came, she took Lennie out for a walk. Stephen watched a Harlequins vs Exeter match and we then watched Episode 4 of *Utopia*. I went up to bed with Lennie around 10.15 p.m. "It's a weird life we're living at the moment trying to cope with Lennie's periods of anger and then suddenly the reverse. She has just said 'Are you alright?' to me in a caring sort of way."

After breakfast on Saturday, I cleared emails and sorted out the remaining grandchildren's saving books before the three of us attended a very prayerful Mass on livestream. Lennie nearly drove Stephen and me mad after lunch when we had non-stop sport, including England vs France women's rugby, Newcastle vs Chelsea, England vs France from Twickenham. Chelsea won 2–0. In the evening, we watched *Mary Poppins*. On Sunday, I sent Gilly an email suggesting that Lennie and I no longer be active trustees. I don't know what we would do without her. Mass was prayerful on the Feast of Christ the King. I put the TV on during the afternoon. By the time *Blue Planet II* came on, Lennie started questioning "where the children were and what the plans for tomorrow were, over and over again". Stephen came downstairs and helped get Lennie under control and made us supper. In the evening, Stephen and I "had to cope with one of her most aggressively angry hours and more until she finally went up to bed after lovingly kissing me around 9.15 p.m."

On Monday, Stephen kindly brought us a cup of tea in bed and Lennie "was delighted and asked, 'Who is that young man? What is his name?' I cleared emails before the three of us attended Mass on livestream. Leanne came and drove Lennie down to Vision Express for her eye test while Stephen and I went to Nationwide, where I paid for my Christmas presents for Douglas, Will and Iris. I then drove Stephen to St. Luke's, where he picked up his prescriptions. Stephen cooked our lunch and washed up afterwards. We had a strangely quiet afternoon until Natasha turned up and cooked us a supper of lasagne. Richard phoned and asked me to stop pestering him about going to Mass."

Tuesday was Andrew's birthday, and after we'd attended livestream Mass, we phoned him to sing 'Happy Birthday'. We prayed that his eye operation would be a success. Thursday started much the same. I started writing annual letters with Christmas cards; a slow business. Leanne came, cooked our lunch and took Lennie out for a walk. In the afternoon, both Stephen and Vicky took Lennie out for walks before Vicky cooked a tasty supper. Stephen put on *Home Alone,* which unusually amused Lennie. Sue phoned, probably in response to my recent email. They've had real family problems isolating because of COVID-19 in Italy. "I am lucky to have two lovely sisters. Lennie went up to bed at 9.30 p.m., after driving me mad for her inability to follow my suggestions about where things were."

My Friday diary noted that last night we couldn't find Lennie's nightie and she went to bed fully dressed. After breakfast, I cleared emails and sent one to our M.P. pleading for a retention of our development expenditure to 0.7%. It seems we'd heard from Sue that she'd had COVID-19. Having given Lennie an Ibuprofen, she was taken for a walk round the river and car park by Leanne. I contacted the parish office to suggest how to allocate a cheque for four different purposes. Vicky came and took Lennie out for a walk. In the afternoon, Chelsea beat Rennes away 2–1 with a late winner. Stephen cooked Lennie a second supper of cheese on toast, and I took her up to bed around 10 p.m.

My Wednesday diary recorded that our lovely son, Stephen, brought us two large mugs of tea and later helped Lennie make decisions about what to wear and fastened her beads, also making the bed for us. After breakfast, I cleared emails and then attended Mass online, praying for Andrew that his eye operation today would be successful. I also sent Sue an email supporting her and her family after COVID. After breakfast, I cleared emails before we attended Mass online, remembering Andrew's eye operation. Later, he phoned us after recovering from his anaesthetic. After Mass, I sent an email to Sue, whose family Andrew told us had had COVID problems. In the afternoon, I did my weekly Sainsbury's shopping online. Naomi was held up by traffic, but after she'd made supper, she took Lennie out for a brief walk. In the evening, I finished reading Ephesians and Isaiah but was unable to watch Luke in *Harlot* because of Lennie's demands. Stephen was talking brilliantly with Lennie. Before Mass on livestream, I managed to prepare another couple of Christmas cards. Before Leanne cooked our lunch, she took Lennie for a walk, as did Marie before she cooked our supper. In the late afternoon we watched the T20 match between South Africa and England, which we won on the last couple of balls. Stephen put on *Home Alone,* but Lennie just wouldn't relax and watch it. Infuriatingly, she kept saying things like she just wanted to have a talk with me. It was halfway through the film before she began to calm down.

"On Saturday after lunch, Lennie was going on and on about taking the children home – totally resistant to the realities that this is our home, and all our children are in their fifties! The argument went on more and more angrily for well over an hour and there was absolutely no reasonable exchange or dialogue. Stephen was afraid I'd have a heart attack and suggested to Lennie the answer might be a care home. Lennie very slowly calmed down."

On Sunday afternoon, we spent some time watching the T20 match, which England won with only a couple of balls to go, and the Chelsea–Spurs game which ended 0–0. Monday was my 88th birthday, but Lennie didn't realise this early on. During the day, I had phone calls from our children and grandchildren and Ann. "Bless them all." On Tuesday 1st December, relations with Lennie were difficult and I was very angry in the afternoon when, in the middle of an interesting French film, she just wouldn't stop talking. In the morning, we complemented Mass with bread and wine, which we offered in parallel to the consecration. Leanne washed Lennie's hair while I spent an hour writing Christmas cards with lengthy letters. To the four oldest grandchildren, I added a copy of *Laudato Si.*

"Lennie seems very difficult these days. Last night she put on her day clothes on top of her nightie, but I managed to persuade her to come back to bed." After breakfast, I cleared about twenty-five emails before the three of us attended Mass online, sharing a piece of bread and glass of wine and water. The Sainsbury's shopping was delivered and later I booked next week's shopping. Leanne and Faye both took Lennie out for a walk before they prepared lunch and supper. In the evening, I managed to watch Chelsea beat Seville 4–0. Lennie wrecked the first half for Stephen. On Thursday, the day passed much as usual with emails, Christmas cards and Mass. Belinda and Faye took Lennie out for a walk, and I slotted in some time reading scripture. On Friday, I recorded that we had made love around midnight. Stephen kindly helped Lennie get dressed and Leanne took her for a walk before cooking lunch. We then drove Stephen over to his apartment for a quick check-up. In the evening, we watched a film based on Shakespeare's *Coriolanus*. For much of the first half, Lennie wouldn't stop talking and demanding answers to her fanciful questions, assuming we were either going 'home' or to Mass.

On Saturday, I sent an email to Mario, who is seventy-nine tomorrow. With help from Lennie, Stephen brought down the Christmas tree from the loft and fixed it with lights and decorations. In the afternoon, we watched Chelsea beat Leeds 3–1. Then, on Sunday, I wondered how I would cope as things got worse and I was frightened by how near we got to hitting each other. This wasn't the first time I'd exploded with Lennie. She seemed to spend all her time gabbling away "throughout all of a TV film which Stephen was watching, or after supper when we were listening to the news. She seems quite impervious to other people's expectations and needs and without a sense of community. I must pray not to explode so easily but Lennie does drive me mad."

On Monday, I took a taxi to and from the Royal Surrey Hospital, where "I had my annual pacemaker check-up" and was told it should last another five or six years. For only the second time since March, we attended the Immaculate Conception Vigil Mass at St. Pius'. Richard came with a present for Lennie, but stayed at the door, due to lockdown.

Tuesday was Lennie's 85th birthday. At Mass, she "was quite strange and went off to look for lipstick in the middle of the Mass." Around teatime, Andrew came with some presents for Lennie, and we had a delightful firework display in the garden. Unexpectedly, Chelsea had a Champions League match that evening, which ended in a 1–1 draw.

On Wednesday, I cleared over twenty emails before Mass and afterwards I wrote about seven charity cheques, which Leanne kindly posted. After lunch, I ordered the Sainsbury's shopping online for both 16th and 19th December. Belinda took Lennie out for a walk before cooking us supper. I read the last couple of chapters of Matthew before moving on to Mark. On Thursday, the cleaners didn't come as usual. Leanne and Faye both took Lennie out for a walk before preparing our lunch and supper. In the evening, Lennie was "a menace, interrupting everybody and not allowing others to watch a programme". During the day I managed to read up to Mark Ch 8. Friday was another very difficult day, during which we were warned that Lennie might become incontinent. She fell asleep during livestream Mass. During the day I read a lot of Andrew's very interesting novel about the closure of the parish church at Kidlington. "Stephen has just noted, for the second time recently, that Lennie had gone into the kitchen to go to the loo in the vegetable bucket. Today we had signs that Lennie's toilet needs might become a more serious issue."

On Saturday, "Lennie had problems finding non-wet knickers and had shambolic drawers. Stephen spent some time sorting it out and arranging a wash in the washing machine." In the evening, "Lennie's behaviour was appallingly provocative. Despite repeated pleas from Stephen and me, she kept mucking around with electrical wiring. In the end, we turned off the TV and became quiet." Sunday was another mixed day. "The Taizé hymn at Mass reminded me it was one of the many places we had been to in our blessed lives. During the evening, we watched a couple of episodes of *Pride and Prejudice*. Monday was my brother David's 85th birthday, but I don't know whether he is alive or dead. Be with him, Lord." Both Leanne and Faye took Lennie out for a walk before they prepared meals. During the day, we watched the final episode of *Pride and Prejudice* and I tried to follow *The Young Victoria* but was frustrated by Lennie's non-stop interruptions. My Tuesday diary recorded: "Last night Lennie came to bed fully dressed and this always means I have to be very persuasive several times during the night and get her back into bed rather than wandering off. Both of us started transferring dates from our 2020 to our 2021 diaries. The three of us then attended Mass along with our offering of a slice of bread and mug of wine and water. I paid Angela Sharpe for next year's 'Bible Alive'. Faye took Lennie out for a walk twice today before she cooked our meals. Stephen put on an interesting French film this evening."

On the third Wednesday of December, I booked Mass at St. Pius' on Christmas morning and at St. Joseph's on our wedding anniversary. "Lennie just isn't 'with us', though, at the moment and doesn't take on board the realities of the lockdown and that she hasn't taught at school for twenty-five years." I paid the Everycare bill online and ordered loads of chocolates to give to our carers for Christmas. It was helpful that we were sent an email with who our carers were going to be. Thursday was a bit of a mixture as we were getting ready for Christmas. Richard decided not to come because of Tier 3 restrictions, but we had cheerful exchanges with Will and Iris. Stephen went out for a short walk with Lennie, "who seems totally oblivious to my physical limitations". I read several articles in *RENEW* which were critical of clericalism and authoritarianism in the institutional Church.

Friday was another fairly busy domestic day. "Last night wasn't easy and I began to wonder whether I needed an extra hour from the carers, for example, 8.30–9.30 p.m., to monitor Lennie's undressing and preparing her clothes for the next day." On Saturday, Bishop Richard celebrated Mass with the investment of a new deacon and John Lamb's retirement. Afterwards, we drove Stephen to Boots to pick up his prescriptions. The Sainsbury's shopping was delivered mid-afternoon. "Lennie worried me by opening the washing machine door and putting a load of food into the oven." Stephen probably sorted it out. Gilly turned up with Christmas presents for Richard and Andrew and news about a new Tier 4. They both came late in the evening with their presents.

On Sunday, we attended a very pleasant livestream Mass. "I had a lovely, sympathetic and supportive letter from Gilly, advising me to get carers involved in dressing Lennie. I am inclined to agree but hesitate." On Monday, I noted: "As usual these days, Lennie went to bed with all her clothes on. Around 4 a.m. I found her a new pair of knickers and persuaded her to return to bed. But I don't think I slept between 4 a.m. and 6 a.m. And Lennie didn't wake until after 7.30 a.m. I then helped her put on a sanitary towel in her knickers with the tights on the <u>outside</u>." Before the three of us attended a peaceful and prayerful Mass online, I cleared emails. Stephen kindly put all the washing on radiators. Leanne came and took Lennie for a short walk. I managed to read Chapters 14–18 of John's Gospel. In the evening, Chelsea struggled to beat West Ham.

On Tuesday 22nd, my diary records "a terrible night. In the early hours Lennie must have gone out of the bedroom and later returned at least ten times. I kept calling her back, but she was absolutely obsessed with the need to go out to school or the children. Eventually, she stayed downstairs with Stephen, who this morning told me she had boiled eight eggs. What then becomes a major concern is that she causes a gas explosion by leaving the gas on." Stephen complains that she also mucked up some wiring for the

Christmas tree. This morning, I wondered about various types of Everycare cover, "but this morning it is obvious that Everycare could not cope with the sort of problem we had last night". The three of us attended livestream Mass and I then, with difficulty with an ageing laptop, managed to complete an online order for Sainsbury's shopping. The evening was pleasant and friendly.

One of our carers had COVID. Stephen fed us and then we watched Chelsea lose 3–1 to Arsenal. "Lennie had problems thinking Maureen was going to call and drive her home." Stephen took her out for a walk. On Sunday, Stephen had a sore throat, so isolated himself a bit. But he joined us for Mass online and later prepared our meals. In the mid-afternoon, Richard, Luke and Ben came and kept their distance outside the house; it was good to see them after so many months. I started reading Joan Chichester's *The Time is Now*. On Monday, the three of us attended Mass on livestream on the Feast of the Holy Innocents. Carers took Lennie for a walk, and it was otherwise a fairly normal day.

Tuesday 29th was Lennie's and my 60th wedding anniversary. "We drove to St. Joseph's, where Mgr. Tony and Fr. Tom both came over to wish us well and quietly give us a bottle of Brut. How very kind of them. There were a good few St. Pius parishioners afterwards and quite a number of phone calls, including from Doug's family. Gilly kindly brought us lunch, which we would have had in her house had we not been in lockdown. At one point Lennie had three blouses on. Stephen got her to take off two of them and then she calmed down. We started watching 'The First Thirty Years' collection of our family photos ... Thank You, Lord, for our 60th anniversary and the love and support we have been given today. Help me be a better husband in the remaining years we have."

On the final Wednesday of the year, I found Lennie had taken my vest and shirt from 'my' chair. The three of us attended Mass, after which I sent out half a dozen thank you messages for presents yesterday. I finished reading Joan Chichester's *The Time is Now*, "in other words to follow biblical evidence that we are all called to be prophets but that includes being persistent in <u>acting</u> on the job and seeking justice and challenging the powerful, including the institutional Church". After the Sainsbury's shopping had been delivered, I spent about an hour ordering next week's shopping online. Faye took Lennie round the block and then cooked supper. Thursday was the last day of the year 2020. Lennie was in a strange mood. The cleaners came. I told Lennie that she couldn't put on a bra over a pair of knickers. Then, for the first time, I put on a large pad in a clean pair of knickers and finished putting on her skirt before going to the other bedroom to attend Mass on livestream.

On the last day of the year, I added that as long ago as May it had seemed to me that this year's diary was chiefly dealing with Lennie's dementia. "As of now, I feel that there is enough over the past six or so months to trace the development of the illness and of the limitations of my attempts to cope with it as a loving and caring Christian. It hasn't been easy, and I've got quite a short fuse. During the whole year we've had carers twice a day, morning and evening, and I've declined in mobility and so become more and more dependent on the carers and Stephen. COVID-19 has limited us greatly this year, but it hasn't bothered me all that much. But it has clearly limited what Lennie expects of life – going out and meeting people. But she really doesn't seem to be at all aware of the consequences of the pandemic and this evening was angry at being asked to go for a vaccine next week, feeling it was an unnecessary imposition. Before I forget, I have suddenly realised that I am eighty-eight and not likely to live much longer. I'm sure Lennie would then need to go into a care home. I also have a sense of guilt that I didn't persist with recommended exercises – so that it is my fault that my mobility has declined, so that I don't go on any of Lennie's walks."

CHAPTER 9

The Year 2021– January 2022

This chapter deals with Lennie's deteriorating dementia in her final year at our marital home at 7 Oak Tree Gardens, before going into a care home, Claremont Court, on 31st January 2022. With hindsight, it was a very difficult year for me, living twenty-four hours every day with someone who was likely to go walkabout any time of the day or night and therefore needed full-time attention, including the locking of all the external doors, the kitchen at night, and the garden gates. In this chapter I have tried to abbreviate, but also provide extracts from my diary of 4–500 words each day to facilitate the distinction being made about attending Mass 'sacramentally' or 'spiritually' with subsequent analysis, using selected detailed accounts.

I noticed that my writing of my diary on Friday 1st January 2021 was very clear. I clearly deteriorated over the next two years. Before we attended Mass on livestream on the Feast of Mary, the Mother of God, I cleared emails and paid the latest Everycare bill. When Stephen took Lennie out for a walk, it gave me the chance to skim the weekend *Tablet* and ponder whether or not to write them a letter protesting at the distinction being made between attending Mass 'sacramentally' and 'spiritually'. During the evening, Stephen put on a DVD about a young hacker. My diary for Saturday 2nd January recorded that Lennie went walkabout several times during the night and even brought me a cup of tea. After attending Mass on livestream, I believe in a period of 'lockdown' because of the COVID-19 pandemic, I finished and sent off my letter to the *Tablet*. In the afternoon, we watched Brighton come back to draw with Wolves 3–3.

Sunday 3rd January's diary noted that, "as usual, Lennie went to bed fully dressed, went downstairs in the middle of the night, eventually returned and rejoined me until we got up at 8 a.m. To my surprise, on a Sunday, there were no parishioners in the livestream, presumably due to 'lockdown' as a consequence of the COVID pandemic." Lennie was still doing the washing-up while I remained on the lounger. Monday 4th January was much as usual, and "the day occupied with the daily chores. Up to a point, I am coping with Lennie's memory loss and putting up with those occasions when she needs to be told that I am her husband, Mike."

0n Tuesday 5th January, Stephen and I watched a film about the young prophet, Greta Thunberg. During the day we heard from all four of our children, who were isolated from us during a period of 'lockdown' as a result of the COVID-19 pandemic. On Wednesday 6th January, the Feast of the Epiphany, I recorded that "Lennie continues to go to bed in her daytime clothes, though this morning she put on her tartan skirt under her blue dress". We attended Mass on livestream from St. Joseph's. On 7th January I found out that the *Tablet* had published my letter, though they omitted the first paragraph referring to Joan Chichester's inspiration. I failed in my attempt to renew my Blue Badge and aimed to get help from Gilly. Our carer, Vicky, took Lennie out for a walk and then invited her to join her in the kitchen where they had a good chat, "the best she'd had for a long time". Today we had the news about the Trump-encouraged attack on Capitol Hill. They sounded like Nazis to me. Our car was returned that afternoon after its annual M.O.T. with SEAT.

My diary of Friday 8th January noted that "Lennie slept all night with her blue summer dress on with her tartan skirt on top. This morning, she was complaining again about pain in her left leg, and she toyed with remaining in bed." Before attending Mass on livestream, I tidied up my file from a company called SMC going back to our purchase of a SEAT in 2014. The readings differed from those recommended in *Bible Alive*. Saturday 9th January turned out to be a somewhat frustrating day. Lennie was downstairs with Stephen until about 4.30 a.m., when she came up to join me in bed. I didn't manage to read any of the Old Testament. In the evening, Lennie was still unclear that this was our house, but she came down to watch TV in a nightie and cardigan. Around 5 a.m. on Saturday 16th January, "Lennie 'wanders' around the house. After four or five wanders, I managed to persuade her to come to bed and we managed to sleep peacefully together until around 7.30 a.m., when I led us with the Mass readings and the prayers." I cleared emails before the three of us attended Mass on livestream. During the rest of the day, we watched cricket and football on the TV, ending with Chelsea's not very impressive 1–0 defeat of Fulham. On Sunday 17th January, I noted that Lennie "is always irritated and picks a fight when she sees me sitting and reading the *Observer*. I've taken out four pages on climate change by an Extinction Rebellion activist. In spite of Lennie's continuous chat and repeated questions, I managed to skim today's *Observer,* with its quite pessimistic analyses of the continuing effect of Trumpism and the failure to face up to the challenge of climate change."

Monday 18th January was fairly stressful, starting with an early visit from Thames Water mechanics, who arranged to come and repair our leaking tap on the 29th. The three of us then attended Mass online. "I did notice what looked like faeces on the stair lift. I've previously noticed it on Lennie's loo and have washed it. But this latest looks as if it is more serious ... Lennie then drove me mad. Firstly, she was unable to make us a mug of tea; then she couldn't find the end of the wire connection later, though earlier she'd switched it on. She is unable to follow instructions about where things are, on the right of the table, etc. When Natasha came Lennie decided not to go for a walk but spent nearly three-quarters of an hour chatting, mainly about primary school teaching. Natasha helped me to cope with Lennie, who persistently wanted to put on her raincoat and 'go home'. Lennie's world is difficult to cope with."

Lennie's anxieties seemed to dominate Tuesday 19th January. She spent much of the night downstairs, but when I suggested she join me, she said she didn't want to go to bed with me. I had difficulties with Google and my laptop, and I was unable to attend the online Mass from St. Joseph's. So, later on we attended online Mass from Alabama, though I didn't like the frequent Latin insertions. Today was Katie's 25th birthday and she had a major job interview, which was successful. In the evening, "I managed to cope with Lennie's permanent questions about her dad, where we are, where her Mum is, and so on".

My diary for Wednesday 20th January noted my concerns that Lennie was showing signs of incontinence. We got no sound from St. Joseph's but followed the Mass as best we could. The bulk of the day was taken up with the inauguration of Joe Biden and prayers in St. Matthew's Catholic Cathedral. I noted in my diary, in some detail, four quite distinct stages in Lennie's and my relationship that night. It ranged from the closest cuddles for some time to refusing to come to bed with me "and also accusing our carers of only being concerned about 'money, money, money'". After lunch, Lennie had one of her awful spells, "threatening both Stephen and me. Stephen is doing well keeping cool". Since Paula left at 1p.m., "Lennie has gone bonkers insisting we go and look after the children, totally resistant to the response that they are all in their fifties. Sometimes Lennie looks potentially likely to hit us, but Stephen and I are aware that with the coronavirus it wouldn't be safe to put Lennie into a care home. Stephen and I are putting up with her persistent harassing, but it means our ordinary lives are destroyed. I managed to see Lennie had her late-night pills. She physically showed me she needed a tampax in her knickers, quite oblivious of the need to be discreet."

On Friday 22nd January, I noted that "Lennie has absolutely no awareness of my mobility limitations since my leg operations last year ... I found it was necessary to help Lennie distinguish between a bra and pants and Stephen very kindly came to help us. There are times when Lennie seems quite sound but other times when she can't distinguish between her bra and her knickers and needs help."

On Saturday 23rd January, I noted that Lennie was sick last night. After clearing emails and the three of us attending Mass online, we spent the rest of the day in front of the TV watching episodes of *Outnumbered* and *Only Fools and Horses*. I was allowed to sit on the lounger all day. On Sunday, 24th January, I noted that Lennie had spent a lot of the night ranting on about the need to pay for her clothes. We had some of the heaviest snow I'd ever seen that morning. I spent much of the day skimming the *Observer* and watching Chelsea beat Luton 3–1 in the Cup. I then had an unexpected explosion of diarrhoea, which took a long time to clear up. Lennie repeatedly asked me to go out for a walk with her and later became angry and wanted to go back to her home. In the early hours of Monday 25th January, Lennie went off fully dressed and only returned to bed around 4.30 a.m. After lunch, we discovered that Frank Lampard had been sacked as Chelsea's manager and replaced by Thomas Tuchel. On a completely different note, recently, I had been ploughing through the Old Testament and today had reached Chapter 15 of Ezekiel. In the late evening, Stephen and Lennie "verbally battered each other over a late supper requested by Lennie".

On Tuesday 26th January, I was pleased to record that "Lennie remained with me all last night together in our bed. Marie came at 8 a.m. She was brilliant on this first of her morning visits. She went upstairs and chatted with Lennie, apparently seeing her have a shower and her selection of clothes." I checked emails and with difficulty amended the Sainsbury's online shopping before getting the online Mass for the three of us. Two young men from the solar company ESE came to check our solar panel system. They found no problem inside the house but recommended a visit to check outdoor connections when the weather improved. Wednesday 27th January was Stephen's 56th birthday. Bless him for all he does for us. We attended Mass at 1 p.m. from EWTN. Andrew visited us and we watched Chelsea only scrape a 0–0 draw with Wolves. During the rest of the day, I managed to read up to Ezekiel 37. On Thursday 28th January, the three of us attended the 10 a.m. Mass before the rest of the day dribbled past. I skimmed today's *Guardian* which Stephen brought home. We and the carers coped with an angry Lennie during the day.

On Friday 29th January, I "just couldn't help Lennie more than find her a pair of knickers and managed to stop her trying to put on a blouse as knickers. That is why we really do need the 8–9 a.m. female help for Lennie ... I managed to clear emails before the three of us attended today's livestreamed Mass from St. Joseph's ... After Leanne's shift ended, Lennie went on and on about going for a walk, quite insensitive to our situation, which included the visit of four Thames Water engineers. Lennie's non-stop talk drives me nuts as I try to read some scripture." In the afternoon, we participated for about half an hour in a Zoom meeting of the Family Group. "Lennie entered one of the combative phases, demanding to go out and find home and went on and on about teachers and parents. She got angrier and angrier and threatened to get the police ... Stephen and I tried to ease things, but Lennie was totally unable to participate in any discussion about facts, such as this is my/our home. A quiet

Lennie came down mid–evening and joined me and said how much she enjoyed being with me."

On Saturday 30th January, "Lennie went to bed in her pyjamas but dressed around 1–2 a.m., calling me something like 'a nasty bad-tempered oaf'. At 7.30 a.m., she brought me up a mug of coffee and a scone! After breakfast, I cleared emails before the livestream Mass was attended by the three of us." During the day we watched TV: *Outnumbered* in the morning, international athletics in the afternoon, and *Independence Day* in the evening. On Sunday 31st January, we had a lovely email from Richard about playing with Will and Iris last Sunday. The three of us then watched Mass online. "When we went downstairs, everything changed. Lennie became aggressively combative and in spite of Stephen and me trying to keep things cool, she was very difficult. Then Gilly phoned and it gave us a break. After lunch the TV stopped working and we missed the Chelsea vs Burnley game, which we won with Alonso's goal. Not an easy day."

On Monday 1st February, "Lennie went to bed last night fully dressed and spent an hour or so 'making breakfast' in the middle of the night". During the day, I paid Everycare online and was concerned that our current annual costs were about £27k, but so far, we had not needed to dig into our savings. During the day I made charitable payments to our trustee children as a token of gratitude for all the work they did for the Trusts.

On Tuesday 2nd February, the Feast of the Presentation in the Temple, I tried to understand at what point the three wise men visited Jesus, after which Joseph took Mary and Jesus to Egypt. I spent much of the day looking up Old Testament quotations. On Wednesday 3rd February, I noted again that Lennie had gone wandering in the early hours and had later slept on this morning as I got up in time for Marie's first shift. So, Stephen and I attended Mass online on our own.

When I was watching the TV, it was always difficult when Lennie would not stop talking with endless questions. At some stage, Stephen switched on Channel EWTN, which was "an impressive illustration of Catholic commitment led by some Divine Mercy Sisters". In many respects Thursday 4th February was a fairly typical day. After a good night's sleep, "Lennie started chatting, saying she didn't feel like going to school". I cleared emails, the cleaners came, and we attended Mass on livestream. Stephen and I took it in turns to cope with Lennie's non-stop chatting. In the evening, after Chelsea had beaten Spurs, Lennie was obsessed with 'the children'.

Friday 5th February was much the same after a reasonably good night's sleep. Two or three of the carers took Lennie for a short walk. I checked a couple of insurances and the three of us watched Mass on livestream before going down for coffee. I continued my reading of the Old Testament and we later played three rounds of 'elevenses'. Later, we put on the DVD of the first thirty years of our married lives. I skimmed through the *Tablet,* which I noted was becoming much more international.

On Saturday 6th February, I checked the battery of our car, which I hadn't driven for some time. As usual on a winter's Saturday, we spent the afternoon watching Six Nations Rugby and in the evening *Independence Day Resurgence*, which Lennie declined, and *Line of Duty*. On Sunday 7th February, I cleared emails before the three of us attended livestream Mass. But my laptop played tricks and went blank just after the *Agnus Dei* on the livestream Mass. This seems to be happening quite regularly these days and I just don't seem to be keeping up to date with all the latest I.T. developments. After Mass, we went downstairs and watched the Test Match and received phone calls from my dear sister, Ann, and from Gillian and Andrew. "Lennie rattled the doors, so Stephen took her for a walk at half-time, with Lennie crying she wanted her mother and father, brother and sister! Lennie was very restless and went to bed around 5.45 p.m." In the evening, Stephen and I watched Chelsea beat Sheffield United 2–1.

On the morning of Monday 8th February, "Lennie was irritated that I hadn't consulted her about our carer Marie coming and got herself up and dressed before Marie came. Upstairs, I cleared emails and put on Mass on livestream on the diocesan Feast of St. Cuthmann. After Mass, we watched the end of day four of the England-India Test Match." Sleet prevented Lennie being taken out for a walk by either of her two carers today. After lunch, I dozed for a while. "When I woke, it was in the middle of angry exchanges between Stephen and Lennie. We struggled through the early afternoon with Lennie in a different world. I wasn't her husband; we hadn't lived here for twelve years; Stephen and I were both liars; and Lennie laid the table for the 'children'." But I insisted I wasn't going to be pushed into going to bed before 10 p.m.

Tuesday 9th February was a strange sort of day. Lennie got helpful support from her carers but she didn't make life easy during the rest of the day. "At one point Lennie's persistent messing around led me to explode. But I apologised within a few seconds, and we survived. Stephen had to put up with some awful accusations and being told to leave this house." In the evening, Lennie decided she wanted to go to bed. "Almost immediately after one of the carers had gone, Lennie was in one of her awful states worrying about where the children were. After over half an hour of getting nowhere we phoned Gilly to see if she could chat with Lennie. But sadly, Lennie was angry with Gilly. Later Gilly phoned back but nothing changed. Strangely, Lennie remained quiet, stroking a wooden painted dog that we had bought her on advice, as we watched a brutal film about cocaine."

Wednesday 10th February was a mixed day. The three of us attended livestream Mass and then three ESE mechanics came, hopefully to repair our solar panel connections. While watching the Lambeth Farm Show on TV, "sadly, Lennie has no staying power and was soon irritating Stephen and me by first asking us over and over again about the next Mass this evening, and then secondly, messing about laying the table for how many over and over again. Lennie seems totally unaware of the reality of COVID-19." We phoned BT clarifying how to use their Halo 2 system. We attended Mass on livestream on the Feast of Our Lady of Lourdes. Afterwards, I managed to complete an online weekly shopping request to Sainsbury's. Belinda came and took Lennie out for a walk and played games of cards with her. During the day, I read Chapters 12–16 of Matthew's Gospel. Chelsea beat Barnsley in the FA Cup. Vicky came and dressed Lennie for bed, who later came down to watch TV, where she "dozed on the sofa and occasionally expressed anger that I hadn't gone up to bed with her". On Friday 12th February, Lennie came down early and Vicky chatted to her and played cards with her so that I was able to go upstairs, clear emails, tidy up correspondence and start shredding files before the three of us watched livestream Mass. As usual, Lennie was very angry when I didn't go up to bed with her at 8.30 p.m.

On Saturday 13th February I noted that, "Lennie has been going on and on about 'waiting for Mike' and 'who are you?' She didn't seem to see me as her husband. Later, she came to me and said Stephen was a lovely young man and she wanted to marry him. My pointing out that he was our son just didn't register." Still under 'lockdown', we watched Mass online this Sunday morning, 14th February. Gilly phoned us and told us Katie had been offered a job as a psychiatric assistant and Douglas had been offered some jobs in P.E. at St. Peter's. In the afternoon, we watched the France–Ireland Six Nations match. In the evening, Lennie "was obsessed with looking after children, sometimes school, sometimes ours, and suggested her husband Mike had walked out on her, and so forth. For over half an hour I let her discuss this and her attractions to a young man who had been friendly and helpful. In the end, Lennie rather damaged Stephen's and my evening."

Monday 15th February appeared to be a typical and somewhat frantic day. Stephen helped me shower. During the day, I read a couple of chapters from Genesis and Mark. In the evening, Stephen and I watched Chelsea beat Newcastle 2–0. Faye dressed Lennie ready for bed, but she came down fully dressed and was then fairly angry with me for not joining her in bed sooner. After emailing Villanova, they replied that they had rejected my paper "because I hadn't developed my own argument but relied too heavily on outlining other people's work".

Shrove Tuesday, 16th February, saw Vicky do a good job with Lennie, changing the underwear and blouse she'd worn all night and showering her. The three of us attended Mass on livestream from St. Joseph's, with Mgr. Tony urging us to use Lent as a preparation for the Easter season to follow. "Lennie was bombarding me with demands to lay the table etc. Eventually, I exploded, and she came over to me threatening to hit me and telling me to get out of the house. Stephen helped calm things down. Then Marie arrived and within a few minutes had taken Lennie, who'd walked over to kiss me, out for a walk ... I tried, unsuccessfully, to read more Mark and Stephen came to the rescue and put on an interesting comedy. But Lennie broke off around 4 p.m. and wanted to lay the table, ready for 'the children' and became quite heated." In the evening, I read as far as Mark 16. On Ash Wednesday, 17th February, I noted that Lennie had gone to bed dressed over her nightie. After breakfast it took me an hour to order next week's Sainsbury's online shopping. I typed another page of Stephen's blog. I managed to read the first five chapters of Luke's Gospel during the day.

On Thursday 18th February, Faye spent around three-quarters of an hour helping Lennie wash and dress while I sent donations to six charities, checked emails and then found the livestream Mass on the laptop. Unexpectedly, early in the afternoon, Richard turned up with Ben, Will and Iris. I tried to persuade Will and Iris to read a chapter of the Bible each day, "but I don't think I persuaded them. Because of the lockdown, they remained outside. Stephen persuaded us to go out into the garden, where I pruned a couple of roses and helped calm things down. Then Marie arrived and within a few minutes had taken Lennie, who'd walked over to kiss me, out for a walk. I walked ten short lengths of the garden, but realised how very unstable I am on my legs at the moment. I then read five chapters of Luke. Lennie was very disturbed and concerned about 'the children'."

On Friday 19th February, "Lennie went to bed fully dressed ... When I came down for breakfast, Faye helped her wash and change some of her clothes." After lunch, we drove Stephen over to Cranleigh to pick up his post. I was quite relieved that my driving seemed OK after several months of the pandemic lockdown. "Physically, I am aware of a rapid decline in my physical energy." I read more of Bill Gates's *How to Avoid a Climate Disaster*. "Lennie was fully dressed, and we went to bed together without any angry exchanges." February 20th seemed to be a fairly standard Saturday with plenty of sport on TV, including Chelsea's disappointing 1–1 draw with Southampton. Stephen put on a DVD, *Little Women,* which Lennie stayed to watch. Afterwards, we went up to bed together. These days we were still saying some prayers routinely in bed before getting up. This included the Mass reading and *Bible Alive's* reflections.

"After breakfast on Sunday 21st February, Jane from Everycare phoned us and gave us the shocking news that one of our carers had COVID-19 and we needed to isolate ourselves." I was concerned about my vulnerability because of my age. The three of us then attended Mass on livestream. In the afternoon, Lennie went on and on about supper and bringing the children home. Then she began to threaten Stephen and me with the walking stick. After some time and in desperation we phoned Gillian. The phone call calmed us down enough for Lennie to go for a walk with Stephen.

On Monday 22nd February, after a pretty good night's sleep, "Lennie was in a pre-retirement time warp". At 'What's On' Catholic daily Masses, "the three of us then attended Mass on livestream" and managed to follow the EWTN Alabama Mass. "Sadly, around Communion, Lennie became absolutely obsessed about the time and what about 'the children' and telling their parents where they were. For half an hour, Stephen and I stressed that I needed help with my laptop." On Tuesday 23rd February, Guiseppe didn't get the laptop back to us in time so the three of us followed the EWTN Mass from Alabama. Everycare carers were still taking Lennie out for short walks. In the evening, I watched an excellent Chelsea team beat Atlético Madrid in the European Championship. On Wednesday 24th February, "Lennie got half–dressed last night. I took the opportunity to tell Gilly and Stephen that I loved them. We celebrated Mass online and, in the afternoon, I managed to get Frances's Zoom meeting of the Family Group. I'm finding it difficult to read five chapters of the Gospels each day during Lent."

On Thursday 25th February, I was woken early "by an insistent Lennie, who wanted to know, over and over again, who would be taking her to school. She was totally resistant to advice that schools were shut because of COVID-19 and anyway, she retired from teaching twenty-five years earlier ... Stephen has taken over with Lennie and is chatting to her endlessly." The three of us attended Mass on livestream from St. Joseph's. Afterwards, we watched the Test Match with India. In the evening, I participated in a diocesan Zoom meeting. On Friday 26th February, I recorded that "as usual, Lennie went to bed fully dressed and then started wandering around the room from 5 a.m. onwards. After clearing emails, the three of us attended Mass on livestream from St. Joseph's. My dear sister Ann phoned this morning. After lunch, Lennie threatened to go for a walk to find Maureen, who died ten years earlier!" Stephen took her for a short walk, after which I sat outside with her on a lovely afternoon. I finished reading Bill Gates's book on tackling climate change, while Lennie's carers took her for short walks or played scrabble with her.

On Saturday 27th February, I was angry when I discovered all my clothes on the chair next to the bed had been nicked. "We had a bit of angry talk and for the first time I can remember she smacked me on the face. Fortunately, I resisted the temptation to headbutt her. Later, we started our day with today's Mass readings and prayers." In the afternoon, we watched some football and the Six Nations rugby match between England and Wales. The main theme of my diary on Sunday 28th February was coping with Lennie's memory loss and reminding her that I was her husband of sixty years and that we had lived in our present house for twelve years.

I have always regarded St. David's Day, 1st March, as the first day of spring and indeed it was a lovely day. It was a busy morning and I phoned ESE to carry out a check on our solar panels and Fr. Tony Lovegrove for an annual chat. The three of us attended Mass on livestream from St. Joseph's and as usual, Deacon Michael gave a thoughtful homily. I recorded that I was having serious problems with incontinence and urine trickling down my legs. The carers took Lennie out for short walks while I read Michael Mann's recent book, *The New Climate War*.

Tuesday 2nd March was a fairly standard day with Mass on livestream from St. Joseph's. In the afternoon, "Lennie was going on and on about looking after our children" so I went out into the garden and spent some time reading Michael Mann. On Wednesday 3rd March, I noted that "Lennie changed last night and wore a pyjama jacket on top of her skirt." The day didn't go smoothly, so I was late in getting livestream Mass. Then, in the middle of the Mass, ESE. phoned to arrange a check on our ten solar panels. I read some of Raymond Brown's commentary on Mark's Gospel.

In the evening, Stephen put on a film, *Charlotte Gray* about an S.O.E agent in Vichy France. Gilly called during the evening, and we struggled to remember what we had been doing during this boring time of lockdown.

I cleared emails before arranging the livestream Mass for the three of us. Thursday 4th March was another fairly ordinary day. Then I remained upstairs, preparing for this evening's diocesan 'invited' meeting. Andrew phoned and sounded quite chirpy, though he confirmed that he and Caroline had serious problems. We watched TV before going to bed. Friday 5th March was much the same. From around 5 a.m., "Lennie was getting dressed and messing around, not keen to get back into bed. Her talk was incessant and eventually, I was cross. This led to a fierce: 'You are bloody selfish; all you ever think about is 'me, me, me.'" She probably added 'I hate you' and more. Stephen had done some shopping at Sainsbury's and brought home a *Guardian* and *Daily Mail*! After clearing emails, the three of us attended livestream Mass. I cleared the downstairs loo, which had become clogged up. Before supper, we watched yesterday's 1–0 defeat of Liverpool by a superb goal by Mount. Stephen and I watched the first episode of *Deutschland 89* before we went to bed.

On Saturday 6th March, I noted that about 3.20 a.m., "Lennie was insisting on getting dressed. She messed around in her drawers for a couple of hours and refused to rejoin me in bed. In the end she wandered off. The three of us attended livestream Mass at St. Joseph's, where Mgr. Tony gave an interesting reflection on today's parable of the prodigal son. We remembered the famous painting in the Hermitage, St. Petersburg. Later, while Stephen took Lennie out for a walk, I drove to St. Joseph's, where I went to Confession with Fr. Roy, who recommended I pray the 'Our Father' slowly and repeatedly ... I felt it could easily be my last Confession and that I'm near the end of car mobility."

On Sunday 7th March, I noted that I'd "had a reasonable night's sleep with a fully-dressed Lennie until nearly 6 a.m. And then I patiently responded to her endless and repeated questioning about school, Mass and what we were going to do today. Two simple responses: schools are closed because of COVID-19 and you retired from teaching twenty-five years ago just didn't have any impact. I had my shower this morning and found myself thinking that it wouldn't be long before I'd need help ... Stephen spent half an hour responding to Lennie's repeated questions about this house and the fact we live there."

The three of us attended livestream Mass from St. Joseph's. "We are very lucky with our carers and IT people. I wasn't very successful reading about Michael Mann's book. In the early afternoon, I got so fed up with Lennie's questioning that I went out onto the patio for the rest of the afternoon. Gilly telephoned to check on us."

On Monday 8th March, Lennie decided to get up around 4 a.m., and eventually wandered off and couldn't be persuaded to come back to bed. But sadly, I couldn't go to sleep again. Stephen took Lennie for a walk and scaffolders came and did a good job. I spent time typing up one of Stephen's blogs. "The three of us then 'attended' Mass on livestream. Lennie was in tears at being told her mother had died thirty–five years earlier. Stephen and I discussed Lennie, but I'm still opposed to a care home. But Stephen was worried about his own health, and I sense he is looking forward to returning to Cranleigh after lockdown ends. During the afternoon, Lennie was bothered about packing a bag full of clothes, but where she was going wasn't at all clear."

On Tuesday 9th March, we didn't have too bad a night, though Lennie went wandering, fully dressed, probably around 3 a.m. She returned to bed, but I didn't get off to sleep after a 5 a.m. visit to the loo. Mandy came at 8 a.m. and helped chat to Lennie and with her help changed the bed linen. The ESE Solar Panel mechanics came late in the afternoon, and I finished reading Michael Mann's book. Stephen is continuing with his blogs and is angry if interrupted. We did an excellent job chatting to Lennie.

Wednesday 10th March was a fairly ordinary, busy day. "But Lennie was totally disorientated getting dressed ... She harangued Mandy for 'pushing her around'. It was quite embarrassing, but Mandy took it in her stride ... Luke phoned. He was finding the isolation difficult ... Lennie was difficult, laying the table for 'the children'." In the evening, "Lennie was locked into a small world before the deaths of her parents and sister. She tearfully expressed no knowledge of them." In the mid-evening Lennie was cross with me for not joining her in bed.

On Thursday 11th March, I noted that just before midnight I was woken by Lennie from a deep sleep, telling me it was time to get up. "Lennie eventually returned to bed and this morning cuddled me and said, 'Oh I do love you; I always will'." Before Mass, I cleared emails and sent a copy of my Villanova paper to Andrew, Mgr. Tony, and the Family and Justice and Peace groups. We drove Stephen to G-Live for his COVID-19 vaccine. The toe specialist came today for Lennie. "Soon after she had gone, Lennie started angrily demanding and threatening with her walking stick to 'go home' and tried to open both doors. Stephen and I repeatedly pointed out that this was our home. But all to no avail. Lennie was getting very angry and threatening. In the end, Stephen, bless him, offered to take her for a walk ... Stephen's gesture had quietened Lennie, who is wondering where all the people are. She is unaware of the 'lockdown' and that her parents died such a long time ago."

On Friday 12th March, I noted that "Lennie went to bed in a nightie but in the early hours got dressed. I managed to persuade her to come back to bed. But a new one this morning was her sudden objection to her attending Mass every day and feeling as if she was in a nunnery!" After reading Matthew's reflection on divorce (19: 11–12), I was worried about both Andrew and Richard, and I prayed for them both. I've given up drinking wine during Lent and haven't been overly impressed by the rather aimless *Invite* diocesan programme. During the day, I managed to do some typing of Stephen's blog. On Saturday 13th March, I did some more typing of it and Lennie "complained about my bad temper ... Gilly turned up and took Lennie for a short walk to celebrate Mother's Day the next day. Later, Richard turned up with Luke, Will and Iris. Lovely to see them." Later, we watched England beat France in the Six Nations rugby match; I went up to bed at 10 p.m. to join Lennie in bed.

On Sunday 14th March, I noted a difficult night when Lennie had opted "out of her nightie and got dressed with her summer skirt showing underneath her blue skirt ... For an hour after 3 a.m., she rummaged around in her drawers, supposedly getting dressed. An hour or two later, I did manage to fall asleep. Later, we managed to keep Lennie with us while I cleared emails, did some typing for Stephen and prepared for Mass on Mothering Sunday on livestream. After some time, we found it difficult to cope with Lennie, who insisted we were or should be preparing to feed 'the children' and cope with the 'other people' as well." Andrew came in the early afternoon, and we had an interesting chat.

He also made it clear he didn't think I was a good driver! Just before going to bed. "Lennie said she loves me but doesn't think I love her. Help me, Lord, to be a loving husband."

On Monday 15th March, we had a rather mixed start to the day before we read the day's Mass readings and said our prayers for the living and the dead. I cleared emails and sent some suggestions for changing the emphasis and focus of *RENEW* and 'Catholics for a Changing Church'. The three of us attended Mass on livestream and I managed to finish typing Stephen's blog. In the afternoon, we watched England's T20 match. Lennie was pretty angry with me for not going out with her. "She seems to be completely unaware of my physical disabilities, and that I have been unable to go for a walk for around two years now."

On Tuesday 16th March, "in the early hours, Lennie was wandering around, not really knowing what was going on. She was irritated by my suggesting she should come back to bed. She was quite switched off and objecting to the 'play' to the crowds! The three of us attended Mass on livestream. When Leanne came, she took Lennie for a walk while I, with difficulty, managed to complete my typing of Stephen's blog." In the afternoon, we watched England beat India in a T20 match. When Mandy came, she took Lennie out for another walk. "Lennie was pretty angry with me for not going out with her. She seems completely unaware of my physical disabilities. Lennie doesn't know what to do and resists being told what to do."

On Wednesday 17th March, Stephen and I enjoyed *The Farming Life* before breakfast. "Lennie was very involved with the children's cards sent to her on Mothering Sunday." Voytek came to tidy up the garden. The Sainsbury's online shopping was delivered mid-afternoon, and I typed out next week's request and corrected Stephen's blog. In the evening, we watched Chelsea beat Atlético Madrid in the Champions League. On Thursday 18th March, I recorded that "several times during the night Lennie wandered off, and several times returned to the bedroom saying, 'Where am I supposed to be going? What am I supposed to be doing?' In the end, I realised I wasn't going to sleep again." The carers took Lennie out for a short walk. Ann phoned, bless her. Lennie's cousin Peter also called and had a strange conversation with her. "Stephen and I struggled to watch the England vs India T20 match with all Lennie's questions and strange claims about what was going on. We watched the news about the coronavirus pandemic, which takes up more than half the news every day." I took part in the diocesan 'Invite' group that evening and during the day managed to read a few chapters of Luke's Gospel.

On Friday 19th March, Lennie joined me in reading Friday's Mass readings and saying our prayers for the living and the dead before getting up. I was exhausted for most of the day, but managed to pay Everycare and was grateful that Lennie's and my pensions enabled us to pay around £25k a year for our carers. We had a very informed conversation with Faye about Lennie's dementia. "Lennie expressed her usual anger that I hadn't gone up to bed with her."

On Saturday 20th March, while Stephen and I watched the Six Nations rugby matches, "Lennie was wondering whether she ought to retire! Over and over again she asked how old she was and suggested eighty–five wasn't a bad time. Her interruptions continued throughout the next game." On Sunday 21st March, I noted that "We didn't have a bad night, though Lennie was fully dressed in a summer dress and needed a wash this morning. Lennie was in a combative mood, but Stephen was at his best as a great conciliator. Today's Mass readings: stick with your suffering because God is with you. Help me, Lord. Lennie was busy finding the right clothes to wear. Gilly came with her two dogs and took Lennie out for a brief walk. She is much less mobile than only a month ago." In the afternoon, we watched Chelsea beat Sheffield United 2–0 in the quarter–final of the FA Cup. In the evening, I watched TV until I joined Lennie in bed at 10 p.m.

Monday 22nd March was much as usual, though the weather was so pleasant that Stephen put the washing out on the line outside. The three of us watched Mass online and were impressed by an excellent homily by Deacon Michael. During the day, I read about half of Wendy Mitchell's *Somebody I used to Know* about dementia, but to me, one of the carers, it made me wonder if I myself had early signs of dementia. In the afternoon, Lennie joined me on the patio for three-quarters of an hour when I was hoping to read. After supper I washed and dried Lennie's hair. "Sadly, Lennie was cross she hadn't put curlers in and was totally resistant to the idea that Hair Partners, shut at the moment, would take two and a half hours to do a perm."

Tuesday 23rd March was typical. "Lennie was also in a different time frame this morning. She didn't recognise our bedroom, which we'd slept in for over twelve years and wanted to be informed about all the other rooms in the house. In my frustration, I told myself that, "I need to forgive seventy-seven times!" Stephen kindly came up and helped me put on my clothes. A challenging article by Polly Toynbee in the *Guardian* about inequalities and lecturers on zero-hour contracts made me realise how lucky we have been with our pensions. Mandy came to get Lennie ready for bed.

On Wednesday 24th March, Lennie was taken up to Newlands Corner for the first time in months. After the Sainsbury's shopping delivery, I ordered next week's shopping online. I was interested in the differences in the experiences of dementia between Wendy Mitchell and Lennie. While Wendy was coping on her own with difficulty, "Lennie is not living on her own but with her family carers, husband and son, plus regular Everycare carers (20 hrs/wk). But many of the illustrations of decline are reflected in Lennie's memory loss and focus on old instances, for example, her parents and sister; the decline of her domestic capabilities such as cooking) but also personal capabilities such as showering; loss of memory of former friends, colleagues, etc. A carer helped Lennie put on her nightie, but by the time I went up to bed Lennie had fully dressed herself and this made me irritable."

On Thursday 25th March, "Lennie got up early as usual, and I didn't get back to sleep again. Guildford Community Mental Health team phoned and after Lennie passed it back to me, I noted an appointment in two weeks' time. When we discerned the alternative, Lennie went ballistic, angrily refused to be dragged into a meeting when "all they are interested in is 'money, money, money'! Faye came about this time and was very handy in calming the row down. The ESE engineers also came and repaired the solar panels." In the afternoon, with Lennie sitting three yards from me, she "several times asked, 'Where is Mike?'" The Everycare carer "got Lennie dressed in her nightie ... At 9.55 p.m. she came down fully dressed but we agreed to go up to bed ... I've just remembered that I forgot to join the night's session of the diocesan 'Invite' fifth session, although earlier in the day I'd spent a good hour preparing for it. *Mea maxima culpa*!"

On Friday 26th March, Lennie was fairly difficult all day. The three of us attended Mass online, after which we spent much of the day watching England beat India in a One Day International. "Lennie is aggressive, and she is cross that Maureen, her sister, isn't coming ... Natasha came and was again very sensitive to Lennie's needs and implicit demands." On March 27th I noted, "Lennie stayed down when I went up to bed at 10.15 p.m. and didn't join me until around 2 or 3 a.m. As usual, I didn't sleep after 4 or 5 a.m. And we started our day with Mass readings and prayers not long after 6.30 a.m. Lennie reacted strangely to a card from her Berwick friend, Rosemary ... Later, she was utterly stressed about the money in her purse and bag. No doubt about her dementia ... Sadly, there was little sport on TV, so I spent much of this afternoon reading today's *Tablet*."

Sunday 28th March marked the beginning of British Summer Time, and I noted: "This COVID-19 has very seriously limited the usual Holy Week services. Lennie kept asking over and over again whether she should have something for Mike!" In the afternoon and evening, I watched the O.D.I. with India, which we lost by a few runs. "Stephen then put on *Deutschland 89,* which requires 100% attention to cope with the complexities. But Lennie never stopped talking and asking where the children were."

On Monday 29th March, I recorded that "Lennie, around 5 a.m., started asking about the theatre visit we were supposed to be making. Although I kept insisting that in the lockdown all theatres were closed, she kept repeating the query and ended up accusing me of lying about not informing her." I drove Stephen to the bus station on his way to Cranleigh for the visit of a BG engineer. Around midday, I noted that "conversation with Lennie is getting a bit fraught and I exploded when she came towards me with knives in both hands in front of Claire ... I complained when she claimed to be able to make lunch when she couldn't even make us a cup of coffee!" This was demonstrated in the afternoon when she kindly offered to make us tea, "but what came out was a pink milky cup with blackberries in the bottom. Lennie is obsessed with the mothers of her 'class children' and their unreasonable demands ... The children and Maureen have supposedly been round, in spite of my denials."

Tuesday 30th March was a rather easier day. I spent some time typing Stephen's latest blog *Why Now?* It was a lovely, sunny day and we spent most of the afternoon in the garden.

In the evening, while Stephen was taking Lennie out for a brief walk, I dropped the supper plates on the floor in the kitchen. Lennie's knee was giving her trouble on Wednesday 31st March. This was an awkward and error-filled day and I had to retype a text which I suddenly lost. I also failed to find the video of livestream Mass at St. Joseph's, but when following an alternative at Cork Cathedral, the screen suddenly went blank. I also failed to check my NatWest online banking. I ended the day by recording that "Lennie wasn't very pleased with me and said she thought all I was interested in was 'me, me, me'. I was a liar and only interested in my wishes."

Thursday 1st April was Maundy Thursday, and because of the lockdown, we only followed the evening service online, though with bread and wine and water. Around midday, Stephen and I drove off to G-Live, where we were scheduled to get our COVID-19 vaccines. To our relief, Marie, who had taken Lennie for a drive, brought her along in time. It was a lovely day, and I managed, with some difficulty, to order our weekly Sainsbury's shop online. "The Mass of the Last Supper was strange in lockdown with no washing of the feet and, to my surprise, no people at church during the service. But we participated as we usually have done, with our piece of bread and glass of wine and water." On Good Friday, we watched the service on livestream, with "not every person kissing the cross and limited numbers at Holy Communion". In the evening, we watched the DVD of *The Passion of Jesus*.

On Saturday 3rd April, Andrew and Caroline came on their Easter visit and we watched Chelsea's 5–2 defeat at West Bromwich Albion. After lunch, "rather by accident, I put on Handel's *Messiah* from the Coliseum and then a Holy Week Meditation from Kings College, Cambridge. Lovely. The three of us then attended the Easter Vigil on livestream. It was without laity, with all three priests and Deacon Michael. It was well orchestrated, but we had to persuade

Lennie to stay for the Holy Communion and our bread and wine."

On Easter Sunday, 4th April, "we watched the Papal Mass at St. Peter's celebrated by the Pope. Then, by fluke, I switched to BBC1, and we celebrated Mass with Archbishop Welby. I was greatly impressed by the similarities in our services and beliefs." After Stephen's lunch, along with Richard's Christmas present of *Châteauneuf-du-Pape*, we watched two hours of Mass on EWTN and BBC1 livestream. During the rest of the day, we had visits from Gilly, Doug and Douglas and their two dogs, and later from Richard, Will and Iris. Telephone calls came from Sue and Ann.

On Easter Monday, 5th April, "Last night, Lennie went to bed in her nightie, but by 1–2 a.m. was fully dressed and insisting on her need to catch a train. She eventually, perhaps 3–4 a.m., returned to bed with me ... Before breakfast, I wrote two information cards, which we put in Lennie's purse and handbag. I managed to clear emails, but the laptop is giving me problems which I don't understand. The three of us then watched today's Mass on livestream. Two carers this morning did a good job as companions of Lennie, and I was very grateful." In the afternoon, I spent some time outside wearing one of the excellent jumpers Lennie knitted some time ago. In the evening, I listened to Classic FM and watched a bit of football. After a mixed night on Tuesday 6th April, Lennie was "obsessed with schools, uniforms, and totally unaware of the Easter holiday". During the day I read the *Tablet*, now regarding itself as an 'international Catholic weekly'. Andrew phoned and suggested taking me down to Southsea for a drive. We watched some Champions League football in the evening.

On Wednesday 7th April, I wrote, "Lennie was infuriating last night, dressing and undressing several times over and over, but eventually she came to bed fully dressed around 10.45 p.m." After breakfast, I cleared emails and wrote cheques from both Lennie's and my accounts (both joint). "The three of us then attended livestream Mass, where Fr. Roy made the point, on the basis of today's readings, that Jesus is always with us." I then had a row with Stephen and "had run out of patience when Lennie couldn't follow what I'd suggested. Lennie shifted gear and we suffered a good half an hour or more of her ranting on and on. Mandy did a great job sewing poppers on Lennie's skirt and calming things down. After she'd left, Lennie was walking up and down between the front and garden doors, rattling the handles, threatening to hit us and get the police and just not accepting that <u>this</u> was our home. Eventually, Stephen took her out for a brief walk." In the evening, Stephen and I watched Chelsea's 2–0 win at Porto. "But we had an awful hour with Lennie interrupting all the time and angrily criticising us for watching the match and not communicating with her at all. Stephen is chatting to Lennie but spewing out his various concerns about secret services (MI5 etc.)."

On Thursday 8th April, I noted that "Lennie took half an hour or so last night deciding what to wear before eventually coming to bed. Then, around 2–3 a.m., she put on her outdoor coat and went off downstairs, where I gathered she slept without waking Stephen. Then, while I was shaving, she put on my shirt, and I had to persuade her to give it back." The rest of the day was rather mixed. Faye twice took Lennie out for a walk around Whitmore Common. In the evening, our neighbour, Giuseppe, came and helped me cope with some of the difficulties I'd been having on the laptop. We put on a DVD, *Anna,* about a KGB/CIA assassin, while trying to cope with Lennie's interruptions.

Friday 9th April was an important milestone in the development of Lennie's dementia. My diary records: "Last night was an unexpected warning. Shortly after 2 a.m., I was woken from a deep sleep by a conversation downstairs attended by Stephen, who'd been awakened by a phone and the entrance through the garden door by two young men who'd brought Lennie back from outside the Anchor and Horseshoes pub on London Road. She'd gone 'walking' in the middle of the night and is quite unaware of it this morning. I'd obviously forgotten to take the key out of the door last night ... Stephen has just taken Lennie out for a walk. She is quite unaware of the problem she created last night and quite unaware that she is retired, no longer a teacher, that this is the Easter vacation, and there are no schools, and so forth. Help me, Lord ... Stephen and I watched today's livestream Mass ... Prince Phillip has died. May he rest in peace ... Belinda took Lennie for a brief walk and, as usual, Lennie did the bulk of the washing and drying-up."

On Saturday April 10th, we spent much of the day watching sport, including England's women's rugby defeat of Italy and Chelsea's 4–1 win away at Crystal Palace. On Sunday 11th April, there was no livestream Mass from St. Joseph's, so we followed it from St. John Fisher's at Merton. I read a few chapters in the New Testament and noted that Abraham's faith was demonstrated by his doing. Andrew then very kindly took me down to Southsea, the town of my birth, for possibly the last time. We had a pleasant day.

On Monday 12th April, I noted that Lennie and I were still regularly reading the day's Mass readings and commentary in *Bible Alive* and the praying for the living and the dead every day in bed before getting up for breakfast. Lennie had gone to bed last night fully dressed, left the bedroom and was persuaded sometime later to return. She looked a bit out of sorts today. Her leg was giving her pain but the carer, Faye, was very helpful. In the evening, we watched a couple of football matches. On Tuesday 13th April, "when I was awakened around midnight, Lennie was fully dressed and went downstairs. I went to the top of the stairs and called her back to bed. This morning, when we had an amicable cuddle, she was wearing shoes in bed." I ran out of ink that morning trying to print Andrew's thirty–page report from A Call To Action and Stephen has given me dozens of poems to type for him. "The three of us then attended Mass on livestream. Later, the Community Mental Health nurse came and Lennie took part in a detailed but provocative survey observing her memory loss. It was challenging to realise that Lennie didn't know the day, date, month or year as well as more general knowledge questions such as the first female P.M. Fortunately, there were no explosions and I hope it will be helpful." In the evening, we watched Chelsea beat Porto 2–1 to get through to the Champions League quarter-finals.

On Wednesday 14th April, when Mandy came at 8 a.m., I drove Stephen down to the bus station, hoping the BG engineer would come on the third attempt. "Lennie joined me for the livestream Mass but was in an angry time warp at the end. Where have I taken the children? It is my selfishness to take them away from her; it's all 'me, me, me'; I'm just a bad-tempered, selfish man." Later in the evening, "conversation was difficult; Lennie wondered when we were going home and kept talking about recent meetings with her parents and Maureen!" After Mandy had taken Lennie for a short walk and made us supper, "Lennie was in one of her most frightening moods afterwards, threatening me with a stick for not opening the front door". Nonetheless, I managed to watch the evening match and "Chelsea will be playing in the Champions League semi-finals".

On Thursday 15th April, it was noted that Lennie had dressed and gone downstairs to lay the table around 1–2 a.m., then returned to bed after earlier angry exchanges. "This morning, we followed Mass online from Cork Cathedral. In the afternoon, Gilly and Doug came around and Doug kindly screwed on a lock on the back gate and also moved the key safe to outside the front door. Gilly keeps suggesting I ought to consider additional Everycare support, given Lennie's developing dementia and regular periods of anger." At the end of the day, I added: "Earlier today, Gilly raised the issue of my needing more Everycare support even if it means digging into our savings. Lord and Holy Spirit, please help me to do Your will and trust in You."

On Friday 16th April, I noted: "Last night Lennie took over an hour to get into bed fully dressed. It tested my patience but eventually we tried to get to sleep about 11.30 p.m. Then about 3.45 a.m., Lennie again started worrying about getting up and that irritation again lasted some time. She wouldn't stop talking about me and our bedroom, which was like a shed! When we started getting up as it approached 7 a.m., she said how much she loved me and always had done, and how much she loved our house. Two contradictions in a matter of hours. I managed to read today's Mass readings and say our prayers together before going down for breakfast." I was getting bogged down typing out Stephen's poems or blogs. The carer "Belinda came at 11.30 a.m. and after quite a feisty discussion – Lennie didn't accept her need to have carers take her out – took her out for a drive." The rest of the day passed much as usual, with Lennie chatting on and making it difficult to read the *Tablet* or watch television.

On Saturday 17th April, we watched the funeral of Prince Philip, Duke of Edinburgh, on the TV. "It was beautiful; a strong affirmation of Christian faith plus environmental concerns and God's creation of nature and a deep concern for it. Lennie is in an angry mood, wondering where 'the children' are and why the gates are locked so that she can't get out. This morning, I did an hour's work typing a few more of Stephen's poems before the three of us attended Mass on livestream." We watched a fair amount of football later.

The 18th April was a fairly typical Sunday. I typed more of Stephen's poems before the three of us attended Mass on livestream. Gilly and Doug came, and Doug kindly strengthened the garden gate and post. Later in the day, we drove Stephen to *Penrose* to allow an electrician to come and address some problems. I didn't feel very well driving back from Cranleigh and, unusually, had a couple of puffs of my Nitrolingual spray. Monday 19th April was a fairly mixed day. After the three of us had attended Mass on livestream, we drove Stephen to the bus station, so that he could sort out a problem with Thames Water and return to us later. I started the day with severe constipation problems but in the afternoon was suddenly taken unawares with a terrible case of diarrhoea. In the evening the phone didn't work; another problem to cope with. We ended the day watching football.

We started Tuesday 20th April reading Stephen's speech to the Sanhedrin and his stoning near Saul. Before we attended Mass on livestream, we watched a bit of our marital DVD of the first thirty years. After lunch, I had a very deep sleep and afterwards found Stephen battling with Lennie's incessant questions. Responding to a phone call from Howell Lewis, I said I didn't think I could manage to attend the Men's Group lunch again.

Wednesday 21st April was another lovely summer's day, and we spent a good part of it outside. Lennie irritatingly didn't help when Stephen tried to use superglue to cope with a loose sole on her shoe. I wrote to the Trustees today; I expect I was suggesting that both Lennie and I ought to retire at this stage in our lives and that the three children take over responsibilities now. "I managed to read the first six chapters of Ephesians, with all their suggestions about love and tolerance." Later in the day, I ordered next week's online shopping in spite of twenty minutes' delay finding 'checkout'.

Thursday 22nd April was again an up-and-down day with Lennie. At one stage in the middle of the night, she got dressed and went downstairs, where she woke Stephen. AOL again did not recognize my name or password. The carers often took Lennie out for a walk, while Stephen prepared our lunch and supper. I noted that Mandy helped Lennie complete postal votes for Councillor and Police Commissioner and then, "Lennie is in one of her viciously angry moods. I am her absolute bully; selfish, etc. Just how ugly and nasty I am, and so on. 'I've never met anyone so cruel and thoughtless.' Dementia is a cruel illness ... Lennie came down after Naomi (carer) left and kissed me three times! It's all up and down!"

On Friday 23rd April, "Lennie started her getting-up routine around 4–4.30 a.m. and her searching included going through all my clothes on my chair, nicking my shirt, vest and possibly underwear ... Mandy went upstairs and clearly helped Lennie to get dressed and sorted out all her underwear issues." The three of us attended Mass online and Mgr. Tony recommended we didn't opt for fish on Friday but celebrate the Feast of St. George (martyr) instead, so I particularly enjoyed a Gin and Tonic later. Stephen kindly repaired the curtain rails in our lounge. In the evening, "Lennie then had one of her angry moods, insisting on going out to meet her mother, and so on. Stephen, bless him, has gone out with her."

On Saturday 24th April, "the three of us attended Mass on livestream after which I spent over three-quarters of an hour typing more of Stephen's poems". He cooked our lunch. Richard, Will and Iris came, and we had a very friendly chat in the garden. Sadly, neither of the two children had read even one chapter in the Bibles I'd bought them at Christmas. We watched Chelsea beat West Ham 1–0. On Sunday 25th April, I recorded that "I had a brief row with Lennie when I went up to bed last night because she was repeatedly changing skirts. She angrily hit me on the right arm and almost immediately I had a huge bruise on my arm. This morning it spread all the way up my arm ... I managed to clear emails before the three of us attended Mass on livestream. Fr. Roy gave an impassioned plea for more young men to seek the priesthood, because the Church and diocese were in urgent need of more priests ... Gillian came round with some sandals she had ordered for Lennie and was taking one pair back to change the size. Bless her, Lord."

Lennie wasn't easy to cope with at times on Monday 26th April. "Last night she'd switched off the Wi-Fi and woke me early. I drove Stephen to the bus station on his way to get his water supply back upstairs in *Penrose*. We attended Mass online, and I sorted out appropriate payment procedures with Everycare. After a quiet afternoon, Gilly and Doug came round and took away the curtains to have them cleaned; again, bless them. Lennie was rather rude with Belinda, who later took her out for a walk around Whitmore Common. Earlier, Lennie had asked at least twelve times when we were going to Mass this evening."

On Tuesday 27th April, when Lennie was about to throw away her orange-juice glass, "I protested, and we had an angry exchange just as Mandy was about to come. She cooled us down and took Lennie for a brief walk, bless her." After breakfast, I checked emails, did three-quarters of an hour's typing for Stephen, and then when there was no 10 a.m. Mass at St. Joseph's, followed Mass with the Bishop of Cork. For reasons beyond me but having something to do with her dementia, Lennie left me halfway through Mass, concerned with holes in her tights. The latter half of the afternoon was battered by Lennie's panic over the plan to take her for a hair appointment tomorrow morning; what should she wear and so forth over and over again for a couple of hours until Belinda came and took her out for a walk.

Wednesday 28th April seemed to be very busy. Mandy took Lennie to Hair Partners for a perm. Lennie was quite "against my reading today's Mass readings, so I said my prayers quietly to myself before getting washed and dressed." After breakfast, I cleared emails but lost the AOL icon. I then spent three-quarters of an hour typing some of Stephen's poems before attending Mass on livestream. I drove over to Burpham to pick up Lennie and pay for her perm. Andie had done a great job. Stephen returned early and cooked our lunch. "After lunch, it was a question of trying to relax, not easy with Lennie's incessant chat." After the Sainsbury's shopping had been delivered, I spent over an hour online, ordering next week's delivery. After paying Everycare, I was relieved to see we had no reason yet to dig into our savings. After supper, "Lennie gave us a rough time insisting on her right to 'go home' and completely ignoring our emphasis that <u>this</u> is our home". In the evening, while I was watching football, Lennie came downstairs, and "didn't know we were married sixty years ago or that Maureen was dead, all repeated over and over again".

On Thursday 29th April, I wrote, "Last night was one of the most difficult yet and really made me wonder if Lennie ought to be in a care home. Although Mandy had seen her dressed in a nightie, by the time I went up to bed, she was fully dressed and had to be encouraged to come to bed. She generally doesn't realise I am Mike, her husband of sixty years, and that this is our house. In the early hours, she moved the chair which I had put in front of the door and was mouthing away outside the bedroom, wondering where everybody was. Her verbal battering then went on for another two hours, 2–4 a.m., and with the grace of God, I didn't lose my temper, but tried to cope with the endless repeated questions about where I was, where we were, and so on. At last, around 4 a.m. I managed to persuade her to stop talking and we had a couple of hours' sleep. *Deo Gratias*." The cleaners came and I cleared emails and typed up two or three of Stephen's poems before we attended Mass on livestream. Lennie was irritatingly wanting to leave Mass before the end, but we survived. Lennie helped Mandy take the washing off the line outside and then put it on radiators.

On Friday 30th April, I observed that it had been a pretty good April, even if Lennie went to bed fully dressed and got up with four blouses on, and unpredictable radiators. In the afternoon, Doug came round and repaired and reset the wooden rings for the curtain` rails. "Lennie was very difficult over supper, insisting that 'the children' had all been invited and laying the table for five people ... I refused to open the doors when she insisted there was an evening Mass and that her father's car was outside. But her weird dreams continued and included murdering her parents and that she'd had a brother as well as a sister."

On Saturday 1st May, I noted that Lennie disappeared in the middle of the night and wandered all over the house. "Lennie is still going on about 'going home' with her parents." On the Feast of St. Joseph the Worker, in the morning we attended Mass online and in the evening at St. Pius' we attended Mass directly for the first time since our 60th anniversary. In the evening, we watched Chelsea beat Fulham 2–0 and then Clemmie's first day at school in *The Yorkshire Farm*.

On Sunday 2nd May, Gilly and Doug came for a chat, in the garden because of lockdown. When they left, "Lennie was obsessed that she had cooked the meal and that they had rejected the invitation", though Stephen cooked lunch as usual. Richard visited us later with an *Observer,* which I skimmed later. I read the first five chapters of Revelation before going to bed. On Mummy's anniversary, Monday 3rd May, Lennie's knee and leg were causing her a lot of trouble and she declined Belinda's offer to take her for a walk. After lunch, "Lennie was talking absolutely non-stop about fanciful engagements with children and so on". I was so frustrated that I put on some warm clothes and went outside to read the *Observer*. Later in the afternoon, "Lennie is now creating all sorts of problems, including burning a water jug and refusing to admit she had any responsibilities". On Tuesday 4th May, I found "Lennie a pain because she insisted on laying the table with knives, forks and spoons in spite of my objections" before reading Revelation and going to bed.

On Wednesday 5th May, although "she said she'd always loved me," Lennie repeatedly asked if she had a boyfriend. Mandy was most helpful with a bolshy Lennie, who at first refused to have her pills. Meanwhile, life struggled on much as usual and I managed to order a week's shopping from Sainsbury's online. "Thank You, Lord, for helping us today."

On Thursday 6th May, there were local elections and Andrew was elected as a Councillor in Reading for two years. "Be with him, Lord." I was concerned about my diaries being deposited in the archives at Farm Street, though I didn't immediately follow it up. "Unusually, Lennie was very against the Mass, suggesting the reading from Acts was rubbish and later angrily walking off in the middle of the consecration ... Emma came to cut her toenails. The next couple of hours were hard going. Lennie just wouldn't stop talking about the 'children' coming for a meal, suggesting that we needed to lay the table for six and totally ignoring my claims that there would be just the two of us. Faye took Lennie off for a drive; she came back full of love and kisses!" It was much the same on Friday 7th May. "Lennie is obsessed with looking after 'the children', but she is utterly resistant to the realities that they are all in their fifties." Lennie was insistent that I should unlock the front door so that she could go off to school, and a desire to 'go home'. The carers who took her for short walks helped me considerably to cope. "Help me to do Your will, Lord, and be a good spouse."

On Saturday 8th May, I was irritated that Lennie appeared to have taken my socks. "Then downstairs the table was an absolute shambles with coffee all over the place in mugs, bowls, saucers, all over the table. How to cope with this?" It was much the same on Sunday 9th May, when "Lennie is repeating over and over again if she ought to go out in the car to get the children. Stephen says she's repeated this at least twenty-seven times!" On the Monday afternoon of 10th May, "Lennie, for the best part of an hour, angrily argued she had a right to have a key out of this house ... and to 'go home' and so forth. Lennie is challenging my patience, which according to Paul means love. Forgive me, Lord, and help me be a better spouse and carer ... Lennie has just put on her coat over her nightie! What next?" My diary for Tuesday 11th May noted: "Today started at 3.45 a.m., when Lennie got dressed and started wandering around. So much so that I told her irritably that it wasn't fair to wake other people up in the middle of the night. Downstairs, I got a verbal bashing for always wanting my own way; it would be better if I went to live somewhere else! ... I do enjoy watching the Owen family, who pull together remarkably on their Yorkshire farm."

On Wednesday 12th May, "I discovered several plates and cutlery in both my study and near the laptop" instead of being taken into the kitchen, "another example of memory loss". The kitchen tap had also been left on, fortunately into the sink. Stephen cooked lunch and coped with the Sainsbury's shopping delivery in the afternoon. "Then another sign of Lennie's dementia. I went to the loo and found Lennie sitting on the high seat spending a penny. I managed to move her to the loo and later Stephen kindly wiped up the urine left under the high seat by Lennie earlier." I then booked next week's Sainsbury's online shopping. Lennie and I said our night prayers together. The 13th May, my mother's birthday, was Ascension Thursday. Stephen set off for Cranleigh before Mass, but the rest of the day passed much as usual. "Please, Lord, let us have a good night. The carers all seem to have a sympathetic view of me in our relationship." Friday 14th May was very much as usual, with Fr. Roy emphasising the theme of mission and evangelisation and our response in his homily in the livestream Mass. In the evening, I enjoyed watching Scandinavian crime dramas.

On Saturday 15th May, Chelsea were beaten 1–0 by Leicester, I think, in the Cup Final. My Bible reading has got as far as Chapter 19 in Exodus. I was tired on Sunday morning, 16th May, and struggled to shave and have a shower. "Mgr. Tony's homily encouraged us to recognise that God is with us in spite of difficult challenges." Gilly and Katie came to visit us in the afternoon. "They both allowed us to cuddle them for the first time for about a year." Monday 17th May was a fairly normal day with nothing unusual. Tuesday 18th May was rather different as Lennie had a painful tooth. Mandy was a great help, taking her to the dentist and chasing up her medication details with the surgery, and so on. Other carers took Lennie out for short walks. I couldn't get livestream Mass from St. Joseph's and ended up following Mass with the bishop in Arundel Cathedral. On Wednesday 19th May, I was a bit miffed to get an email from Gilly, who'd had a conversation with Jane (Everycare), "where they seemed to suggest I ought to learn from the carers how to handle a difficult Lennie".

On Thursday 20th May, I noted: "Last night was the third night running that Lennie had had a full night's sleep, not getting dressed and going downstairs. She remained with me as we read today's Mass readings and said our prayers for family and friends, living and dead. After online Mass, Lennie needed me to help make coffee. I'd done so and she moaned about too little milk ... for the first time I can remember, I smacked her physically. *Mea maxima culpa.* Frightening. Please help me, Lord. I have a sense that Lennie has forgotten it. *Deo gratias.* Her memory loss was obvious when over half a dozen times she asked me what my name was when we were getting up ... In the late afternoon, Lennie was going endlessly on and on about preparing an evening meal for all the family."

On Friday 21st May, the carers put on a load of washing, which they later put out onto the radiators. During the livestream Mass, Mgr. Tony stressed "the sending out of the apostles after the resurrection and sending of the Holy Spirit, and our call to respond to the Lord's call". Mandy took Lennie for an X-ray of her tooth. Before going to bed, I prayed, "Help me to be a better person, Lord". On Saturday 22nd May, "Stephen joined us before the end of the homily and brought us up bread and wine to offer up for Jesus to accept if He wanted to", as I indicated in my letter in the *Tablet* on 9th January.

On Pentecost Sunday, 23rd May, "the three of us drove off for our first Mass at St. Pius' for some time. It was good to see familiar faces again. The Pastoral Letter from the Bishops' Conference strongly emphasised justice and peace issues, especially environmental." Today's meeting of the Trusts "manifested the excellent professional financial competence of Gillian and the maintenance competence of Richard on building issues etc. Andrew, too, made some very helpful contributions and we will be exploring further the ways we may recruit two new trustees because of uncertainties in the original trust documents."

On Monday 24th May, in the early afternoon, "Lennie has gone upstairs after half an hour of marching up and down rattling the front and garden doors and hitting me slightly with her stick as she tries to get me to get up and open the doors, so she can go and see 'the boy next door' and if I don't she will report me to 'the Head'". The rest of the day passed much as usual. On Tuesday 25th May, we followed Mass on livestream from EWTN at 1 p.m. In the afternoon. we coped with Lennie's often strange behaviour, which led to my having to switch off TV programmes. On Wednesday 26th

May, Lennie's dental appointment was cancelled, and Mandy took her to Jackman's Garden Centre for a coffee. Stephen came with me for my cardiology check-up at the hospital. We then attended the livestream Mass from EWTN at 1 p.m. I did a fair amount of typing of Stephen's poems. After the delivery of the Sainsbury's online shopping, I ordered next week's online delivery. "Gilly phoned to prompt me to add to our current Everycare cover and not to bother about digging into our savings when necessary."

On Thursday 27th May, I noted that we hadn't had a bad night. "Lennie went bonkers after Mandy left, claiming she'd left without telling her. Her anger led her to threaten me and the window with her stick ... The four or more hours of the afternoon passed by OK with no feisty or angry sessions from Lennie. Faye has taken her out to take her home to Mike. *C'est la vie*!" On Friday 28th May, I recorded that we hadn't had a bad night. It was so warm that I'd slept on top of the blankets and eiderdown on the bed. Stephen left early to get his vaccine for COVID-19. Mandy put out the washing machine clothes put on for a wash earlier by Stephen. I asked Everycare to provide an extra hour's cover on four afternoons each week. We managed to have a quarter of an hour's chat with Marie over the fence after the long lockdown. My diary for Saturday 29th May noted that Lennie had gone wandering in and out of the bedroom several times in the night. In the evening, Chelsea won the European Championship. Richard, Will and Iris phoned to shout their heads off!

On Sunday 30th May, we attended Mass on livestream. Gilly visited with her lifelong friend, Alison, and we discussed some of the uncertainties about the Trusts. In the afternoon, we sat out in the garden. "Lennie talked about giving up teaching; I suddenly had heart problems." I managed to read up to Deuteronomy 27. The 31st May was a beautiful Bank Holiday Monday. We watched livestream Mass on the Feast of the Visitation. We spent much of the afternoon outside in the garden and I read to the end of Deuteronomy. I persuaded Stephen to water the roses and bushes in the garden. On Tuesday 1st June, I noted that "after Faye left at 9 a.m., Lennie and I had an angry exchange, probably following Faye's ironing of my trousers and shirt. I was angry and irritated that Lennie had probably taken my shirt upstairs and it has disappeared. She bashed me on the arm with two Sunday missals and I have proof with a 3–4-inch purple bruise on my right arm!" I coped with Lennie's wafting two knives and cleared the table of superfluous cutlery when she went out for a walk with Leanne. Late in the afternoon, "I discovered Lennie had let water flow onto the kitchen floor and hadn't turned off the gas on the hob. I mustn't just leave her without checking what she is doing. So much for freedom for me!"

My diary for Wednesday 2nd June recorded that "from about 12.20 p.m. last night Lennie angrily woke me for being so lazy and wanted me to put on one of three skirts she'd put out, one of which she threw at me as we exchanged angry arguments, and I fearfully thought I wouldn't be able to cope with this if it became regular. She wanted me to get dressed in a skirt and complained that I never did anything. I tried to argue that it was black outside, the middle of the night when we should be sleeping. I gradually realised that I'd better shut up and keep out of the argument. Eventually, Lennie put on one of the skirts and came to bed. She stayed there until we started our day with today's Mass readings and prayers."

The Sainsbury's weekly online shopping was delivered, and I then sent off next week's request. On Thursday 3rd June, I wondered, "Should I put locks on the kitchen and bedroom doors? Or would this fire up Lennie's anger?" When I had problems with my laptop, we watched Mass on livestream from Newry Cathedral. "During Mass, Lennie drove me mad a couple of times and apart from shouting I banged my hand on the table." She wouldn't listen to my suggestion that a broken necklace needed to be taken to a jeweller's. But she was very loving after Mandy had taken her up to Newlands Corner for a drive.

Friday 4th June was a fairly typical day, which included clearing twenty emails, chasing up British Gas for *Penrose* and a Thames Water bill, and playing cards with Lennie. On Saturday 5th June, I noted that Lennie had wandered off during the night, though I managed to persuade her to come back to bed. I selected the eight charities to give donations to this month. In the afternoon, we sat out in the shade in the garden, and I skimmed the *Guardian*. On Sunday 6th June, we attended Mass at St. Pius' for the first time in quite a while and people were very friendly. Gilly and Doug visited later, and Doug fitted an internal key box while Gilly arranged to replace zips on two of Lennie's skirts. Richard came in the afternoon, and we watched an uninspiring 1–0 defeat of Romania.

Today was seventy-seven years since D-Day. On the afternoon of Monday 7th June, "Lennie accused me of wandering off for an hour leaving her alone. This fantasy continued after the carer came and continued in spite of her offer to take her for a drive, for example, to the river. Lennie's crazy anger persisted until she ordered the carer out and insisted she never wanted to see her in this house again. This is the first time this has happened. Somehow, we survived the rest of the afternoon." After the carer left, we "sat in the garden for a while and Lennie told me how much she loved me. But when we came in things changed. At least eleven times she asked me if I wanted any food and totally denied she'd had any food since breakfast. Her anger got worse, and I thought she was going to hit me. Eventually, another carer turned up and she gradually got Lennie to cool down. But it didn't outlast her hour. Lennie has just said she'd never met such a bloody liar! She took off the nightie that the carer had put on her. She dressed back into day clothes, threw a toilet roll at me and threatened to smack me ... She's been a nightmare for much of the afternoon and evening."

Tuesday 8th June was a bit better, though Lennie did wander off through the front door. Thankfully, a neighbour kindly escorted her to the end of the road and back. "She is impossible at the moment ... Lennie is repeatedly walking from the garden gate through the house to the front door. Please help me, Lord." I managed to negotiate a reduction of our payments to Sky. An ESE mechanic came to check our solar panel equipment. It was a lovely day and Lennie and I enjoyed sitting out in the garden all afternoon. Wednesday 9th June was much the same. The quarterly *RENEW* of the Catholics for a Changing Church published my letter with a rather ancient photograph of me. I ordered next week's Sainsbury's shopping online. Today's mail included one from our M.P. responding to my complaint about the reduction of our national contribution of aid for developing countries and I pondered responding to the Jesuit Refugee Service's urge to write and complain about the treatment of asylum seekers. On Thursday 10th June, I finished reading thirty-five pages of Stephen's poems before he returned to Cranleigh. "Lennie went on and on about feeding the children and looking after them, etc. (thirty plus years ago?)."

On Friday 11th June, I recorded "a pretty good night together, but Lennie was angry when I tried to get her to put on a bra before a jumper. She has a 'thing' at the moment about our care workers only being 'in it for the money'. For nearly an hour, Lennie has been concerned about the children being picked up by their parents and then insisting that the plastic garden chairs are taken inside to prevent them being stolen! Life isn't easy. Lennie's time frame seems thirty years ago ... Lennie took up three plates of sweets 'for the children coming for a meal'!" On Saturday 12th June, I spent much of the day skimming the *Guardian* outside. On Sunday 13th June, we were still following Mass on livestream and found it "very peaceful and pastoral". Afterwards, Gilly and Doug came, and Doug fitted a lock on the kitchen door. In the afternoon, England beat Croatia in the European Championship. Afterwards, "Lennie started screaming in a loud voice about going to look after 'the children' but is quite oblivious to our pointing out that all our children are in their fifties. And she hasn't taught in a school for twenty-six years. The argument got quite noisy with the door open."

On Monday 14th June, it seemed that "this is the world of a poor old guy trying to cope with his wife's dementia". The afternoon after the carer had left "was awful. Lennie was totally unable to recognise this as her house and kept complaining about not being allowed to walk to her home and at one stage shouted 'Help! Help!' by the back garden gate. How much more difficult is this going to become? So far, she hasn't hit me with her threatening stick." On Tuesday 15th June, I wrote, "Last night for the first time I locked the kitchen door with Doug's key. The lock is intended to safeguard the gas on the hob in case Lennie starts using it when she gets up in the middle of the night and then forgets to switch it off. But Lennie was furious that I wouldn't give her a key for the front door to enable her to go to her 'home'. Our anger led to a sort of wrestling match and her arms gripped over my arm, creating a 5–6" purple bruise and tore open the skin on my arm, which oozed blood all over the place. I managed to put a couple of plasters on it." Later, I phoned the surgery who told me to go to the Woking drop-in centre and they told me there were often two-hour queues. "Somehow, Lennie feels she is being left out of decision-making." In the afternoon, I read as far as Chapter 14 of 1 Kings. In the evening, we drove Frances to the Yvonne Arnaud for about the first time in two years and saw an interesting play about the friendship between Graham Greene and Tim Philby. "I wasn't too comfortable driving home and it made me think perhaps it is time for me to think of giving up driving." Wednesday 16th June had an angry start, with Lennie wearing my vest and shirt and the shorts Gilly had bought me falling off. Lennie has put some "weeds into the water butt; in my anger I banged the table and knocked some gel onto the floor. Come on, Mike! Love is patient!" Both Andrew and Richard felt I needed a proper plaster on my arm to avoid infection. Andrew kindly drove Stephen back to Cranleigh.

Thursday 17th June had a bad start when I discovered a damaged knee had bled all the way down to my ankle. Mandy, one of the carers, arranged an appointment for me in the surgery and later, with difficulty, I drove there. Dr. Cross arranged for me to see a nurse, who put on an NHS plaster and, in the end, arranged for me to have it checked for several weeks. Most of the evening was spent looking through the Jesuit journal, which had interesting references to St. Aloysius in Glasgow where I went to school and was confirmed around 1941. Friday 18th June was rather mixed, with international football matches on much of the day. England and Scotland drew 0–0 and Gilmore was the Man of the Match. Saturday19th June started badly with a fall by Lennie, which resulted in blood all over the floor. Stephen was a great help. I also had a very sore neck and was miffed when it was largely ignored by Mandy when she came. "I/we need to plan for Lennie going into a care home at some point if we are to avoid serious conflict. I'm very wary about this. Richard, Will and Iris turned up." The European internationals took over much of the day. On Sunday 20th June, Ann's 87th birthday, I drove us to Mass at St. Pius', but "Lennie wouldn't wear a mask". I had problems controlling my urine. "Gilly phoned me to wish me a happy Fathers' Day; bless her." Richard bought me the *Observer* and I skimmed it for much of the afternoon.

On Monday 21st June, an interrupted night with Lennie led me to reflect that "poor sleep is now fairly regular". The new CEO of Everycare came with Jane "to discuss the development of care for us. They seemed to be unduly concerned about me and the need for peace and space. We discussed possibilities of Lennie going to local social services 9–4 p.m. Days out with others; choir singing; and possible need of sleeping tablets; etc. I did point out that I had no cover for the twelve hours at night from 8 p.m. to 8 a.m. I was unsuccessful in reading the *Tablet;* Lennie was disgruntled at having no conversation." Belinda came and played cards with Lennie while I drove off to the surgery to have my plaster updated.

On Tuesday 22nd June, soon after livestream Mass, "Lennie became aggressively angry that I'd allowed Emma (toenails) to bring a colleague along. Lennie was furious and said she didn't want any job doing. Emma was excellent and gently talked Lennie into cutting her nails while her colleague quietly disappeared. Lennie also agreed the next session in eight weeks. So, all ended well ... The afternoon has not been easy. Lennie never stops fussing, but it is never quite clear what she is expecting or trying to do." The carers looked after Lennie during the rest of the day. After a 1–0 win from a rather lifeless England, we went up to bed, though "Lennie didn't recognise me as her husband and wouldn't come and join me in the double bed. For the first time, as far as I can remember, she went off into the other bedroom and slept in the other bed." Wednesday 23rd June was a lovely sunny day, and we spent some time outside. We managed to battle through the rest of the day without there being any serious rows. As always, the carers helped by taking Lennie out for a walk or a drive, singing or playing cards with her, and so on. It was rather different the following day.

My diary for Thursday 24th June notes that "it was just after midnight when I was awakened by an angry Lennie asking what I was doing in her bed! I talked with her for over half an hour until I finally persuaded her to come to bed to get some sleep. The rest of the night was friendly and loving."

I had an early hair appointment with Dennis, and Stephen remained at home until I returned since there was no carer that morning. The periods between carers were frequently difficult, but it helped when one of them took Lennie for a walk around Whitmore Common. On Friday 25th June, I didn't have the best of nights and after breakfast I had a disastrous three-quarters of an hour and failed to get St. Joseph's Mass on livestream. In the end, I managed to get an African priest in a Dublin parish. When checking emails, there was one from Sylvie Collins-Mayo, who was being ordained as an Anglican priest the next day. "I sent an immediate reply and also phoned the parish office to ask for a prayer at that night's meeting for her. Bless her, Lord, and keep her close to You." In the afternoon, I went to the surgery to have my plaster replaced and was told it might take weeks to finish it. Lennie was difficult most of the evening and I was unable to interest her in any TV. There were times when she banged the door for it to be unlocked and a few other times when she came downstairs to kiss me and tell me how much she loved me!

On Saturday 26th June, I prayed for Sylvie and watched her ordination and was struck by how similar our liturgies were. I skimmed today's *Guardian*. Gilly kindly drove us to and from her house for supper, the first time for a year as a result of the lockdown following the Coronavirus pandemic. On Sunday 27th June, I noted that Lennie had got up in the middle of the night and gone downstairs to sleep on the second settee without waking Stephen. We followed Mass from St. Joseph's on livestream. As always, Stephen cooked us lunch. In the afternoon, I struggled to skim the *Observer,* "but we then had a couple of hours of verbal battering from Lennie, who went on and on about fanciful arrangements with parents and children. Stephen was excellent, participating in chat with Lennie, whereas I was angry and sometimes explosive."

Monday 28th June was a bit of a mix. "I was increasingly aware of my advancing inadequacies associated with ageing. Into Your hands, oh Lord, I commend my spirit. Later, Lennie wasn't terribly interested in watching Wimbledon tennis", but later Faye took her out for a walk around the block, around three-quarters of a mile. My diary for Tuesday 29th noted that "around 2.15 a.m., I was awakened by knocking on the lounge windows. Lennie was outside the lounge, banging on the window outside, not being able to move the door and 'return home'. Last night I'd obviously left the key in the patio door and Lennie had aimed to go wandering. Fortunately, the garden gate was locked." Lennie spent the rest of the night in bed with me. During the day on Wednesday 30th June, I drove off to the surgery to have my plaster updated while Mandy took Lennie to the dentist. Bob Durston then drove me to and from the Men's Group lunch for the first time in a couple of years. It was good to meet so many old friends after the lockdown.

On Thursday 1st July, I was puzzled by Lennie's repeatedly going downstairs every night. "Her response was basically 'I don't know; I just want to do something!' In other words, I presume I'm not doing anything wrong. But it is still unclear how I ought to respond and show patience and love." While Marie took Lennie out for a walk, I was able to begin reading Mark's book on the S.O.E. and its references to my Aunty Pat as a 'red-headed sledgehammer!' Late in the afternoon, there was panic when Lennie couldn't be found anywhere. It seems she had found the garden gate unlocked since Voytek, our gardener, came yesterday.

Friday 2nd July wasn't a bad day. Lennie didn't wander off last night. I was very taken by Solomon's prayer in 2 Chronicles 5–6. The weather was pleasant and encouraged us to sit out in the garden. I went to the surgery to have my plasters and bandages on my left arm updated. After being taken for a walk around Whitmore Common, Lennie watched some of the Wimbledon tennis and we went up to bed just before 10 p.m. On Saturday 3rd July, Mandy helped sort out Lennie's clothing. I spent some time after we'd attended Mass on livestream skimming the *Guardian* and the *Tablet*. In the late afternoon Richard, Will and Iris turned up but only stayed until half–time in the Denmark–Czech Republic match. Later Stephen and I watched England win 4–0 and reach the semi-finals.

My diary for Sunday 4th July shows that "Lennie remained with me practically all night, still wearing her nightie." I had a rather obscure email invitation from Prof. Francis Davis, which needed clarification. The three of us then attended Mass on livestream, after which Gilly came and stayed just over an hour. We gave her a birthday card and present. I found the *Observer* disappointing today. In the evening, we watched a Harry Potter film. On Monday 5th July, there was a rough start to the day. Stephen and Faye put out a load of washing on the line before he set out for Cranleigh. Deacon Michael gave his usual challenging homily at the Monday morning Mass, which we watched on livestream. Faye and a new carer took Lennie out for a much shorter walk than a few months ago. The evening carer was a bit clumsy and authoritarian when taking Lennie to bed and "Lennie's freedom instinct came out, as she insisted she didn't need anyone to undress her and get her ready for bed".

On the morning of Tuesday 6th July, I wrote, "It has taken me a good hour to recover from a sense of exhaustion, dependent on my zimmer frame, simply busying myself around the kitchen putting out cereal bowls and trying unsuccessfully to tighten the screw holding the handle of a saucepan". At this stage in our lives the carers did not regard me as one of their clients. Howell Lewis phoned to try and get me to attend the Men's Group lunch on Wednesdays. "Marie was doing a supervisor's check-up and confirmed that both Lennie and I had deteriorated significantly, physically and possibly mentally, over the past six months."

On Wednesday 7th July, I had problems getting the livestream Mass until the gospel. I was finding it difficult getting our breakfast when dependent upon the zimmer frame. In the afternoon, I read more of Mark's book on the S.O.E. and then managed to book next week's Sainsbury's shopping online, in spite of difficulties over checkout. England beat Denmark 2–1 to go through to the final of the European championships. Thursday 8th July 2021 was Gilly's 58th birthday; bless her, Lord. Around 8.30 a.m., Stephen left us. "Bless him for all he does for us, caring for us three days every week. I miss him greatly when he is not here. I managed to skim 2 Chronicles 28–31 before going upstairs to get livestream Mass from St. Joseph's after clearing emails." In the afternoon, Lennie was insistent on her coping with children and their parents (over thirty years earlier). "Lennie's demands are incessant, and she is totally resistant to my suggestion that they are no longer her responsibility since she retired twenty-six years earlier. Ann and Andrew both phoned for ten to fifteen minutes each. Douglas called to join Gilly before they returned home." I managed to read up to Chapter 41 of Mark's book before going up to bed.

Friday 9th July seemed to be a regular sort of day corresponding to Jesus's commands. I read a lot of Andrew's novel. I drove to the surgery for the weekly replacement of the dressings on my left arm. Saturday 10th July was much as usual. I managed to get to Chapter 55 of Mark's book. In the afternoon, we watched the British Lions and then England beating Pakistan in a 50-over match. On Sunday 11th July, I had sudden and unexpected diarrhoea and made quite a mess. Stephen kindly helped clear everything up afterwards. "Bless his heart; he did a great job clearing it up and cleaning the carpet. *Deo Gracias.*" In the evening, we watched Italy beat England 3–2 in the penalty shoot-out.

In my diary for Monday 12th July, I admitted that "increasingly these days, I am aware of having to cope with ageing and declining physical abilities". Stephen was very helpful before he set off for Cranleigh. Before we watched livestream Mass, I cleared emails and read more of Andrew's novel. "Lennie no longer automatically washes up even simple piles of plates after meals. The carers frequently take Lennie out for a short walk." On Tuesday 13th July, we followed our usual routines, including livestream Mass. In the afternoon, Belinda took Lennie for a short walk and then for a drive up to Newlands Corner. In the afternoon and evening I read more of Mark's book on the S.O.E. as well as Andrew's novel. On Wednesday 14th July, I noted that "around 6.45 a.m. a loving Lennie joined me as I read today's Mass readings, and we said our usual prayers. Stephen brought up bread and wine and this made all the difference to our sense of involvement." My reading of Andrew's novel was limited by my tendency to drift off to sleep. In the afternoon, I was unsuccessful in attempting to order our weekly shop from Sainsbury's. Stephen made a tasty but over-large supper. "Obviously my appetite is not as great as it used to be, though I still try to adhere to my boyhood guidance, eat everything put on your plate. Lennie was awful at this stage, working on the assumption that we should be preparing meals for the children." In the evening, Stephen and I watched South Africa beat the British and Irish Lions.

Thursday 15th July was "a rather pleasant day. Lennie didn't wander off last night. I ordered next week's shopping from Sainsbury's online. Voytek came to do our garden. Stephen got some money from the ATM for me. I drove to St. Luke's surgery to have my plaster replaced. There was a lovely concert on Classic FM this evening which attracted Lennie." Yet my diary for Friday 16th July noted that "after a very pleasant and peaceful evening, Lennie suddenly, around 11.30 p.m., started being aggressive about the fact that I was lying on the bed, and she was trying to adjust the blankets. In the end we spent a whole hour sparring. Then again, an hour or so later, she woke me with my Medisure medicine, and I feared that they were hers and that she'd taken them in the wrong order or something ... I had to persuade Lennie to take off a bra she'd put on the <u>outside</u> of her blouse and re-dress in the proper sequence." After the online Mass, Marie took Lennie to the Hair Partners for a cut and blow-dry. In the afternoon, while Belinda took Lennie up to Newlands Corner, I spent an hour reading Andrew's novel. "Lennie's mobility has rapidly declined very seriously, and she has difficulty just walking to the loo ... I tried, unsuccessfully, to persuade Lennie to come out and enjoy a summer's evening in the shade, but she is bothered about her job of looking after a group of children and is totally resistant to suggestions that that might have been in thirty to forty years ago but is not the case today." Saturday 17th July had a beautiful morning. When I explained to Lennie why I couldn't carry my breakfast, "she called me a 'nasty brat' ... Stephen came in time for Mass, after which I spent around one and a half hours reading Andrew's novel." Later, I got to Psalm 29. Lennie signed a birthday card 'GRAMA' instead of 'NANA'.

On Sunday 18th July, I wrote: "After a peaceful night, while I was shaving and showering, Lennie nicked my socks and clean shirt and was wearing them. Then she tried on three different dresses." Gilly drove us to Mass at St. Pius' and afterwards there was a meeting of the three children. "I'm feeling rather depressed that Stephen's two days have ended rather suddenly." On Monday 19th July, I noted that Stephen "hasn't said much about the four children's natter about our ageing yesterday. They were just exchanging updates. I always miss Stephen when he is not here." This seems to have been a very confusing day, with Lennie worried about having lost a baby she was looking after and being advised by Claire that as nobody had phoned it was probably safe with its parents. "Stephen warned me that he'd found several spoons in the refuse bin." On Tuesday 20th July, I noted that "Lennie was violently sick around 1–2 a.m., all over the bathroom mats and floor". As I wasn't mobile enough to clear it up, Mandy coped when she came at 8 a.m. She took Lennie to the surgery for a blood test and learned that I/we could arrange for 'district nurses' to visit us. I did manage to email Andrew about his book. I suggested that "his book is really the result of a serious sociological study rather than a novel".

On Wednesday 21st July, I recorded that "we had a reasonably good night last night, but Lennie was up and 'getting dressed' around 6 a.m. This was a provocative shambles. Lennie struggled, with my help, to get her nightie off but after I'd folded it to put under her pillow, she put it on again. As I was struggling to dress myself, this was very irritating." Later, I ordered next week's online shopping from Sainsbury's. "Lennie makes criticisms of Stephen which can be quite ugly and provocative. Stephen doesn't find it easy to 'switch off'. Lennie is quite awkward in undressing 'in public' and gets quite cross when we insist that she doesn't."

Thursday 22nd July seemed to be a busy, awkward and not an easy or comfortable day. Early in the day, I wrote, "I have already lost my temper as Lennie has failed to respond to my guidance ... Mandy says she couldn't comment when I admitted I was a bad-tempered oaf. Amongst all the day's uncertainties, I had the last change of my plaster at the surgery." My diary for Friday 23rd July opens with evidence of severe incontinence in 'my' loo. "It seems that things are deteriorating quite rapidly. Life is a bit of a shambles at the moment, but gradually things are getting done ... Today we prayed for Benedict on his 26th birthday. Help him to get ever closer to You, Lord." Lennie only ate a fraction of her meals and later broke a glass in the kitchen. I read the weekend *Tablet* and a couple of carers took Lennie out for a short walk or trip up to Newlands Corner. The Tokyo Olympics started that day.

Saturday 24th July was the first day of the Olympics and I watched various sports much of the morning, apart from attending Mass online. Stephen cooked us lunch, after which we watched the Olympics and a Hundred cricket match and then boxing selected by Stephen. My Bible reading took me as far as Psalm 109. On Sunday 25th July, the women's cycling was gripping. Gilly drove us to St. Pius' for Mass and then back home afterwards. I wasn't terribly interested in Stephen's DVD about the SAS and read to Psalm 124 and skimmed today's *Observer* before going to bed. On Monday 26th July, Stephen set off early for Cranleigh. I noted that Deacon Michael had again given a very challenging account of the parables we'd read at Mass in the last week. Gilly then took Lennie to St. Luke's. We watched more Olympics and I read as far as Psalm 145. It seems that "Gillian and Everycare are worried about Lennie's sudden loss of mobility and problems with her knees and general deterioration. I personally am increasingly aware of my deteriorating mobility. Today hasn't been easy, but I pray that I will learn to control my temper. Please, Lord, give me the grace to control my irritation and bad temper and cope with Lennie's illness."

My diary for Tuesday 27th July noted signs of Lennie's incontinence on the lavatory seats and top blanket. Otherwise, it seems to have been an ordinary day with livestream Mass in the morning. Much of the day we watched the Olympics. The carers were good as usual; Claire put out the washing on the line and Faye took Lennie out for a drive and 'to go home'. My diary for Wednesday 28th July records "a 'pretty good' night. Lennie and I had a cuddle and we then read today's Mass readings and said our prayers together." After breakfast, I cleared emails and sent several birthday and anniversary cards before attending Mass on livestream. After lunch, I ordered next week's Sainsbury's shop online. I felt knackered after putting away some of the Sainsbury's shopping delivery. Stephen, bless him, did the bulk of it. In the evening, we watched the

Olympics and a historical documentary. "Lennie is going on and on. I just can't follow two parallel conversations: between Lennie and Stephen, and the TV. It drives me nuts ... Lennie has been demanding all evening. It is impossible to relax with her incessant discussions, which prevent us watching anything ... She has just come down with her nightie on back to front after Stephen and I had objected to her beginning to undress in front of us. She is also demanding help with her necklace, which she has popped on and off."

On Thursday 29th July, I wrote: "Lennie was awkward and left three-quarters of her lunch and was just difficult afterwards. She never relaxes. She brought in half of the washing on the line, then denied she had done it." In the afternoon, Faye took Lennie out for a drive and arrived after we'd had one of our worst explosions so far with threats to hit each other. "She'd accused me of lying when I pointed out that she'd left over half of three or more meals. It looked as if she was going to get into the Medisure packets, and so on. Tensions got higher and I lost my cool, at least verbally. Lennie needs 100% care to prevent problems and I haven't reached that requirement yet. How best can I explain the challenges she creates?"

The Olympics continued to be an important background on Friday 30th July, and I cleared emails before we attended Mass on livestream. An electrician came, but I didn't want to be talked into making yet another substantial payment, for example to control my voltage. In the evening, "at Lennie's request, after her third visit downstairs after 'going to bed', I went up for about the first time. I helped her undress and put on her nightie. She is no longer able to respond automatically to 'your nightie is under your pillow'."

On Saturday 31st July, "Stephen was here well before Mass, to which he brought us bread and wine." Again, the

Olympics dominated much of the day and, as always, I enjoyed Stephen's Saturday G&T. "In the early afternoon, I dozed a bit and skimmed through today's *Guardian*." Richard came for a couple of hours in the afternoon, and we watched South Africa brutalise the Lions in the second Test. On Sunday 1st August, "Stephen kindly volunteered to help me put on my socks, vest, shirt and trousers. After Mass, Gilly came with a load of washing, since they are in the early days of replacing and redesigning their kitchen. The rest of the day was divided between the Olympics and my attempt to skim the *Observer*."

On Monday 2nd August, I noted, "we didn't have a bad night. Stephen kindly came upstairs and helped me dress – a great help putting on my socks and shirt, etc. Stephen left at 8 a.m. when Mandy arrived, and I managed to phone the Pharmacy and order our medication." We attended Mass online. Deacon Michael gave another thoughtful homily. When I was clearing emails before Mass, "there was confirmation of our bookings for three or four at St. Pius' for the next three Sundays". As we watched a Hundred cricket match, "Lennie continued to behave strangely, talking about pyjamas. On Tuesday 3rd August, I couldn't get a livestream Mass from St. Joseph's but managed to get it from a parish in North London. In the late afternoon, "Lennie was certainly very unsettled and at one stage I found her undressing in the lounge and putting on her nightie and then her dress on top of it. But we survived." Before going to bed, after watching a T20 match, I read to Isaiah 10.

On Wednesday 4th August I noted, "We had a good night last night ... I nicked myself shaving this morning and it continued to bleed for quite some time. It took me ages to dress myself – an exhausting chore and I'm not sure how much longer I can cope with it." We watched some Olympics before attending Mass on livestream. After the Sainsbury's shopping was delivered, I ordered next week's shopping online. Apart from watching *Baptiste,* I managed to read up to Isaiah 17. In my diary of Thursday 5th August, I wrote: "Last night I lost my temper when I went upstairs and found Lennie messing around in my study. Stephen cooled things down ... Mandy helped Lennie get up after the cleaners had come. Stephen had taken bread and wine upstairs for the livestream Mass." Mandy advised me to put all our medications in a bag behind a locked kitchen door at night. I read up to Isaiah 41 before going up to bed. "Help me to be open to Your prompting, Lord."

Friday 6th August was not a very happy day. We didn't have a bad night. I didn't shave for about the first time, to take care of the cut I'd had on Wednesday. Fr. Roy gave an interesting homily at livestream Mass on the Feast of the Transfiguration. Lennie and I relaxed in the garden or watched the Olympics on TV. "The afternoon was a nightmare, with Lennie driving me mad for over an hour, as I mentioned to Leanne. Sadly, I blew my top. I must have been critical of Leanne and the need to make our meal during her shift. She walked out of the house. Later, she said she was in tears, and I told her I'd put a box of chocolates out to thank her for what she had done for us before our row. I hope we ended reconciled."

My diary for Saturday 7th August started: "A strange start to the day after a peaceful night." Jane helped Lennie get up and dressed. I cleared emails and prepared for the livestream Mass from St. Joseph's. Stephen came and "brought us up bread and wine for the Mass." We prayed for Doug's father, whose anniversary is tomorrow. We watched the Olympics. Then, after lunch, the Lions rugby Test in South Africa, "while Lennie nearly drove me mad with unreasonable demands". Andrew phoned in the evening. On Sunday 8th August, I noted that "last night was pretty quiet and Lennie stayed in our bed". I asked Stephen "to come up and help me dress quickly. He then helped Lennie to get dressed and we both had our pills and breakfast before I drove the three of us, with my zimmer frame, to St. Pius' for the 9.30 a.m. Mass." In the afternoon, I mostly skimmed the *Observer*. "Then, unexpectedly, we had a lovely loving and warm visit from Richard, Iris and Will. It is always lovely to see them. They are so loving towards us."

On Monday 9th August, I noticed bloodstains on the back of the loo and raised the issue with Mandy. "I cleared emails and then got St. Joseph's Mass online. Afterwards, we killed time as I read the *Guardian* Stephen had bought." Claire took Lennie for a brief drive and in the afternoon, Faye took her for a walk. I managed to read up to Isaiah 55. Belinda came in the late afternoon, "much to my relief as Lennie suddenly took off her dress and tried to put on a pair of tights over her head! Belinda sorted this out and then made us supper. In the evening, we mainly listened to Classic FM." I managed to read Isaiah 56–59 before we went up to bed.

Early in the morning of Tuesday 10th August, I found myself thinking I wasn't being a kind spouse cuddling Lennie. "I feel a bit guilty but find it difficult to turn over sideways in bed. After breakfast, I went upstairs and cleared emails, including one from our solicitor Joanna Mason, clarifying issues relating to the appointment of trustees." The carers, as always, helped us when they came on their hour-long shifts. "I was a bit shaken at one point when it seemed Lennie was going to swallow a one-pound coin in the same way she had her pills." Another worry.

On the morning of Wednesday 11th August, "I had an irritated exchange with Lennie, when I put out her pills and suggested she picked up the glass of water on the table to take them with her. But she looked all around the room, although her hand was almost on the table with the water. As I usually do, I got more and more frustrated that she didn't respond to directions such as 'it's just behind you' or 'by your right hand'. I exploded as I usually do. *Mea maxima culpa.*" The three of us attended Mass online and I struggled down the back passage to open the garden door for Voytek. We then had a visit from one of the numerous companies claiming to look after our solar panels that I might have confused with another organisation. After lunch, I had a good sleep until Sainsbury's delivered the weekly shopping. I went upstairs and ordered next week's shopping online. I found time to read Isaiah 63–66. When it became a bit chilly, I came in and we watched a Hundred cricket match and then Chelsea losing 6–5 on penalties in the UEFA Super Cup.

On Thursday 12th August, I suggested that "we had a reasonably good night." Stephen went off home at 8 a.m. and the cleaners came at 8.30 a.m. In the afternoon, I watched the Test match until it rained, and I switched to Classic FM. Lennie was a bit restless in the evening, but Faye had taken her to the Clandon Garden Centre. I read Jeremiah 7–9 before going up to bed.

On Friday 13th August, I started my diary: "Happy 55th anniversary, Ann and Peter. God bless you both and your family. Last night, Lennie started getting dressed around 1 a.m. and it was around 2 a.m. when I persuaded her to come back to bed." It was a bit of a mixed day. We spent some of it outside, where I managed to read about half of the weekend *Tablet*. We also spent some time watching the Test Match on TV. "Belinda did a good job easing Lennie through strange concerns about the sale of our house, her dad, and other issues." On Saturday 14th August Gilly joined us, having "brought her washing while her kitchen is being redone. After Mass, she kindly helped me submit online my application to renew my driving licence. We then watched the Test Match and I skimmed the *Guardian*. Lennie was very demanding. Stephen handled her pretty well, before cooking us a huge supper."

On Sunday morning, 15th August, "Lennie came downstairs with her blue dress on, but with Stephen's waistcoat and a skirt on under her dress and she had no bra on. We tried to persuade her to dress more respectably, and Stephen was more helpful than me. Fortunately, we got her dressed properly by the time Gilly arrived to drive us to St. Pius' for Mass." I spent much of the afternoon skimming the *Observer*. With her endless dressing and undressing, "Lennie destroyed a peaceful evening".

Monday 16th August seemed to be another mixed day, with routine domestic and everyday chores clashing with some aspects of Lennie's dementia. Belinda took Lennie out for a walk in the morning and in the afternoon drove her up to Newlands Corner. I had a dreadful and unexpected dose of diarrhoea. The carer helped Lennie go to bed early. I managed to read Jeremiah 20–23 before going to bed. On Tuesday morning, the 17th August, Mandy explained that Lennie probably had what is commonly referred to as Sundown Dementia. Halfway through livestream Mass, I remembered Lennie had a dental appointment at 11a.m. Marie drove her to the dentist, but she refused to have her tooth removed. In the evening, I reflected that "it is difficult to explain how Lennie completely destroyed three to four hours". I managed to read as far as Jeremiah 45 before going to bed.

On Wednesday 18th August, I struggled to take myself to the surgery for an annual check-up and reflected that in future, given my deteriorating mobility, I needed to have someone with me to help open doors and lifts. "Back home, Lennie was a nightmare – unable to find the loo by the front door or respond to 'door on the right'; or insisting on going home in spite of being told this is home; and so on, over and over again." St. Joseph's wasn't on livestream, so I found Thornton Heath for Mass today, which we watched with the bread and wine brought up by Stephen.

On Thursday 19th August, I started with "Life seems to be getting more and more difficult." In fact, it was essentially a day of coping with Lennie all day. "Last night she went off downstairs and I persuaded her to come back, though she was very restless. I failed to sleep again after 4 a.m., much to my frustration." In the late afternoon, the toenail cutter came to cut Lennie's nails. We then watched the Hundred cricket final, and I read as far as Jeremiah 51. Lennie was very loving on the morning of Friday 20th August, which followed a usual pattern: "get up early; read today's Mass readings and say prayers together; check emails and follow Mass on livestream before mid-morning coffee. In the afternoons, we sit out in the sun if we can and have a snooze. Carers come for three or four hour-long sessions and are helpful, taking Lennie out for a walk or for a visit to Newlands Corner. Stephen and I try to watch TV in the evenings, but Lennie is usually difficult and disturbed." Saturday 21st August started with worrying chest pains, which made me realise that if I had a heart attack, I didn't think Lennie would be able to help. At one stage I thought I needed at least one of the children to be with me every night, but later that didn't seem very realistic.

On Sunday 22nd August, "I was helpful in ensuring Lennie had on a bra and took off her nightie. I shaved and showered this morning and then Stephen came up and kindly helped me get dressed, which was much appreciated. Gillian kindly picked us up and drove us to St. Pius' for Mass. After Mass, Gilly stayed with us and helped Lennie by filing her nails and very professionally rubbed Zerobase on my arms, legs and forehead." After Stephen's lunch of roast chicken, "Lennie had one of her strange spells, expecting 'the children' to arrive soon". I skimmed the *Observer*, which had several articles on the 'Afghanistan disaster'. Chelsea beat Arsenal 2–0 to go top of the table. In the evening Lennie was 'maddening'! On Monday 23rd August Lennie was reported as going to sleep downstairs on the sofa the previous night. After breakfast, I sent a copy of Sylvie's and my paper on the Young Christian Workers (Y.C.W.) by email to Pat Jones. I finished reading Lamentations and then Chapters 1–8 of Ezekiel. "Thank You, Lord; it's not been a bad day."

On Tuesday 24th August, my diary noted: "This morning when Lennie started getting dressed, it was a shambles: no bra and a vest <u>outside</u> a cardigan." Mandy helped sort it out and Lennie came down in a blouse and skirt. I went upstairs and cleared emails before Lennie and I attended Mass on livestream. It was a very hot day, so in the afternoon we came inside and watched the opening ceremony of the Paralympics in Tokyo, which was very moving. In the evening, "Lennie was obsessed that I was wearing sandals and not shoes. She also thought I wasn't being generous to our children, especially Stephen. I coped pretty well with her aggressive line for the best part of an hour. But I eventually snapped and smashed my zimmer frame down when she couldn't put her garden chair on the others as we came in."

On Wednesday 25th August, when checking emails, I found "a sixteen-page essay on Pat Jones's mother's involvement with a Women's Y.C.W. I found it a fascinating outline of Catholic working-class life in the early post-war years in a mining community, and also of the particular battles women had to achieve justice at that time ... We attended Mass on livestream and Stephen came in time to bring up bread and wine before the offertory." In the afternoon, after the Sainsbury's shopping had been delivered, I struggled to order next week's Sainsbury's online shopping. I then watched England in a Test Match with India. In the evening, I wrote, "Lennie is going through a difficult period. It is difficult for Stephen and me to cope without getting angry." After quite some time, we managed to get her to put on her nightie, take off her skirt and go up to bed.

On Thursday 26th August, I opened my diary with a prayer: "Oh Lord, teach us the shortness of our days (Psalm 89), a theme I've become more and more aware of as I've struggled to do basic things like getting washed and dressed. Things seem to have changed rapidly over the past year. It is only a few months since Lennie used to walk round the block every day, but now she barely walks beyond the end of the cul-de-sac. I haven't exercised regularly and now am almost totally dependent on my zimmer frame, even to walk to the loo. Be with us, Lord and help us to cope with our last times as You would have us." After a relatively peaceful night, "Lennie had one of her strange periods when she wouldn't stop messing about and utterly failing to relax". The evening was difficult: "Lennie was 100% restless and I couldn't do anything apart from try to cope with her hallucinatory problems." It was helpful when Mandy came and took her up to dress for bed. But after Mandy left, she came up and down the stairs half a dozen times. I watched a T20 match and 1 read Ezekiel 10–13 before going to bed.

I had a strange start to the diary of Friday 27th August: "We had a pretty good night's sleep but then something strange happened after we'd read today's Mass reading and said our prayers. Lennie came out of the loo with a pile of loo paper with faeces on and put it on the dressing table. I expressed horror and eventually took it and flushed it down the loo. She seemed to be saying it was necessary for cooking for the children. Incomprehensible, but I suppose one of the strange byproducts of mixed dementia." The rest of the day included checking emails and attending Mass on livestream. After supper, "I struggled to cope with a disturbed Lennie trying on various cardigans and refusing to leave the basin with clothes potentially to be ironed. In trying to cope with Lennie's persistent unreasonable demands, and with the washing, I've been battered with 'I hate you' and told I never do anything." Before going to bed, I read Ezekiel Chapters. 14–21, dozed a bit and listened to Classic FM.

On Saturday 28th August, I noted that we'd had a good night and friendly start to the day. I had quite a discussion with Mandy, who was suggesting cutting our hour-long sessions with carers to three–quarters of an hour. I was interested because I was aware that our bank balances were declining, and I was trying to avoid digging into our savings. Richard came in the afternoon as we watched an impressive Chelsea battle to retain a 1–1 draw after James was sent off for handling the ball in the 48th minute. I managed to read Ezekiel 22–26 before going up to bed.

It was a lovely morning on Sunday 29th August when I drove the three of us to St Pius' for Mass. I'm afraid I acknowledged incontinence today, the latest problem of ageing. We sat outside most of the day. Gilly came and spent an hour with us this morning before they go off on holiday. During the rest of the day, I skimmed the *Observer* when I wasn't dozing. I tried to respond to the Burpham Neighbourhood questionnaire before joining Lennie upstairs."

On Monday 30th August, I didn't get back to sleep after 4.30 a.m. "In spite of my continuous pleas to the Lord, Lennie started getting up around 6 a.m., and put a bra on over the outside of a cardigan. Eventually, I got up and went and washed, but I needed Stephen's help to get a shirt and pair of trousers out of the wardrobe. I can't reach up high and was enormously grateful to him for his help." Stephen did a mini shop at Sainsbury's, Lennie did some ironing, and I went upstairs to check emails and get livestream Mass on the laptop. After Mass, "Lennie is, as usual, fussing about the washing on the line outside. Drives me nuts! After watching one of Stephen's DVDs, I sat outside and read Ezekiel 33.3. I noted two references in Ezekiel (18.20 and 33.20), which stress that God judges us by what we do."

Tuesday 31st August was an ordinary day, when Stephen went off early to spend the day in his apartment in

Cranleigh. We watched the Paralympics a bit before we attended Mass on livestream. "Lennie observed that we both had bad tempers. She was demanding all afternoon with many nonsense questions such as 'Where are my parents?' and claims that she'd seen them in the last couple of days. I invited her to join me outside, but she can't relax for more than a minute or so." When the cleaners had gone, we went upstairs, cleared emails and then attended Mass on livestream. "We were grateful for the piece of bread and the wine Stephen had brought up. He'd taken on board that Lennie's dementia might make it difficult to distinguish between 'left' and 'right', for example. Again, 'Your raincoat is in the cupboard under the stairs' ... Lennie's carer had put it out for us." Afterwards, I typed some of Stephen's notes. After Natasha had gone, we "entered a difficult spell. It drives me mad that Lennie cannot find the toilet when I say 'down the corridor and just after the radiator on the right'." Faye did a great job with Lennie, who was quite aggressive at times.

Friday 3rd September was a fairly typical day at this stage of Lennie's dementia. It seems that last night "we'd had a row and she said she hated me and didn't want to come into the same bed. But later she said she loved me, and we held hands." Lennie had painful legs that morning and didn't join me for livestream Mass. In the afternoon, Dr. Barnado came and added codeine to her list of medications. Faye took her for a drive while I "watched a bit of the Test with India. In the evening, Lennie was very mixed up; she wouldn't relax but felt she needed to be looking after the children. Help me, Lord, to behave as You would wish me to."

Saturday 4th September was another typical day for us at this stage in our lives. I had "a shower. Lennie is getting angry that she can't go 'home' and is walking up and down asking how she can get home. My insistence that this is home has no impact whatsoever." I cleared emails and did some work amending some of Stephen's poems before putting on the livestream Mass. We watched the Test Match with India before lunch. Andrew paid us a quick visit in the afternoon. We sent apologies that we wouldn't be attending the Oak Tree Gardens meeting. In the evening, we watched Stephen's TV selections, and I skimmed the *Guardian.*

On Sunday 5th September, "Lennie is moaning about her sore knees". I drove us to St. Pius' for Mass and back. "Then Gilly came and was pleasantly helpful and friendly before she left." In the afternoon, we watched England beat Andorra 4–0. I tried to skim the *Observer* in the evening with repeated interruptions from Lennie. On Monday 6th September, Stephen put on a week's load of washing before he set off for Cranleigh. I then "forced myself to go upstairs and clear emails before watching the livestream Mass from St. Joseph's with Lennie." I declined an invitation from John Wijngaard to join an academic group on the grounds that I was increasingly immobile and was the main carer for my wife, who had rapidly deteriorating mixed dementia. In the afternoon, I wrote, "Lennie's demands are endless. Mandy kindly got us a wedding anniversary card for Gilly and Doug."

On Tuesday 7th September, I struggled with my zimmer frame while Lennie came downstairs "saying she is in pain and 'can't do this anymore'." Lennie was in a lot of leg pain and didn't join me until halfway through the livestream Mass. I realised that we'd soon have to dig into our Fidelity savings. We sat outside much of the day. I expressed horror when Lennie started undressing in the lounge. On Wednesday 8th September, I noted that we'd had another seriously broken night after which I didn't get back to sleep again. So, I got up early and wrote out my September quota of cheques for charities, especially those for refugees and the homeless. I noted that Lennie's account had declined by £2,000 over the past year. We sat outside much of the day, but there was too much chat to allow me to read the *Guardian.* I managed to order next week's shopping from

Sainsbury's online. On Thursday 9th September, practically half of the day's diary dealt with the period before breakfast and Mandy's` coming to help dress Lennie and calm things down after I'd had a terrible night trying to cope with her interruptions. The diary also showed how evenings are generally lost in the same way.

On Friday 10th September, Lennie was in considerable pain after being dressed by Mandy. At this point in time, I was still trying to lay the table for breakfast with my zimmer frame before Mandy came at 8 a.m. But it was hard going. Louise took Lennie out for a short walk before cooking our lunch of fish fingers and chips. We had a row over locked doors, but fortunately Lennie was taken by a documentary about orang-utans. After Leanne left, "it didn't take long before I lost my cool. Again, Lennie wanted to go to the loo and didn't follow my directions: 'straight down the hall, past the radiator and on your right.' When she stands outside and doesn't even look right it drives me nuts, especially if I have to get up from the lounger, which is difficult these days given my limited mobility, and I shout angrily. Lord, please forgive me and help me do better." When Marie left at 8 p.m., "Lennie came down briefly to kiss me and tell me she loved me".

Saturday 11th September had a typical start, and I was "down just in time to wheel out the pills for us both." Mandy was a great help and earned a box of chocolates. I cleared emails before putting on livestream Mass. I spent the bulk of the rest of the morning and the afternoon skimming the *Guardian*. We watched some of Chelsea's match against Villa. On Sunday 12th September, we drove to St. Pius' for Mass. "I felt I had to sit through much of it; I find standing very difficult these days." On the way home, I noted I was having difficulties with incontinence and noted my need for special pants. Back home Lennie and I had a pleasant half-hour chat with Marie over our garden fence. Later, Marie "said she only occasionally heard me shouting and said she thought I was doing OK with a difficult situation. Help me, Lord, to do what You want me to do."

On Monday 13th September, I wrote that Lennie: "doesn't seem to be cleaning her bottom sensibly but is pulling out the loo paper used for wiping her bottom and putting it down all over the place. When I tried to get her to drop it into the loo she didn't respond, and this led to a shouting match and Stephen's helpful intervention. How relieved we were when Mandy came." Later, Marie took Lennie to the Park Barn Hive for social interaction, which gave me five hours of freedom. I listened on a CD lent to me by Frances Allen, to an excellent speech given at the National Justice and Peace Network Conference (NJPNC). I also cleared emails and attended Mass on livestream on my own. Tuesday 14th September was another mixed day with the usual routines such as checking emails and attending Mass on livestream. I was quite struck by the contrast between the Old Testament God, who seemed to encourage the genocide of Esau's descendants and the New Testament Jesus, who was so merciful and taught us to love our enemies. Wednesday 15th September was another difficult day with Lennie. She walked out of Mass halfway through. Stephen and I watched a couple of rugby internationals and a Champions League match.

On Thursday 16th September, Stephen left early to spend two days in Cranleigh. "Lennie went to bed last night fully clothed and we had a pretty good night's sleep." Mandy took her upstairs after breakfast to have caring company. "With my limited mobility these days I'm not much good as a cuddler." I did some work on Stephen's poems, cleared emails and set up livestream Mass. In the late afternoon, I wrote: "Lennie is pleading for someone to help her. I've spent the last hour responding to calls to move her chair into the sun, into the shade, get a cushion to ease her bottom, take her to the toilet and put up with all her refusals and denials, and that I am a bloody lazy oaf and never do anything to help. Then suddenly Lennie came in from outside and said, 'I do love you' and sat on my lap for a while. Lennie was unsettled as always, changing shoes and sandals over and over again and going outside into the garden and back half a dozen times."

Happy 55th birthday to Richard on Friday 17th September. "May the Lord be with you always and be important to you in the final stage of your life." I had a strange night last night and when I didn't "get to sleep after 4.30 a.m., I decided to get up and do an hour's work typing up Stephen's amendments to his poems." I opened the door for Mandy, cleared emails and got livestream Mass.

I had constipation problems that morning. "I came out to find my zimmer frame gone. Faye found it behind the shed. Another sign of the times. Lennie had one of her evening spells, first messing about with her bag, taking things in and out. Then she messed around with a blouse although she was perfectly dressed." In the evening, I enjoyed watching England's Women footballers draw 1–1 with Macedonia. "Before going to bed I read some more of Matthew's Gospel." As usual, on Saturday 18th September, I put out Lennie's pills before breakfast. "Eventually we went upstairs, and I cleared emails before we attended livestream Mass from St. Joseph's." Most of the rest of the morning and afternoon I spent outside in the garden trying to skim the main sections of the *Guardian.* In the evening, "Lennie came down and was a pain. I had to go upstairs, take her skirt off and put on her nightie. Time to go to bed. Please Lord, help me tomorrow morning ... I feel we need carers both morning and night on every day. Forgive my bad temper, Lord." On the morning of Sunday 19th September, "I was relieved to have some female help from Louise" when Lennie was finding her bra too tight and was putting it on over a vest. I drove the three of us to Mass and sat during much of it. Later, I watched Chelsea beat Spurs 3–0. "Lennie was a pain in the neck over the next couple of hours

… Stephen was a bit depressed by all the demands on him this weekend."

On Monday 20th September, I started my diary: "It was a very disturbed night. Around 1–3 a.m., Lennie refused to return to bed, repeatedly dressing and undressing. Stephen helped me get dressed before he set off for Cranleigh. We'd both had a difficult weekend with Lennie." And sadly, for the first time, "Lennie did not attend any part of the livestream Mass. I sent a congratulatory email to Gilly and Doug on their 35th wedding anniversary and cleared emails." I also got out lists of Christmas cards sent in 2019. Louise then put out the washing on the line. I spent much of the afternoon sitting outside in the garden, trying to read today's mail and the *Tablet* in spite of Lennie.

On Tuesday 21st September, my online banking wasn't working. The vapour trails in the sky were intriguing. I phoned my cousin Pat's daughter to say we wouldn't be able to attend Pat's funeral but phoned our parish office to book a Mass for her. I did manage to finish reading Matthew's Gospel and the first six chapters of Mark. Lennie was awkward and brought the medical chair from the toilet to the lounge. "Yet later she came and kissed me and said how much she loved me." Wednesday 22nd September was much as usual, but I did manage to clear emails before Lennie joined me for livestream Mass. Afterwards, I paid an Everycare invoice on Nat West online banking. Voytek came to do a session of gardening and helped Lennie stumble back without her falling. After Sainsbury's shopping had been delivered, I went upstairs and ordered next week's shopping online. In the evening Andrew visited in time for Stephen's supper of cauliflower and macaroni cheese and stayed for an hour's chat. His relationship with Caroline seems to be breaking down. He'd shaved off his beard. "Lennie was coping with nasty bites from a spider this afternoon." We watched Chelsea beat Villa 4–3 in the

Carabao Cup. Lennie went into the other bed upstairs but joined me in the early hours.

On Thursday 23rd September, Stephen helped me get dressed before going off to Cranleigh for the next two days. At this stage we stayed downstairs while the cleaners did their stint upstairs before we went up to clear emails and then attend Mass on livestream. Jane's daughter, Natalie, came to assist us at lunchtime and threw away some food which was out of date and potentially a health hazard. In the late evening, I struggled with fairly uncontrollable diarrhoea. On Friday 24th, we attended Mass on livestream, after which I cleared emails. I didn't feel like any lunch that day. I had another bowel eruption, which took some time to clear up, and I changed my clothes and put on a load of washing. On Saturday 25th September, after online Mass and clearing emails, Gilly unexpectedly came with her two dogs. She was very critical of the cleanliness of the house and went off to Sainsbury's to buy disinfectants. "Lennie walked up and down the house and garden all afternoon. Later, Lennie behaved awkwardly for Stephen and me by dressing with new pants or taking off her jumper or cardigan downstairs. With much anger, we gave her her pills and then persuaded her somehow to go up to bed and undress upstairs."

On Sunday 26th September, I wrote that I was finding it increasingly difficult to shave and shower myself and recognized the need soon to dig into my Fidelity savings. Stephen helped me get dressed and I phoned Laura Anderson to say we wouldn't be able to attend Mass at St. Pius'. Stephen took Lennie for a walk before we watched Mass online from St. Joseph's. Much of the day I spent skimming the *Tablet*. Richard came and cuddled Lennie. In the evening, I watched *Vigil* with Stephen, but this was interrupted by a very difficult Lennie who wanted to undress in front of us. Stephen persuaded me to continue wearing shorts on Monday 27th in the garden a lot of the day. "Gillian phoned and laid down the law. Just because she was a woman, there was no reason why she should do more to help with the family finances." I went to bed before 10 p.m. On Tuesday 28th September, I was grateful that Fidelity was prepared to switch £30,000 to my NatWest account over the phone. It was otherwise a rather ordinary day, which ended with my watching *Line of Duty* and enjoying the Karelia Suite.

On Wednesday 29th September, after breakfast I sent a 55th birthday wish to Sylvie before clearing emails and attending Mass on livestream. Afterwards, Stephen came, and we watched Keir Starmer's Labour Party Conference speech, which was quite impressive. We enjoyed going out in the garden in the sun. After the Sainsbury's online shopping had been delivered, I went upstairs and ordered next Wednesday's shopping online. In the evening, we watched Chelsea lose 1–0 to Juventus. On Thursday 30th September, while I was washing, "Lennie put on my vest and short-sleeved shirt I'd put out for tomorrow. I was furious but Stephen came up to give some calm." After lunch, "the next three hours were pretty awful; Lennie just never stopped. I would have loved to be allowed to doze off but walking up and down, she repeatedly woke me up. I gave her codeine and paracetamol, but she couldn't pick up the water glass in front of her. Absolutely infuriating. It means I must get myself up physically – not easy these days." In the evening, I watched another episode of *Line of Duty* and listened to Mozart and Brahms on Classic FM. It looks as if Friday 1st October was when I first tried on pants for incontinent males. After breakfast, I went upstairs, cleared eighteen emails and got us livestream Mass from St. Joseph's. In mid-afternoon, Victoria drove us to Godalming, where we had our booster jabs. In the evening, I watched a T20 match and then found the next episode of *Line of Duty*.

On Saturday 2nd October, our carer was unwell, so I had to serve both medication and breakfast using the zimmer frame. It was the first time I'd had nobody to help with Lennie. Around 11 a.m. I realised we'd forgotten to go and get our flu jabs at the cathedral. So, I drove the three of us there and there was no trouble. I dozed a lot of the afternoon. Lennie was awkward as usual. In the evening, Chelsea beat Southampton 3–1 with two late goals and were now top of the table. On Sunday 3rd October, I noted, "I am struggling more and more with getting up, shaving and showering. Stephen, bless him, came up and helped me dress. I drove the three of us to Mass, where I spent the bulk of the time sitting down. I can't stand for long these days. In the afternoon, Richard turned up and was a delightful visitor for an hour or two. On Monday 4th October, I recorded that on the whole we had a good night's sleep, and in the end, we even managed to say some prayers together for the first time for quite a while. Andrew came to drive Lennie to the dentist in Kingston. Back home afterwards, we were lucky that on her afternoon shift Louise had brought in the washing on the line as it was chucking it down when we returned home. In the evening, Lennie was irrational for a time.

On Tuesday 5th October, when paying my Everycare bill, my account confirmed that Fidelity had transferred £30,000 into my Nat West account. After clearing emails, I found livestream Mass. While Faye took Lennie for a walk round the Clandon Garden Centre, I listened to some of the recordings from the NJPNC talks which Frances had lent me. They included "three youngsters who spoke up excellently on behalf of their generation". The rest of the day seems to have been a bit of a mix. I watched some David Attenborough films before going to bed. On Wednesday 6th October, Mandy, as always, took Lennie upstairs after breakfast and dressed her. I wrote another letter to the DVLA about renewing my driving licence, which was due to run out in a month's time. I cleared emails before getting livestream Mass from St. Joseph's. Voytek came for probably the last time of the year and left both the front and back gardens looking fine. In the afternoon, after the Sainsbury's shopping had been delivered, I ordered next week's online, with the usual difficulties with Sainsbury's checkout. "Richard suddenly appeared, unexpectedly. But the two boys and I had a very interesting hour chatting, mainly about David's family."

On Thursday 7th October, I put on a pair of the new pants Stephen had bought me recently and he came up to help me dress. One of the emails I checked afterwards was one between Andrew and Gillian, "who are committed to exploring local care homes in the event, for example, of my death. Mandy came at 8 a.m. when Stephen left for home." The cleaners came and when they'd finished upstairs Lennie and I went up, checked emails and put on livestream Mass. Another rather mixed day with Lennie a bit disorientated. I was considering the incontinence pants, "all recorded because it is a sign of what our difficulties are at this stage in our lives. Lennie asked for a paracetamol, but when she didn't know where the dining room table was, I had to get up and take it to her, but she then refused to take it and, as usual I exploded, unhelpfully. During the day I managed to read Luke 14."

On what was my father's birthday, Friday 8th October, I wrote, "I didn't have a bad night and Lennie was very affectionate. But I don't think I slept after 3.30 a.m." The day proceeded much as usual. I checked emails and arranged livestream Mass from St. Joseph's. I wrote my first Christmas card to Lennie's friend, Rosemary, in Berwick. The rest of the day just dribbled away. On Saturday 9th October, a lot of time was spent seeing whether Richard or Gillian could drive Lennie to her two dental appointments in Kingston the following week. In the afternoon, after my usual doze, I joined Lennie outside in the sun and skimmed the *Guardian*. On Sunday 10th October, I wrote that I'd had a pretty good night's sleep, though I went to the loo more frequently than usual. Gilly drove us to and from St. Pius', where the Mass was said for my cousin Pat Loring, whose funeral was in two days' time. The day ended with Stephen's choice of fight, which Tyson Fury won.

On Monday 11th October, Gilly confirmed arrangements for NHS transport to take Lennie to and from Kingston for her dental treatment. She then came to drive Lennie to Milford for an overall check-up. Several arrangements for taking Lennie to Kingston seem to have been altered late on and the whole issue was time-consuming. I finished reading John's Gospel before going up to bed. Tuesday 12th October was a nightmare. Lennie wandered off after I'd opened the door for Mandy. Then Richard phoned to say Iris had COVID-19, so he couldn't drive Lennie to Kingston. Stephen reluctantly agreed to come and take Lennie in a taxi. Lennie wasn't impressed that I hadn't gone to Kingston with her, even when I pointed out that I was too immobile to push a wheelchair.

Wednesday 13th October seems to have been another typically busy domestic day, getting up before Mandy reached here at 8 a.m. Then the three of us attended Mass on livestream, and afterwards, printed some of Stephen's amendments to his poems and wrote a few Christmas cards. After a spell in the garden after lunch and the Sainsbury's shopping delivery, it took me one-and-a-half hours to order next week's shopping online, mainly because of the ageing of my laptop. Lennie's interruptions destroyed our attempts to watch serious TV in the evening. Andrew phoned after being released from hospital.

On Thursday 14th October, I was having big problems because I had a very painful elbow, which made it almost impossible for me to push myself out of my chair. "Jane and Gilly phoned me later and seemed to be pressing towards a full-time carer or a care home, which I'm trying to avoid." For some reason, I didn't get through to the online Mass until halfway through St. Paul's epistle. "After Mass I cleared about eighteen emails and responded to two questionnaires before going downstairs." I sat in the garden during the afternoon until it became chilly. "There was a phone call from Andrew saying he had returned to hospital where he expected to get further treatment for his kidney stones the next day. I phoned Richard to keep him up to date and to ask for his prayers ... Lennie has just kissed me and told me I am 'a lovely man'!"

Friday 15th October was another fairly mixed day: "potentially an important day for our family with Lennie's potential tooth extraction, Andrew's potential operation, and his isolating with COVID-19. I pray for them all, Lord and thank You that my right arm seems to be improving. I had a reasonably good night last night ... It was quite hectic getting dressed; I missed Stephen's help." We attended Mass on livestream before Stephen turned up. He took Lennie to Kingston in a minibus. During the afternoon, I went upstairs and wrote about seven more Christmas cards. On their return, Lennie and Stephen gave the impression that the organisation at Kingston was appalling. On Saturday 16th October, the three of us followed Mass on livestream. In the evening, we watched Chelsea fortunately beating Brentford after a Chilwell goal and some excellent goalkeeping from Mendy.

On Sunday 17th October, Gilly drove us to Mass at St. Pius'. Fr. Roy brought us Holy Communion on the front row. Mary Fox said she "was trying to resuscitate the Justice and Peace group and it was interesting that Catherine and Alan Hughes were promoting a parish refugee project. Gillian took us home and spent an hour catching up with our news and telling us about Andrew." We watched Newcastle lose 2–3 to Spurs. "We started watching an episode of *Succession,* but Lennie was as disruptive as usual ... It's not been a great week."

On Monday 18th October, I wrote: "Happy 70th birthday dear sister, Sue. May the Lord give you peace, joy and love always." Before he set off for Cranleigh, Stephen had put out a load of washing on the line. I had difficulty getting livestream Mass and managed to arrive halfway through the epistle from St. Joseph's. "After carer Holly left, things became very difficult, with Lennie wanting to 'go home', mucking about with a skirt which had been out on a radiator to dry; and so on. After another carer had left, we then had another two-hour spell when Lennie created difficulties non-stop. She took off her jumper and blouse and put them on again, over and over again. The result was that at times I had a half-naked Lennie next to me, but she was totally resistant to any of my suggestions and saw me as a selfish guy only concerned about myself and unwilling to give her any attention. Not an easy day." A physiotherapist came and gave Lennie a number of exercises to do, recommending that I did them too.

On Tuesday 19th October, the livestream Mass was a funeral, the first I could remember in well over a year. In the evening, we watched a variety of episodes, including *Our Yorkshire Farm*, one of my favourites, with six-year-old Clemmy pulling lambs out of sheep! Wednesday 20th October wasn't an easy day. "Lennie isn't taking her pills easily and has insisted with Jane that she will decide when she has them. It is difficult to pray consistently with life so disorganised as it is at the moment ... I checked emails and paid the Everycare bill before the livestream Mass from St. Joseph's." In the downstairs loo there were signs of dirty seats and I assumed Lennie was responsible. I only managed to write about five Christmas cards that day. In the evening, Chelsea beat Malmo 1–0 to win 4–0 on aggregate.

Thursday 21st October was Sue and Mario's 49th wedding anniversary. "God bless you and keep you close always." I wrote a few Christmas cards. After watching the livestream Mass from St. Joseph's, there was a lovely ecumenical service from Armagh Cathedral. Marie took Lennie for a short walk. When she'd left, Lennie "started wandering in and out of the room and the garden and then repeatedly said 'I want to go home' or 'Where are my mother and father?' My comments 'This is your home' were completely ignored and it got more and more difficult to cope." In the late evening, "I stuck to my decision not to go to bed before 10 p.m. as pushing me to do so is a form of bullying."

On Friday 22nd October, I recorded that "I had a pretty good night's sleep and Lennie was as loving as usual, though we nearly 'had words' when she couldn't turn off the bathroom light." We went upstairs to check emails and get livestream Mass. "For the first time, Lennie muttered something about the approach of death." In the late afternoon, we watched some fantastic gymnastics from the World Championships. Andrew phoned from Kidlington; it seems that his relationship with Caroline is over. On Saturday 23rd October, after I'd cleared emails, we watched Mass from Arundel Cathedral because the Mass at St. Josephs was a Confirmation Mass with Bishop Richard. Afterwards, I started to skim the *Guardian*, which I found disappointing. We then watched Chelsea beat Norwich 7–0. In the evening, I wrote a few more Christmas cards.

On Sunday 24th October, Gilly came and drove us to St. Pius' for Mass. "I couldn't stand for long and spent nearly all the Mass sitting down." After Mass, Gilly drove us home and we had an hour's chat and raised the issue of Christmas, so that we could make appropriate arrangements with Everycare. We watched a T20 match between India and Pakistan and then Liverpool's 5–0 defeat of Manchester United. In the evening, "Lennie just wouldn't stop and relax. Instead, she kept interrupting a programme about a bank heist. It drove Stephen and me mad. In the end, to our relief, Holly came and took Lennie upstairs to bed."

On Monday 25th October, I noted that "I was lucky that Stephen was here and offered to help me dress, especially putting on my socks ... After Mass, I photocopied Stephen's five-page report on his visit to Kingston with Lennie." As usual, the carers took Lennie for a short walk to the end of our cul-de-sac and back. During the afternoon, "Alan Hughes came round to discuss the parish's refugee assistance project." In the evening, after the carer had left, "Lennie changed gears. First, she took off one of the TV's remotes and I nearly went ballistic. Secondly, she started seemingly destroying one of her artificial wallflowers. Somehow, we cooled off. She is concerned about the wellbeing of the children in her care (as thirty years ago). Eventually, I managed to cope by turning off the TV and shutting up." I enjoyed Classic FM later in the evening.

Tuesday 26th October had the same sort of problems. I told Mandy that when I had told Lennie that she was coming "to help her dress, she was furious and said she didn't want her in this house. Mandy clearly has great carer's skills and ended up doing the physio's exercises with her. In the early hours, I found myself wondering how to cope with the approach of our deaths. I wondered about parcelling off all my diaries to the archivist at Farm Street." After Mass, I managed to check emails and eventually pay Everycare on online banking. "As usual, I dozed off after lunch and put on T20. Lennie was her usual self, unable to sit and relax, but also to leave me alone and let me sleep. It was very annoying." I phoned Ann and asked her to pass on my birthday wishes to Mary. She also told me that Emily and Steve had come over to help Peter get up after a fall. I went up to bed about 10 p.m. "I feel this has not been a good day for me and I haven't done as much as I should have done."

On Wednesday 27th October, I managed to put out our pills before Mandy came at 8 a.m. "She is helpful with Lennie and always manages to encourage her. I feel so limited and sleepy and am not sure what I ought to be doing. I pray that my guardian angel will guide me." I cleared some emails and wrote some Christmas cards before we attended livestream Mass. Stephen came before the end of Mass and Lennie joined him downstairs. I then cleared the rest of the emails and sent apologies to a couple of charities for not attending their meetings because I was so immobile. The weekly online Sainsbury's shopping delivery came in mid-afternoon, after which I went upstairs to order next week's shopping online, coping with problems of checkout as usual. We enjoyed another episode of *Our Yorkshire Farm*, with the Owen family coping with lambing in the snow in May. We also watched episodes of *Location, Location, Location* and *Shetland* before bed.

On Thursday 28th October, it seems I had a confused night, not being clear what the time was. Stephen gave me some toast and marmalade before setting off for the library as Mandy came. When the cleaners came, we stayed downstairs while they cleaned upstairs and swapped over about 9.35 a.m. I cleared emails before Lennie and I attended livestream Mass. During the afternoon, we watched *Escape to the Country* and then *Escape to the Château* while I worked my way through the *Tablet*.

On Friday 29th October, I discovered I'd forgotten to lock the garden gate, so I had to hurry downstairs to stop Lennie wandering off. Before Mass on livestream, I cleared over twenty emails. "Victoria has put on fish and chips and taken Lennie out for a short walk before lunch. I suppose I was naughty or lazy during the afternoon, watching a couple of very interesting T20 internationals, including the West Indies win over Bangladesh by just three runs on the last ball. Andrew then came and brought a very tasty cherry cake. But his patience with his mum is a lot less than mine and I think he just decided that he couldn't cope with Lennie on a lengthy Christmas Day with lunch. Dr. Barnado phoned and we discussed whether or not I should continue driving. He hadn't been contacted by the DVLA, but said he couldn't see any medical reason why I should stop driving. But considering how little I drive, he raised the issue of what would happen if I had an accident. He pointed out that getting taxis on the odd occasion would be much cheaper than the considerable cost of driving at that moment. Lennie was pretty awkward when Andrew was here, cutting up his cake for all the people she fantasised were coming for a meal. Thank You, Lord, for all the support we have had today and help me get closer to what You wish tomorrow."

On Saturday 30th October, I wrote: "I had a pretty good night's sleep ... Lennie seemed to be asleep most of the time. Around 7 a.m., I got up and had my weekly shower and washed my hair, but again I didn't shave ... Mandy got Lennie up and dressed and also put on a load of washing, which Stephen later put on the line. Lennie and I managed to watch the Mass from St. Joseph's." Neither Gilly nor Stephen had strong views about whether or not I should continue driving. "It was a relief to see two Chelsea goals from Reece James lead to a 3–0 win in Newcastle. After supper, I continued to skim today's *Guardian*."

On Sunday 31st October, we put the clocks back an hour at the end of BST and I was awake at 2 a.m. when our bedside clock went back an hour. I drove us to St. Pius' for possibly the last time. "It was good to see so many of our old friends who were all very warm ... Stephen made us a very tasty lunch, sadly interrupted by Lennie's incessant moaning. We watched some women's rugby. I read 1 Cor..13–16 and fiddled around with the last few Christmas cards."

Monday 1st November seemed like an ordinary, busy day. It was the first day of the COP 26 meeting in Glasgow, so a large part of today was spent listening to news updates and responses to the frightening evidence about climate change. Stephen had taken up some bread and wine for our livestream attendance at Mass on the Feast of All Saints, where Deacon Michael gave another thought-provoking homily. This morning, I sent an email to our children "asking them not to buy me any Christmas presents. I put it in the context of two major global problems: COVID-19 and climate change." In the evening, I skimmed the *Tablet,* which I felt was getting "increasingly international but not quite so interesting as before."

Tuesday 2nd November was the Feast of All Souls, so I remembered my parents in my prayers. "Lennie is saying she is waiting for her parents, whom she saw recently! She still thinks she is a teacher with responsibility for 'the children', whose parents have had no notifications about their children." It was a lovely day, so Lennie and I spent some time on the patio enjoying the sun. Mandy came and coped well with "Lennie's illnesses, rudeness and authoritarianism. In the evening, Lennie became more and more angry with me as I pointed out we were at home and so on. But she 'hated me' and complained that I never did a thing." But later, after carer Naomi had left, she "came down to join me and tell me how much she loved me!"

On 3rd November, I put on my new incontinence pants for about the first time; another sign of my ageing! "Stephen turned up just as Mass was coming on livestream. He brought up some bread and wine for us. Later, I spent the best part of an hour looking at information about the Legal Power of Attorney and finding Nationwide cards before going there with Douglas to pass on his account book to him. It took me two hours to do the Sainsbury's shopping online. When I went up to bed, Lennie was very against my getting into the bed and denied we had been sleeping together for sixty years. But she quietened down and I soon slept."

On Thursday 4th November, I tried to find something appealing to Lennie on TV. Much TV seemed trivial to me, though there was an interesting documentary about climate change before I went up to bed. On Friday 5th November, "I cleared emails before we celebrated livestream Mass, with the strange parable about the shrewd manager. Outside, the sky is fascinating with numerous vapour trails." In mid-afternoon, "Lennie was in a mood because both doors were shut and she was going on and on about fantasy needs ... Lennie just wouldn't stop, including bringing in two dessert dishes with a drying-up cloth and a dustpan and brush."

On Saturday 6th November, Stephen came just in time to bring us bread and wine for the livestream Mass. In the afternoon, we watched South Africa beat England in a T20 match while I tried to skim the *Guardian*. More football in the evening until Stephen's boxing took over. On Sunday 7th November, "Stephen came up to help me dress, which was very kind of him". Gilly drove us to and from Mass. By now, it seemed to be accepted that we would sit on the front row, where Deacon Michael would bring us Holy Communion. Gilly also seemed to be under pressure and exploded in a row with Stephen. Both Andrew and Richard visited during the afternoon and evening. On Monday 8th November, I was seriously considering cancelling my DVLA application, my AA insurance, and selling our car. The rest of the day seemed entirely domestic with nothing much to remember; the first part of the day was much as usual with Lennie wearing my sandals. After the online Mass, we watched TV. The carers usually take Lennie out for a short walk or drive in the car.

I was cross that I hadn't heard from the DVLA since August. At one stage in the early evening, "Lennie wandered about and then, relatively unusually, started to pray out loud. She complained that she couldn't talk to Jesus. At one stage we had a row, and she was full of denials." Later, after Naomi had come and taken her upstairs to dress her, she "came down, very friendly" for a kiss and to say 'good night'. I enjoyed watching *Our Yorkshire Farm* with the Owen family. On Wednesday 10th November, the lights were on downstairs, so it seemed clear that Lennie had been there during the night. Early in the morning, we tried to sort out a variety of medical appointments before clearing emails and attending Mass online. Later, I wrote: "Lennie is driving me mad, refusing to take the paracetamol given to her. I exploded and that simply increased her defiance. Later in the day I cancelled my AA membership and insurance and arranged to sell the car. Richard agreed to drive me over to Slyfield to sell it on Sunday. After two hours' slog, I managed to book next week's Sainsbury's shopping online."

On Thursday 11th November, the first part of the day was much as usual, except for concerns about insurance cover for the car while we took it on Sunday to sell it to 'We Buy Any Car'. When I went up to bed, Lennie was messing about, and I wasn't very sympathetic. In the middle of the night, she wanted to chat and get dressed. I was a bit irritable and wanted her to shut up and let me get to sleep. She just didn't seem to be aware of what she was doing to other people.

On Friday 12th November, the news from COP26 was a bit depressing. I phoned Richard to urge him to get insurance cover for Sunday. I couldn't get livestream Mass from St. Joseph's and ended up getting it from Cork Cathedral with no homily. In the afternoon, I watched the Scotland vs Moldova football international, which Scotland won 2–0. In the afternoon, England beat Albania 5–0 at Wembley. "When I went upstairs, Lennie was fully dressed and went to bed like that, no transfer to her nightie." On Saturday 13th November, after my shower, and at 9 a.m. Stephen arrived and came to Mass with us. "Gilly and Douglas came and drove us to Nationwide" and watched a rugby international and later Anastasia came, showered Lennie and helpfully got her dressed for bed. On Sunday 14th November, Gilly drove us to and from Mass at St. Pius'. The shoes she had bought Lennie were too tight, so she took them away to change them; bless her. In the afternoon, Richard drove me to Slyfield where we sold my car. It was the end of my driving.

On Monday 15th November, Gilly came and took Lennie off for a hospital appointment. Stephen came early and brought up bread and wine for the livestream Mass before he left to go to Cranleigh. After Mass, I tidied up some files after the sale of the car. Marie took Lennie out for a drive in the afternoon. When she left, "I had to cope with two hours of Lennie going on and on about going home, although I repeatedly told her that this is our home! She complained I never helped and when I challenged her, she shouted repeatedly that I was a liar. She has just hoped that her dad would come back and is saddened when I remind her that he died fifty-six years ago. Earlier, she'd brought in the food bucket from the kitchen. She wants to be 'doing' something all the time and isn't interested in watching TV. Help me to cope, Lord." After being changed by a carer, she came downstairs and watched some international football until we both went up to bed.

Tuesday 16th November opened with an admission that I'd "just had a verbal explosion with Lennie who earlier, in bed, said 'I love you' and ended up saying 'I wish I'd never met you'". After we'd read some scriptures and come downstairs, "Lennie had one of her mood changes, telling me off for 'inviting' loads of people and accusing me of lying. I managed to keep reasonably cool, but Lennie was extremely angry with me for things I hadn't done!" When Vicky came, she got her to help make lunch. Later, she refused to have her toenails cut by Emma. Faye drew my attention to an excellent documentary about care workers by Ed Balls, which was most impressive. We were phoned to tell us a recent carer had COVID-19. On Wednesday 17th November, I stupidly pulled a scab off my arm and cut myself shaving. Later, Lennie was angry when she realised I'd sold the car. After losing St. Joseph's on livestream, we were joined by Stephen to attend Mass at St. Columba's in

Ireland. I was sleeping in the afternoon when the Sainsbury's shopping was delivered and I then spent some time, and with difficulty, ordering next Wednesday's online shopping. In the evening, we watched the first Ed Balls episode which contrasted the NHS care for cancer patients with care workers.

On Thursday 18th November, I wrote that I hadn't had a bad night, though Lennie had gone downstairs in the middle of the night in what looked like my woollen jumper over pants, and I encouraged her to come back to bed. Stephen kindly came up to help me dress before he set off for Cranleigh. After the cleaners had finished upstairs, we went up and I cleared emails before we switched to livestream Mass. Dennis then came to cut my hair for the first time in months. In the evening, we watched a fascinating documentary about the origins of the universe, the 'big bang theory', and life on our planet. On Friday 19th November, I wrote that I'd had a pretty good night. "But it was a struggle getting down in time to open the door for Mandy." Before she left, I booked a dental appointment, checked with Everycare and cancelled one of two cardiology appointments. "I'm always aware of Paul's 'love is patient' and my need to control my irritability with Lennie." The carers took Lennie out for short walks or drives in the car, and I managed to read much of the *Tablet* during the afternoon. Lennie came downstairs for most of the evening with the *Children in Need* programme.

My diary for Saturday 20th November suggests we had a sort of mini love-making spell last night. "But I found myself wondering whether Jesus would see it as lust. A couple of hours later I woke to find Lennie mucking around with my shoes and socks. Our mutual anger left me pushing her, almost close to hitting her. Another warning: I need to watch my temper and remember 'love is patient'. Help me, Lord. I went upstairs and cleared twenty emails before Stephen arrived and the three of us watched the Mass at St.

Joseph's on livestream. Stephen got me a G&T and I skimmed the *Guardian.*" For much of the rest of the day, we watched football, including Chelsea's 3–0 win at Leicester. Before going up to bed, I read Revelation Chapters 3–4.

On Sunday 21st November, I wrote that I'd had "a reasonably good night's sleep. When I couldn't get easily to sleep in the early hours, I said the rosary." Gillian drove us to and from St. Pius', where I sat during most of the Mass. She asked whether we would like to go for coffee afterwards, but I declined because I needed to go to the loo. Much of the rest of the day was spent watching football and rugby on TV, an episode of *Dan Brown* and then Stephen's boxing.

On Monday 22nd November, when I asked Lennie "why she didn't want to sleep with me, she said I was too old!" Marie came to the dentist with me. Unexpectedly, the dentist said the tooth needed to be extracted by a professional! The rest of the day passed much as usual before we watched a David Attenborough documentary. Before going to bed, I read as far as Revelation Ch. 15.

On Tuesday 23rd November, I noted that "today I finished reading Revelation, i.e., I've read the Bible from Genesis to Revelation this year". Chelsea beat Juventus 4–0 today; I was tempted to email Sue and Mario! "Some final reflections on my relationship with Lennie. There are times when she sounds lonely and not getting the close attention she feels she used to have. And with her time warp she feels she ought to be <u>doing</u> a great deal more for her 'children' and their parents. Be with her, Lord, and help me be more sympathetic and caring than I think I have been."

Wednesday 24th November was our oldest son, Andrew's, 60th birthday. "Be with him, Lord, and keep him close to you." I only just managed to get the livestream Mass on the Feast of St. Andrew Düng-Lac. "The thousands of

Christians persecuted and executed, tortured and killed by the Emperor in the 19th century makes me wonder whether I would have had the guts to resist physical persecution. Please God, I never deny You." Andie came and gave Lennie a perm; he did a good job. Stephen put away the Sainsbury's online shopping delivery. It was late that evening, after help from our neighbour, John Campbell, that I managed to order next week's shopping online.

On Thursday 25th November, Stephen kindly came up and helped me dress. After the cleaners had finished upstairs, I went up and cleared about twenty emails before we watched Mass on livestream from St. Joseph's. There was quite a lot of mail today which needed wading through thoroughly. Stephen put on *His Dark Materials,* but it didn't appeal to me. This was another strange day. On Friday 26th November, Stephen helped me dress and then came with me for my check-up at the Royal Surrey for my pacemaker, which seemed to be OK, though there was some concern about my third wire. After returning home, Stephen went off to Cranleigh, bless him. We watched the EWTN Mass before the rest of the day disappeared with watching Test cricket and putting up with Lennie's obscure musings, such as her parents being around and so on. Marie took Lennie for a drive and then dressed her for bed. After Marie had gone, "Lennie came downstairs to express her love for me before returning to bed". I watched some football before going up at 10 p.m.

On Saturday 27th November, we watched livestream Mass from St. Joseph's. Fr. Roy emphasised two themes: the proximity of our deaths and the second coming of Jesus and the end of the world. "After Mass I sent an email to Frs. Tony and Roy, asking if they would be prepared to visit and hear our confession." Afterwards, I skimmed the *Guardian* before Stephen's lunch. Then I dozed off for a bit. Ann phoned to exchange gossip about our families. During the day I read the first forty-one paragraphs of *Laudato Si*.

On Sunday 28th November, I noted that I hadn't had a bad night, though I didn't sleep again after 4 a.m. Around 7 a.m., I shaved, Stephen helped me get dressed and I cleared emails. Gilly came and drove us to Mass, where I sat most of the time. Mgr. Tony brought us Holy Communion. Back home, Gilly raised the matter of whether or not I had booked a burial plot. Andrew and Richard both visited with birthday presents and we watched Chelsea draw 1–1 with Manchester United. In the evening, we watched a couple of episodes of the first series of *Downton Abbey*.

On Monday 29th November, Stephen went off to Cranleigh shortly after Mandy arrived at 8 a.m. We had some snow overnight. I read another section of *Laudato Si* before going upstairs to clear emails and putting on the livestreamed Mass from St. Joseph's. Faye took Lennie out for a drive while I wrote some of my monthly donations to charities. Andrew phoned for probably over half an hour, telling me that he'd started moving out of Caroline's house. I tried to persuade him to keep his cool and avoid conflict and thought I'd better do so myself with Lennie. Later, Lennie was difficult, undressing in the lounge and putting a jumper over a raincoat.

Tuesday 30th November was my 89th birthday. Andrew arrived about 8.30 a.m. and helped sort out the presents and had a slice of my birthday cake while he was here. I cleared emails, arranged a visit from a British Gas engineer, and took phone calls from Sue, Ann and Michael Wheeler. Stephen was with us for livestream Mass. After lunch, I plodded through the *Guardian* and was pleased to find an article by Polly Toynbee, who is always more interesting than the younger women. In the afternoon, Sylvie phoned, and Maureen Durston brought a cake. Will and Iris phoned to wish me a happy birthday.

Wednesday 1st December seemed to be a mixed sort of day, much as usual. Stephen arrived in time to join us for the livestream Mass. Later, I ordered next week's online shopping from Sainsbury's, which was quite expensive because of the chocolate boxes I ordered for Lennie's birthday and also to give as Christmas presents to the carers. We put on *Downton Abbey*, but Lennie never stopped talking, interrupting and going with Stephen into the kitchen.

My diary for Thursday 2nd December opened with: "It was shortly after midnight that Lennie started dressing and then undressing continuously for over two hours. I tried to get her into bed, but she was very resistant. We had an angry exchange, including slaps, which worried me a bit, so I just tried to shut up. Stephen told me later she'd slept on the lounger. Stephen set off for Cranleigh soon after 8 a.m." We watched livestream Mass and then listened to Christmassy music on Classic FM, which Lennie seemed to like.

On Friday 3rd December, I wrote: "Last night, Lennie did walk about and probably spent the whole night downstairs. Why she won't sleep with me I don't know, but it seems that she doesn't know or realise that I am her husband. I cleared emails in time to get to Mass online. Lennie was very sleepy, and I caught her in time to prevent her falling off her chair sideways." The rest of the day was taken up with domestic chores, such as, on Richard's suggestion, cancelling a cheque to Luke because he had not received it by post.

My diary for Saturday 4th December reported that "we had a good night's sleep; Lennie didn't go wandering. I got up early and had my shower. We went upstairs for Mass just in time. A major theme was evangelisation and our mission to find people to pass on the tradition ... Stephen joined us halfway through the Mass. Later, Gilly came with Lennie's birthday present and news that Douglas had been accepted for a position as a trainee PE teacher. In the afternoon, we watched Chelsea being defeated 3–2 by West Ham. Afterwards, I skimmed the articles in the *Guardian*. Natalie gave Lennie her pills and got her dressed for bed but she came down several times. I read as far as Paragraph 221 of *Laudate Si,* but it has taken three-quarters of an hour of Stephen talking non-stop to Lennie to keep her quiet. Not a good evening."

On Sunday 5th December, Chris and Sue Richardson kindly drove us to and from Mass at St. Pius'. Back home, I tried to relax by skimming the *Observer,* Richard's birthday present to me. Chelsea beat Arsenal 3–0 in the Women's Cup Final. "Lennie was very awkward and intrusive, but later helped Stephen unravel the tree lights he'd gone to Sainsbury's to buy early this afternoon. So, it all ended well, and I finished reading *Laudato Si.*"

Monday 6th December was Doug's mother, Peggy's, funeral. "May she rest in peace. Also, Mario's 80th birthday. God bless him and give him peace, joy and love always." I put out laundry for Stephen to put into the washing machine. Later, a carer put them out on the radiators. The three hours in the afternoon "weren't easy. Lennie was concerned at first with getting a dog or cat. I strongly resisted on the grounds that we were both too immobile these days. She then shifted to other themes, and I battled to keep peace and my reading of the *Tablet* had to be largely given up." After supper, the carer dressed Lennie for bed, but unexpectedly she came downstairs and watched the second half of the Everton vs Arsenal game. "When I went upstairs, I was astonished to find Lennie fully dressed and unwilling to come to bed with me."

On Tuesday 7th December, I started my diary: "But she did come within a short time and we didn't have a bad night ... But Lennie didn't stay for Mass." I finished transferring birthday and anniversary dates into my 2022 diary, while outside the weather was stormy. I read more of David Attenborough's book, *Living Planet,* which Andrew had bought me for my birthday. Lennie came downstairs after having been dressed for bed by the carer. She demanded another meal, but I'd already locked the kitchen door (for safety reasons). "Lennie remained downstairs, all night in the end."

Wednesday 8th December was Lennie's 86th birthday. "I sang 'Happy Birthday' from the top of the stairs. Mandy dressed her in the jumper I'd bought her via Gilly and at the Offertory we were joined by Stephen for the livestream Mass. Gilly, Richard and Andrew all phoned and there were visits from Norma and Frances. Andrew also came. His relationship with Caroline has ended, his financial situation seems dodgy and at sixty he's not finding it easy to get employment. In the evening, we watched Chelsea draw 3–3 with Zenit in the Champions League and in the final two hours I managed to order next week's shopping from Sainsbury's online."

On Thursday 9th December, Stephen set off at 8 a.m. for Cranleigh. "Lennie was intrusive, and in my opinion, rude to the cleaners and I struggled to stop her interfering with them. Eventually, we watched the Mass from St. Joseph's." The carers took Lennie out for a couple of short walks, and I tried to read the latest issue of the quarterly *RENEW*. In the early evening, "Lennie is at her most challenging. She won't stop and listen to the news, and she is full of devices and threats the rest of the time. She threatens to hit me with her walking stick. Earlier, she walked back to the lounge from the loo with the loo paper. At one stage she said she wished she had a boyfriend but within a couple of minutes denied it." After she'd been taken upstairs and dressed for bed, she came downstairs "no fewer than four times. I reiterated my position that I wasn't going to be bullied into going to bed before 10 p.m." In the last hour, I finished reading the *Tablet* and nearly finished the latest *RENEW*.

Friday 10th December was in many ways very similar. "After Mass, I paid last week's Everycare bill and my account is slowly declining. After our lunchtime carer left,

"I think Lennie was again anxious and disturbing. I tried to read the *Tablet* and *RENEW* but quite often dozed off … Earlier, I'd waded through today's mail ... Unexpectedly, there was a lovely message from Sara Arbor thanking me for helping her through her early years in the Sociology Department. Quite unexpected. I just wasn't aware of it. Gilly came to take me to see Dr. Barnado, but he surprised us by not following the Milford appointment up with Gilly but was really focused on what he'd noticed was my deteriorating health and the need not to delay arrangements for a care home for Lennie until there was a sudden crisis like a serious fall or a heart attack. Gilly and I were more or less agreed to pursue the possibility of respite care for a week or two for Lennie in the Spring." Later, I had a chat with Marie who, "like Faye, has given me very friendly support".

My diary for Saturday 11th December noted, "a good night's sleep ... Stephen came around 11a.m. After lunch, Stephen and Lennie went outside and collected two bin bags full of leaves on the lawn, as I watched Chelsea Women lose 1–0 to Reading." On Sunday 12th December, "Gilly came and drove the three of us to St. Pius' for the 9.30 a.m. Mass. I gave in to my sense of weakening energy and sat during most of the Mass. Back home, Gilly stayed for coffee but left quickly because Douglas was recovering from a serious fall on Friday, which had left him unconscious, and he'd been taken to A&E. I tried to skim through the *Observer*. During the afternoon, Lennie had one of her awful episodes, angrily interrupting anything we were watching on TV. She and Stephen battled for over one and a half hours, and it was good when Richard came, cuddled Lennie, chatted away and gave us a break."

On Monday 13th December, Stephen had to set off early for Cranleigh because he had a doctor's appointment, but before he went put a week's washing on and helped me dress. Before we attended Mass on livestream, I cleared twenty-one emails. When the carers came, they usually took Lennie out for a short walk or a drive, but between shifts she was always a bit difficult. In the evening, she came and settled with Classic FM largely playing Christmas carols and *The Vicar of Dibley*.

Tuesday 14th December was my brother's 86th birthday. It is sad that we've had no contact for several years. I couldn't get livestream Mass from St. Joseph's, but I managed to get it from Limerick. "As often happens at this time, Lennie lost the last three decades of her life, was concerned about 'the children', denied that this was our home, and accused me frequently of lying about the fact that we bought this house which is our home." While Louise drove Lennie around the Christmas lights on Bushy Hill, I managed to read a bit more of Attenborough's book. "When Mandy left, it was a question of what will Lennie do now? She is obsessed with fiddling with the numerous vases of flowers. She just won't leave them alone. I'll try and get back to Attenborough while ignoring Lennie's 'Can someone come and help me?'"

Before Mandy came on Wednesday 15th December, I noted, "I had a good night's sleep last night ... Lennie put on her dress over her nightie ... Mandy took Lennie upstairs to re-dress her." The rest of the time passed more or less as usual, watching Mass on livestream. I then had some difficulty ordering the next week's shopping from Sainsbury's online.

On Thursday 16th December, I was rather depressed in the morning. We gave out chocolates and wine for Christmas to our carers. We watched a struggling Chelsea in the evening. On Friday 17th December, Lennie's demands were seemingly implicit all day. I'd forgotten my pills the previous night, so I had them that morning along with the usual morning medications. After clearing emails and attending online Mass this morning, we were driven to St. John's Church Hall, where Everycare staff gave about seven or eight clients a very pleasant meal with a quiz game afterwards. We were then driven home where "the next two hours with Lennie were very difficult; she insisted on plans for supper, often with the family, all afternoon. It nearly drove me mad." Gilly came in the evening to help Lennie get ready for bed. I managed to read to Luke 4 or 5 before joining Lennie upstairs.

Saturday 18th December was much as usual with difficulties getting up before livestream Mass, for which Stephen brought up bread and wine around the Consecration. Later, we watched two episodes of *Downton Abbey* and then "a very interesting version of *The Saviour*, i.e., the life of Jesus. Lennie, as usual, interrupted everything that interested me." I managed a preliminary skim of the *Guardian* before going up to bed. "Help me be patient towards my increasingly strange and unhinged Lennie."

On Sunday 19th December, Gilly drove us to Mass at St. Pius' but we had a taxi take us home afterwards! "But the rest of the day wasn't easy. Lennie complained about my not sitting next to her at meals. I sat in the lounger because it has relatively high arms, which are necessary to help me get up." Later, we watched a bit of football and *Bridget Jones*. "A strange sort of day."

On Monday 20th December, Stephen put a load of washing on and later, "Mandy put them out on the radiators". I cleared about twenty emails and accumulated mail before livestream Mass. "Lennie joined me but at times her concentration dissolved." Later, "Jade, the new carer, did a good job chatting with Lennie and taking her through the 2008/9 photo album, which depicted several overseas visits. When Jade left, I had to cope with nearly two hours of Lennie taking off some pearls, putting them on again, then taking them off which led up to my loss of temper when she just wouldn't leave off the pearls for safety's sake." Mgr. Tony came to hear "my confession about anger, and lack of patience; laziness, limited prayers and occasional lust ... I feel I'm only inviting this confessional visit because of a Church rule possibly put on hold in these times ... To my surprise, he reacted very generously and focused on my general chat to Jesus, which he seemed to suggest was an important theme in the older years." Just before going to bed, I wrote: "For all the wrong I've done, Lord, please forgive me and help me come ever closer to You".

On Tuesday 21st December I wrote, "I had a pretty good night's sleep with fewer visits to the loo than usual". Before our carer came at 8 a.m., I had to wash and dress myself, get downstairs to open the door, and put out Lennie's and my medications and breakfast on the table. After breakfast this morning, I was a bit slow and only managed to get to the livestream Mass after the first reading. "Lennie's attention was a bit limited and I'm not sure she saw herself at Mass. Afterwards, she just doesn't seem to comprehend the arrangements for Christmas and Boxing Day. In the afternoon, Lennie came down with her walking stick used as a hanger with a dress, my shirt and a jumper all attached as if testing them for suitability. But when I refused to let her wander outside, she became quite threatening with her stick and two knives." In the afternoon, Lennie was driven to Whitmore Common by one of the carers. But afterwards, "Lennie complained that she'd been 'dumped'!" Nothing I could say modified this. "When I point out that this is our home, pointed to the three photos on the wall (engagement and marriage of sixty years) and say I am her husband, she denies this and says I am a liar. She carried on a bit aggressively all early evening. Lennie again put water on some of Stephen's latest artificial flowers, brought in a dozen bits of cutlery and was generally aggressive." I read to Luke 12 and skimmed the *Tablet* when Lennie went up to bed.

On Wednesday 22nd December, I wrote: "When I went up to bed last night, I was annoyed to find that Lennie had put on her best dress over her nightie. She messed about putting on clothes and then taking them off for a good hour, during which I kept my cool but didn't get to sleep ... Lennie is very uncomfortable with her leg pain this morning ... I put on Mass from St. Joseph's on livestream. Stephen, bless him, arrived from Cranleigh just before Mass started." After supper, we watched a documentary about carols and then André Rieu. "Lennie was fully dressed when I went up to bed and came to bed fully dressed. We said our three prayers together at 10 p.m.

On Thursday 23rd December, Natasha came and sorted out Lennie's clothes. Stephen's pharmacy was short on one of his medications; very irritating. I had difficulty getting Mass and eventually we followed one from Canada. I watched another episode of *Downton Abbey* showing the difficulties the aristocracy had after WWI. Ben had coronavirus and this modified all arrangements for Christmas.

Christmas Eve, Friday 24th December, was full of uncertainties because of the coronavirus. I showered and dressed myself with difficulty. I hadn't realised there was no 10 a.m. Mass from St. Joseph's that day, but I found a very pleasant Mass in Ireland. "Lennie walked away at the Offertory for a jacket and also with a very sore leg." After Mass and clearing emails, I put on Classic FM and Lennie joined in, singing some of the carols and other Christmas music. Just after the carer, Louise, had left, "Gilly unexpectedly turned up with a pile of Christmas presents. She told us that Katie and Douglas were fighting each other. Katie, she suggested, was very like Andrew in her rigid determination to 'do her own thing in her own time'." Unfortunately, we raised the issue of Lennie's dental appointment in January. "Lennie was furious, feeling she was being pushed into it. It made me wonder if it wouldn't be a good idea to cancel her appointment. She is very worried by the pain in her knee. I don't know how to ease it beyond the two paracetamol we gave her at midday. During the afternoon, Faye took Lennie for a drive." In the evening,

Stephen put on EWTN, and it was the Pope at the Easter Vigil at the Vatican. Andrew came around 9.30 p.m., and we discussed arrangements for Christmas Day.

My Christmas Day diary admitted that I'd "not had a great night. In fact, Lennie, around 4 a.m., started an hour-long session of searching for clothes to wear. Eventually, around 5 a.m., she put on a nightie and dressing–gown and was persuaded to remain in bed. But I never got to sleep again ... Andrew then drove us to St. Pius', where the four of us felt it was a peaceful occasion. Afterwards, Andrew drove us home and then went off to take some presents to Richard. Stephen did the preparation for lunch." In mid-afternoon, we all watched the Queen's speech and then Andrew fired three fireworks in the garden. The boys did the washing-up and then we watched another episode of *Downton Abbey*. After an hour of trying to deal with Lennie's awkwardness when he was trying to give her her Christmas present, Andrew blew his top and made no bones about Lennie's behaviour and the need to get her into a care home. Unlike Stephen, who collaborated with her all evening, Andrew does not have the care-vocation skills that Stephen has ... bed about 10 p.m."

On Sunday 26th December, my diary noted: "I'd had a pretty good night's sleep ... After shaving, Stephen came up and kindly helped me dress ... Gilly picked us up around 9.05 a.m. and drove us to Mass at St. Pius'." Desmond Tutu had died, and we included him in the bidding prayers. "Afterwards, we said goodbye to Andrew, who drove off as usual to see his old friend Vicky and her partner. Gilly drove us home and I skimmed some ordinary comments in today's *Observer*. Gilly then, just after midday, came to pick us up and drive us to Whipley Close. We were attending their lunch as we often do on Boxing Day. It was good to see our grandchildren, Katie and Douglas. They were fully supportive and loving. Bless them ... Gilly drove us home." We watched Chelsea beat Villa 3–1 away. Before going to bed I had a half-hour talk with Stephen, who said he "wished he could have a break on Wednesdays".

On Monday 27th December, "Stephen helped me get dressed – something I'll not have if we drop Wednesdays." After we'd attended Mass on livestream, I spent an hour typing the first page of Stephen's poetry. We tried to have a quiet afternoon, but "Lennie was occasionally demanding and set about dressing and undressing downstairs. I just tried to chill out and spent the time doing a final skim through yesterday's *Observer*. These last few days I've thought more and more about how I am going to cope during the next twelve months with my declining mobility and energy and how to deal with Lennie's developing dementia and her endlessly demanding actions, which drive me more and more mad. Lennie's anxieties and aggressiveness are something we have just got to get used to."

My diary for Tuesday 28th December says we had "an uncertain start to the day." I then phoned Everycare to arrange for further cover while Stephen remained in Cranleigh on Wednesdays. "Please, Lord, help me to do what You want me to do ... I do feel Mgr. Tony's homily at the livestream Mass was a call on the younger generations to fight our country's nasty anti-immigrant policies and detention camps, etc." After livestream Mass, I struggled to type more of Stephen's amendments to his blogs for an hour. Later, we watched a couple of episodes of *Downton Abbey*. "Gilly turned up with flowers and a card for tomorrow's anniversary."

Wednesday 29th December was Lennie's and my 61st wedding anniversary. Stephen kindly "came up and helped me get dressed, particularly socks and slippers." After livestream Mass, to which Stephen brought up bread and wine to simulate what Jesus did at the Last Supper, I phoned Kingston Hospital and cancelled Lennie's two appointments for the next week. "But Lennie wasn't always helpful and at times was a menace, largely undressing herself in front of us in the lounge. She was so utterly resistant to requests not to undress in public that at one stage I hit, or more likely pushed her, onto the settee. I must be careful not to be provoked by her in future ... In the evening, we try to watch TV, but it is impossible to watch TV programmes when Lennie <u>never</u> stops talking. During the afternoon, we had several phone calls from Gilly, Ann and Andrew, wishing us a happy anniversary. Has it been a happy day? Not really. It has been OK, but relations with Lennie are not what they used to be. These days she doesn't have the memory to recall much about our previous life and she often, possibly most often, doesn't recognise me as her husband of sixty-one years. Be with her, Lord, and give me the grace to love her with patience during the rest of our lives."

On Thursday 30th December, I wrote that "I didn't have a bad night, though Lennie did a fair amount of wandering". Before Mass on livestream from St. Joseph's, I cleared emails and paid the Everycare bill. Lennie kept asking me to 'go out', saying "that she had to look after the oldest children. I told her that it was the Christmas holiday and there were no children around, but it fell on deaf ears ... When Lennie struggled to go to the loo, I suggested she take the walking stick. But infuriatingly, she neglects my suggestions as to where the stick is; it may be only one foot away but she doesn't notice it, as if she is totally blind. I'm not good at coping with this ... I was focused on *Downton Abbey* when I found Lennie just behind me, having taken off her nightie, standing there in her knickers and bra–less top. Why does she do this? I am totally unable to understand why she is doing this."

On Friday 31st December 2021, I wrote: "I didn't have a bad night, though again I didn't sleep much after 4–5 a.m. I missed the help Stephen often gives getting me dressed. Lennie was quite friendly in bed before I got up, but she is struggling to walk a few yards. What a big change over the past few months." Lennie and I attended online Mass with the diocesan themes: prayer, formation, and mission emphasised. "During the afternoon, Lennie was at times quite difficult with her aggression and interruptions."

"So, my 2021 year is coming to an end. What a strange year this has been. Thank You, Lord, for all You have done for me and us and help me cope as You would wish next year." On Saturday 1st January 2022, I concluded my diary by observing that: "It's been a fairly busy New Year's Day. I wonder whether I'll meet my 90th birthday and see out the rest of this year. Lennie's 'periods' of anger and irritations are getting more regular, and her knees are causing her a lot of pain. Both of us are increasingly immobile. I'm finding it more and more difficult to get up, even with the arms of the lounger. In other words, I'm going to need lots of Your grace to help me cope with this year, Lord. Please help me do what You want me to do."

On Sunday 2nd January 2022, I noted that: "It was between midnight and 1 a.m. that Lennie dressed and undressed about six times and, of course, I didn't get to sleep with her mucking about. I don't think I slept after about 5 a.m." Lennie was in a lot of pain, so Stephen stayed at home with her while Gilly drove me to Mass at St. Pius'. Gilly phoned Queen Elizabeth Care Home to enquire about respite care. Later, Lennie was "in one of her awkward moods, dressing and undressing in the lounge. Forgive me, Lord, for all my faults and failures to follow Your intentions as well as I should."

On Monday 3rd January, Stephen put a load of washing in the washing machine and helped me get dressed. Lennie remained in bed and didn't join Stephen and me at the livestream Mass. Gilly phoned to tell us that Everycare were concerned about the possibility of Lennie falling down the stairs. "How I am supposed to control that reality when Stephen is no longer here, I'm really not sure. I am coming round, earlier than I had expected or hoped, to the probable need to put Lennie into a care home, where we anticipate she will forget she is married to me for large chunks of the day. When the aggressive violence of Lennie emerges, when she feels she is being pushed around ... I pray to the Lord for the grace to follow His wishes with Lennie during the final time of our lives."

On Tuesday 4th January, I admitted "there had been another disturbed night". Stephen, after a phone call with Jane (Everycare), agreed to remain at home. "Lennie going into a care home is beginning to seem likely fairly soon." The day dribbled away and in the early evening Lennie asked, "'Where is my mother?' … Strange life. Going up to bed with Lennie around 10 p.m., we said our three prayers together and went to sleep."

On Wednesday 5th January, I noted, "We didn't have a bad night." Lennie and I watched the livestream Mass. Faye took Lennie out for a brief drive before the hairdresser came to give her a 'cut and blow-dry'. "But it didn't work wonders for her temper and for much of the evening she was angry and combative." Later, I managed to watch some of Chelsea's 2–0 win over Spurs in the first leg of the Carabao Cup Semi-Final. On Thursday 6th January, I recorded that I was still managing Lennie's large list of medications. "But as I handed her a pill, she pulled off her wedding and engagement rings. The latest problem of an awful evening. Most of the time, I managed to keep cool, and I answered every question she asked as best as I could. But it didn't stop her accusing me of lying, being called an 'awful sod' and other things and several times threatened with a fist or shoe."

On Friday 7th January, I noted that it was a fairly mixed day with lots of interruptions. Jane (Everycare) asked me whether I'd like domiciliary help from 11 a.m. to 9 p.m., which I estimated would cost an extra £25K per year. As usual, I hesitated and later wrote: "Lennie is accusing me of being a 'damn nuisance!' Lennie was very provocative and brought a loo roll from the loo and threw it at me and called me more names and accused me of laziness and more ... After Faye left, Lennie became very aggressive and her bashing me with her stick has left me with a nasty bruise on my left calf." In the evening, I struggled to read a chapter of Naomi Klein's recent book before going up to bed.

On Saturday 8th January, I noted that it had been a difficult night with Lennie "messing about, dressing and undressing". Stephen came from Cranleigh and joined me at the livestream Mass. I'd had a good night, but then had problems with the laptop and just managed to follow the livestream Mass in time. "Lennie was very disturbed and concerned about 'the children' and totally resistant to my repeated instructions that there were no children in our house." I struggled with my laptop but in the afternoon managed to order next week's Sainsbury's shopping delivery. Lennie was quite difficult in the evening, refusing to go upstairs on the stairlift.

On Sunday 16th January I noted that going to the loo last night, I'd banged my leg against the urinal and it bled quite badly. Gilly drove us to Mass, and I wondered "if this is one of the last Sundays that Lennie will attend Mass there. I don't seem robust enough to last much longer." On our return home, we had the six-monthly meeting of the Trustees, with John Dean attending for the first time. He survived Andrew's furious explosion with me after failing to accept a 'joke'. In the afternoon, I skimmed the *Observer*. I also managed to read a bit of the *Tablet* as well as some more of Klein.

Monday 17th January was a lovely day. A book review in the *Tablet* again raised the possibility of writing a book about Lennie's dementia, from the time I wrote a denial to Dr. Barnado in 2014. Lennie didn't attend livestream Mass with me because she was suffering pain in her knee. In the afternoon, she was quite interested in one of the Yorkshire Farm programmes. Faye took her out for a drive and she and Mandy prepared supper, singing in the kitchen. "After Mandy left, it was almost impossible to keep Lennie focused on either Classic FM or any TV. I tried to interest her in Attenborough's *The Green Planet,* but she was focused elsewhere, walking round the room, pulling out odds and ends from under the table, and asking me to put buttons in the holes of her cardigan, and so on. I had just over an hour to read Klein before going to bed."

On Tuesday 18th January, I wrote that "I didn't have a bad night and Lennie was quite loving". I spent some time selecting about eight charities out of requests from fourteen for our monthly charity donations. My main choices were for refugees and the homeless; Lennie's were for children in Africa. She joined the two carers making lunch in the kitchen. In an exchange in the afternoon, "Lennie said 'I hate you' but a minute later she suddenly said, 'I do love you!'" Louise took Lennie for a walk around the pond at Whitmore Common. In the evening, I wasn't very successful finding something Lennie liked on the TV, but we ended up watching Chelsea's unimpressive 1–1 draw with Brighton.

On Wednesday 19th January, Lennie struggled with her osteoarthritis and went downstairs "bashing the front door, saying she wanted to go home". After the lunchtime carer had left, "Lennie is a complete menace and hates me, etc., as I suggest over and over again that she sits down and relaxes, only to be threatened by her fists and spat at, telling me she hates me! ... It didn't take long after Mandy's departure around 5.35 p.m. for Lennie to become impossible ... She is walking round with the zimmer frame and has threatened me with it and called me 'a nasty pig'. Please Lord, help me."

On Thursday 20th January, I noted that "Lennie occasionally fills the vases with Stephen's artificial flowers with water. She didn't seem to be in as much pain with her knee as recently and the day ended quite peacefully." On Friday 21st January, I finished reading Naomi Klein's book and was disappointed she didn't have many suggestions about how to cope with the global problems of climate change "and failed capitalism and commercialism". In the evening, Lennie drove me mad, messing about on the table and putting Stephen's bunch of artificial flowers in the loo. For safety reasons, I locked the kitchen door before going to bed.

On Saturday 22nd January, Lennie slept in until the carer came. I had real problems with the laptop, both before and during the livestream Mass. I later watched Mass from EWTN. During the day I skimmed the *Guardian* and the Salesians' 'Maroon, Blue and Gold' magazine. On Sunday 23rd January, Gilly drove us to Mass, where the front row had been reserved for us. I sat down until the 'Our Father'. Gilly drove us home and we had a pleasant hour with her. In the afternoon, I managed to complete an online weekly shop with Sainsbury's. The laptop wasn't giving me the same problems as yesterday. Lennie was upset when Richard returned home and "she just didn't understand that children grow up and leave home just as she had done".

Stephen went off early on Monday morning, 24th January, and was, I think, being taken by Andrew round the Van Gogh exhibition in London for his birthday. This turned out to be quite a difficult day with Lennie. After lunch, "when I woke up, I went to the loo and put a letter wrongly delivered to us by the front door. Lennie moved it but totally denied it. I'm afraid I lost my temper and banged the zimmer frame half a dozen times on the floor, angrily accusing Lennie of lying. A few minutes later I apologised and said she'd got an illness which she again denied. This all made me think it really was time for Lennie to go into a care home. This morning, she apparently spread faeces all around the bathroom and Mandy cleared it all up. Faye then took Lennie out for a drive and drink."

On Tuesday 25th January, an email from Gillian "confirmed that Lennie was going into Claremont next Monday. It is a worrying warning of a dramatic change in our lives. Please, Lord, help me do as You will. As I write this, she is wobbling to the toilet, but I do fear she will fall at some point." Lennie didn't join me for the online Mass. "A little to my surprise, Lennie point-blank refused to take her pills and the bulk of her lunch." Later, she denied she'd made an appointment to have her toenails cut. "Lennie and I had an angry exchange and later, I cleaned up her faeces all over the loo seat." Lennie was struggling to put her pills into a water glass, but Mandy came and managed slowly to persuade her to "take her pills and then a glass of water. I've not found Lennie easy today, nor have some of our carers. She is defiant and aggressive in her resistance to suggestions about pills or toes or bed."

On Wednesday 26th January, I noted that Lennie had left the lounge lights on all night. I helped her complete a form, which aimed to follow whether or not our signatures have changed as we have aged. I read a bit more of the third book on climate change I bought recently, by Kolbert. "On the whole I had a better day than yesterday, and Lennie wasn't quite so angry and insistent as on previous days. Lennie and Mandy are singing together (in the kitchen) 'whatever will be, will be'. Gilly unexpectedly turned up with a birthday present for Stephen ... She also told me she was due to have a hysterectomy ...Be with her, Lord."

Thursday 27th January was Stephen's 57th birthday, which "he has decided to celebrate with us on Saturday. Be with him, Lord, and never let him have a serious relapse of his psychosis ... Lennie was very warm and friendly, and we had some brief cuddles ... Faye came and soon was easing

Lennie's tears, as she complained that no one was listening ... At bedtime, Lennie was singing cheerfully and beautifully."

Friday 28th January seemed a fairly typical day. Lennie didn't join me until the 'Our Father' for the livestream Mass. I had to add a pile of kitchen needs to the Sainsbury's shopping list. In the afternoon, after my usual sleep, I read more of Elizabeth Kolbert's book. "Victoria took Lennie for a short walk to the end of the cul-de-sac and back. Lennie is very upset that she can't go out and go 'home' and my repeated 'this is your home' is just ignored ... Lennie just won't sit down and relax ... Lennie has just called me a 'stupid cow'. Charming! ... It is a life-changing event on Monday and I'm not sure if I should be feeling guilty. But Marie said she thought it was the right thing to do."

On Saturday 29th January, I noted that "early this morning Lennie was very loving as she often is at this time." I helped get in the Sainsbury's shopping delivery just before Stephen arrived to put it away. I emailed Sue to thank her for her Christmas card dated 29th November! Ann then called for a chat. It was a fairly typical weekend, with my skimming the *Guardian* and trying to please everyone with the TV. "Please God help us to do the right thing for Lennie. Be with her and help her enjoy the various games and group activities available."

Sunday 30th January seemed to be a busy day. Stephen kindly helped me dress. Lennie was very aggressive and indeed rude to Jade, who complained about it. Gilly came to drive us to St. Pius' for a pleasant Mass, which was probably Lennie's last in the parish. She "called me a 'cock-eyed cow' as I struggled to lift my zimmer frame past her chair". Back home, Richard arrived with a carload of Stephen's paintings, as he was clearing his home in Albury ready to move into his new house in Guildford. During the rest of the day, I managed to skim the *Observer* and before going to bed I read Matthew 16–18.

My diary for Monday 31st January records that Lennie went to bed fully dressed and was awkward in the morning. We attended Mass on livestream with the bread and wine Stephen brought up. It was the Feast of St. John Bosco, and I recorded my gratitude for my four years at Battersea Salesian College. "It was a strange morning because we hadn't told Lennie in advance that she was going to be taken to Claremont. She was taken to a 'girlie lunch' and as she was driven off by Gilly, she looked sad I was not with them. I'm not sure she guessed something more serious was being initiated." Before she left, Gilly told us that the police had been informed that there was potential conflict between Lennie and me. "The kind lady, Jean, at Claremont Court, phoned to let me know after lunch that Lennie was happy cuddling a doll and enjoying watching the children at the adjacent primary school play outside."

This was the end of the ten-year development of Lennie's 'mixed dementia' and how I struggled to cope with the increasing range of challenges over the decade. Lennie remained in the Claremont Court care home for thirteen months before she died, holding hands with me and with Andrew and Stephen kissing and stroking her. The final chapter of this book gives something of the flavour of our relationships during this time.

:

CHAPTER 10

Claremont Court, January 2022–March 2023.

This chapter provides a brief account of our contacts with Lennie during her fourteen months in Claremont Court. It follows the years she had spent living with me, her husband, as her 'mixed dementia' carer based on the reflections I had made in my diaries over this period as her dementia developed. This chapter records the occasions when members of our family visited her. My personal plan was to visit her twice each week, usually on Sundays and Wednesdays. On several occasions I wasn't able to do this because of safety restrictions arising, for example, from various rounds of COVID-19. But it is clear that all our children used to visit her regularly. There was also continuing support from my two sisters, Ann, in Royston, and Sue in Ivrea, Italy.

My diary recorded that my first visit was on the Wednesday after Lennie had been taken into Claremont and seemed to indicate that Lennie was quite comfortable. My carer and I had to take lateral flow tests (LFT) before we were allowed in. She was brought to us from the common room, and we chatted to her for the best part of an hour. I recorded that "Lennie seemed a bit unexpectedly at ease with the care home. It seems she has joined in some of the games, etc. ... We said a usual 'see you soon' or whatever, but she didn't seem particularly upset that I was going. In other words, relief that she seemed settled, if a bit sad that our marital relationship is no longer prominent."

On Sunday February 6th, my carer and I saw Lennie walking down the corridor, not for the last time. "I sat with her for about three-quarters of an hour, which in some respects I found hard going. Lennie looked older to me and it was difficult sometimes to follow her train of thought ... She went to the loo and when she came out, she was feeling pain in her legs ... I was quite ready to come home and told her that all the family sent their love and best wishes." That evening, I reflected "on my nooky wife seemingly quite enjoying the opportunities to walk along the corridors, play games and so on, and mix with people without having any noticeable sense of loss about not being at home or with her family".

On Wednesday 9th February, Faye gave me a Lateral Flow Test. At Claremont we also had to wear a plastic shawl and gloves before being taken up to Lennie's room by Lennie's tall carer, Tom. "I suppose I only had about half an hour on my own with her. She looked fine, though with very limited mobility. Physically, she seemed to have deteriorated rapidly over the past week ... Lennie refers to Stephen with a great deal of affection." On the following day, Lennie's doctor, Dr. Baker, phoned and "observed that Lennie seemed to be settling in contentedly". Faye drove Stephen and me to see Lennie on Sunday afternoon, 13th February. We still had to wear plastic covers. I noted: "Stephen read the Valentine's card I'd bought Lennie and then persuaded her to open the chocolate box I'd bought her so that he could have one! I'm looking forward to the time when I will be able to give Lennie a hug and a cuddle."

The following week, Gilly planned to take Lennie a load of things she'd been tidying out in Lennie's room at home. In my diary of Wednesday 16th February, I wrote, "I wasn't really looking forward to the visit because I was tired and sleepy. It started alright, but then Lennie spread five or six hobnobs around the table, in spite of my saying it was half-term. But at the lift Lennie and I had a brief cuddle. On

Sunday afternoon, Stephen and I took his 'Lowry' painting to remind her of Berwick. While we chatted for about three-quarters of an hour, Lennie had, several times, drifted off to sleep. But she seemed disappointed as we were leaving.

On Wednesday 23rd February, when Louise took me to Claremont Court, "Lennie was walking past me as if we didn't know each other. I was finding it difficult to hold a conversation with her and was counting the time to leave (within my carer's shift). When for a second time she wandered off, I followed her for a bit, managed to pull her close for a kiss, and said my goodbye and set off for the lift." Andrew visited Lennie on Saturday 26th and Stephen and I on the following day, Sunday 27th. He had taken a list of photographs which Andrew had put on last year's calendar. "Lennie looked quite happy, though she wasn't all that aware of who we were. But I felt it quite reassuring after yesterday's rather negative assessment by Andrew."

On Wednesday 2nd March, Faye pushed me in the wheelchair for the first time. "She helpfully played several hymns on her audible phone and Lennie was able to join in. Both Faye and I felt she had deteriorated badly over the past few weeks. She was badly bent over her zimmer frame. Almost no conversation with her, though we both tried to keep things going."

On Sunday 6th March, Richard drove Stephen to see Lennie while my carer, Louise, drove me to Claremont, where Stephen wheeled me to Lennie's room and placed me next to her chair. Lennie "was very bent again, but was quite friendly, especially when Richard gave her a little cuddle. Both boys kept her in engaging conversation and gave her the little woollen puppy, Billy, to cuddle. Our three-quarters of an hour passed surprisingly quickly ... I confess I did not really feel 'up' to today's visit because I was tired ... But on the whole, I think it was helpful that the three of us went."

On Wednesday 9th March, "Faye came and we were no longer required to wear plastic aprons and gloves. Faye helped the conversation to keep going." Lennie looked a bit better that day with her head a bit higher. Faye put on a songsters disc and Lennie immediately joined in the songs. "On Sunday 13th March, my carer took Stephen and me to visit Lennie, pushing me in a wheelchair. We chatted to Lennie for about forty minutes. Stephen was very helpful, taking her through the calendar family photos and chatting to her. I never felt I was very successful in sitting next to Lennie. It doesn't help that I'm immobile when I'm sitting in a wheelchair pushed by Stephen. Lennie looked very bent, but she had a smile on her face, seemed pleased to see me and was friendly and seemed at peace in the home."

As a result of Andrew's and Gillian's criticisms and concerns about my original first chapter, I changed the focus of my book from the 'Catholic Family' to 'A Catholic Husband'. So, from Wednesday 16th March, this book became more of a memoir of the last decade of Lennie's life and how I coped or failed. On that day, Faye took me to spend forty minutes with Lennie, who "looked in pretty good shape, smiling and chatting to us, enjoying a chocolate. Faye was a great help, especially when she put on some music to get Lennie singing. There was no prolonged conversation. But Lennie clearly appreciated our visit and was very sorry to see us leaving." Andrew phoned on Friday 18th, having been to see her. "He noted how small she seemed to have shrunk to and again thought she hasn't too long to live now."

On Sunday 20th March, "I was disturbed that, in her five or six weeks in this care home, she is walking with a zimmer frame with an L-shaped stance, looking at her feet and practically unable to make eye contact with me. I don't know how I would cope if Stephen didn't attend to keep chat going. Lennie says practically nothing and has been unable to tell us anything more about her stay there. It is difficult after sixty-one years of married life together, though strangely I'm not deeply upset ... It is as if I am aware that we are both rapidly approaching the end of our lives. And we are aware of everlasting life with the Lord, given His infinite forgiveness."

On Wednesday 23rd March, Louise drove me to visit Lennie. "It was a difficult three-quarters of an hour. Lennie was bent very badly, and Louise helped her get up from her chair, as she wanted to walk around with her zimmer frame. I felt a bit depressed, but Louise said Lennie knew I'd been there."

On Saturday 26th March, Andrew was told we had been unable to get Lennie's signature witnessed. He set off to see Lennie "and later phoned to let us know that Lennie had been very pleased to have the Mother's Day card from her husband, Mike. She was quite taken by it ... She'd earlier had a fall and had a nasty bump on her head." Later, Gilly phoned and said she thought Lennie would die before me. "Lennie apparently had another fall – the fifth, I think, since going into Claremont."

On Sunday 27th March, Richard and Stephen drove off to visit Lennie for Mothers' Day. They returned "a bit quiet. They both thought Lennie had deteriorated very quickly. Their description of their hour-long chat seemed familiar to what my last experience was." On Monday, Claremont Close called and told me that "Lennie had had one or two further falls. I don't quite know how to respond, immobile as I am."

On Wednesday 30th March, Louise drove me to see Lennie and we had roughly an hour with her. "She was very stooped as she came down to her room with a carer. Louise pushed me (in my wheelchair) close enough to be able to hold Lennie's hand and put on DVDs so that Lennie could sing Taizé or other hymns. Both Louise and I felt that this visit was better than last week's." On Friday, Andrew phoned to say he had COVID-19 and so wouldn't be visiting Lennie.

On Wednesday 6th April, Faye drove me to Claremont. "I thought it was a difficult three-quarters of an hour, but Faye was a great help. Lennie seemed cheerful and had a grin on her face. She seems to be at ease in the care home ... She remembered Deacon Michael's visit." On Friday afternoon, Frances Allen kindly drove us "to Claremont Court, where we had a bit of a difficult three-quarters of an hour with Lennie, who kept pushing herself out of her chair". This seemed to dominate our visit, but Frances took Lennie for a walk with her zimmer frame down the corridor, "where I did manage to give her a brief cuddle". On Palm Sunday, 10th April, Shawn drove us to and from Claremont, where there seemed to be concern about clients falling out of their beds. We estimated that yesterday Lennie had her eighth fall.

On Wednesday 13th April, Shawn again drove us to visit Lennie and again, our main concern was to stop her sliding off her chair. On Maundy Thursday, 14th April, Claremont phoned to inform me that Lennie had seen Dr. Baker and had a urinary infection. On Saturday 16th April, "Andrew came with Easter eggs, having spent an hour with Lennie and taken her out for a while into the garden. He told us that she had had yet another fall – her 10th (?) at Claremont and has a sore eye and a cut on her face. Dear Lord, please may she get the attention she needs to stop this repeated falling."

On Easter Sunday, 17th April, several of us visited Lennie at Claremont. Louise drove me there and later in the afternoon Richard drove Stephen to see her. Later, Andrew also went. On Bank Holiday Monday, "Gilly and Katie popped in in the middle of lunch and told us they had been to see Lennie".

On Wednesday 20th April, "Jane MacHay took me to Claremont in the wheelchair and after a brief natter we managed to organise a visit to the garden with a care home assistant. It gave Lennie a change and she sat up straighter and looked quite friendly and talked a bit with Jane and me. She had a friendly grin on her face, and we even managed a sort of exchange of kisses. In sum, it was the best visit to her in Claremont that I can remember. Her bruising was down and for the first time I was able to see her whole face. Thank You, Lord, that Lennie seemed to have recovered a bit and looked more at ease and aware of us."

On Sunday 24th April, we were driven by Everycare to visit Lennie, whom we took out into the garden for a brief spell as I misjudged the timing of the carer's shift. Lennie "was warm and seemed pleased to have seen us and looking forward to our next visit".

On Wednesday 27th April, Faye drove me to Claremont, where she "wheeled me close to the bed so that Lennie and I could hold hands and enjoy occasional face contact". Probably because of COVID-19, I was wearing a mask. "Thank You, Lord, for the gentle love Lennie and I shared through handshakes and gentle cuddles. It was good to have a good amount of eye contact with Lennie and to share with her the occasional grin and mutual love." On Saturday 30th April, Claremont phoned to let us know that Lennie had had another fall, about her twelfth since going to Claremont. On the next day, Natasha drove Stephen and me to see Lennie. We did manage to hold hands, but a big concern was to stop her sliding off her chair and suffering potential damage.

Louise drove us to Claremont on Wednesday 4th May, where we found a sleepy Lennie. We tried to keep chatting by reading her the Claremont Easter card. "Louise showed her some of Stephen's photos of Lennie and me in the garden a couple of years ago. Between us, we tried to get her to respond. Not greatly successful but her smiles and eye contact did suggest she was pleased to see us and we were reasonably pleased with the visit, although Lennie didn't say much." It seems that Deacon Phillips visited Lennie during the week and then on Sunday 8th May, Shawn drove us to Claremont. "So, Stephen and I had three-quarters of an hour with Lennie. I felt my contribution was negligible. It was Stephen who provided all the chat, drinks and chocolates and a DVD from Taizé. He felt the afternoon had gone quite well, but all I'd done is hold hands with Lennie, make eye contact with her and tell her that Michael Phillips might try and visit her next week."

On Wednesday 11th May, "Faye drove me to Claremont to see Lennie". It seems we had quite a job preventing Lennie sliding off her chair. "While Faye was trying to involve her in looking through old (1960–88) photos, I was holding her hand and trying to make eye contact with her. At the end of our three-quarters of an hour, I read my Mother's Day card to her again. Tears welled up in her eyes when I read it to her. So, God bless her, Lord." On Sunday 15th May, Richard drove us to Claremont, where "we were with Lennie for about three-quarters of an hour. Richard was great and kept Lennie participating and responding to all his suggestions. Richard involved her and managed to have a couple of nice cuddles with her." On Monday 16th May, Claremont phoned to say Lennie "had had another fall in the corridor, I gather without the zimmer frame. I suggested she needed more care to see she only wandered off with a zimmer frame. I don't know what else I can do."

On Wednesday 18th May, Faye took me to Claremont, where we found Lennie with her zimmer frame but no shoes on. Her carer, Daniella, decided "she was too restless to go out into the garden. Faye adjusted the bed and Lennie relaxed. We held hands and made flirty eye contact." On Sunday 22nd May, Claremont only allowed two visitors, so Richard took Stephen. Later, Andrew phoned and arranged to take me. "Lennie was quite friendly and occasionally flirty. I held her hand and we made eye contact."

On Wednesday 25th May, Louise drove me to Claremont, where we found Lennie asleep. After chatting to Lennie, "I think she said she's enjoyed seeing me!" On Sunday 29th May, Gilly drove Stephen to see Lennie. On Wednesday 1st June, Ralph drove me to Claremont, "where he wheeled me up to Lennie's room, where we chatted to Lennie for three-quarters of an hour with his help and that of her nurse, Daniella. I thought Lennie was livelier and more amiable than she has been previously in Claremont. I was able to hold her hand and even to kiss her once, difficult from a wheelchair, but she had a smile on her face and made nice eye contact.

On Sunday 5th June, Richard was our chauffeur and drove Stephen and me to Claremont, where Stephen wheeled me to see Lennie. "She looked unstable to me, but I managed to hold her hands, tickle her under the chin, and get her to smile." Later that afternoon, Claremont phoned to tell me that Lennie had had another fall and got a bump on her head.

On Wednesday 8th June, Louise drove me to Claremont. "It was one of the least satisfying sessions we'd had. She was very disturbed today and spent the whole time sliding down the chair and Louise and I spent the whole time urging her to push herself back to avoid slipping onto the floor. Her left knee was very swollen, but she had a lovely smile on her face." On Sunday 12th June, "Richard and Andrew drove off to visit Lennie". Later, Shawn took Stephen and me to see her as they left. "Lennie was lying on her bed. Stephen wheeled me next to her and we held hands, but I couldn't kiss her. A carer adjusted the bed so that she was sitting up and Stephen helped her with cake and tea. He put on the CD left by Andrew, and we spent half an hour or so singing hymns. She said 'goodbye' with a lovely grin on her face."

On Wednesday 15th June, Faye wheeled me next to Lennie's bed. "I held her hand while she was fast asleep. We left her after half an hour with a load of chocolates, which I hope her nurse will give her. Lennie's visit was a bit limited, but she did smile, and we held hands." Around this time, there was little evidence of our children visiting their mother. Sunday 19th June was Fathers' Day and Stephen and I were taken out for lunch by Richard and his family. So, we only had a short visit to Lennie in the afternoon. "So off we went with only an hour of Shawn's shift left. Stephen wheeled me in the chair. Lennie was awake and although she joined in singing a hymn on the DVD, I wasn't able to do much beyond hold her hand and tickle her chin. We were only with her about twenty minutes before we had to leave."

At the end of my diary on Wednesday 22nd June, I wrote: "I pray for Lennie, with whom I felt there was not a great meeting this afternoon. It is often a bit depressing not managing to have a conversation with or any responses to my questions about her life in Claremont." Claremont phoned the next day to say Lennie had had another fall. "Apparently, she is OK. I asked them to please help her use her zimmer frame to avoid falling." It looks as if Gilly took us up to see Lennie on Sunday 26th June after driving us home from Mass.

On Wednesday 29th June, "Jane B. turned up to drive me to Claremont, where we saw Lennie in her room for about three-quarters of an hour. I held her hand at times, but she was more interested in Jane, who was very helpful with questions and chat, but also used her phone to play some hymns and songs, which Lennie responded to quite positively with a smile on her face. I managed also to ask Daniella about the TV, which was showing some excellent games from Wimbledon." After Mass on Sunday 3rd July, Richard drove Stephen and me to Claremont. "Richard did most of the talking, but all three of us had a sort of cuddle with Lennie, who has aged quite rapidly and seems to have lost a lot of weight in the five months since she's been in Claremont."

On Monday 4th July, Lennie had another fall, and they were giving her two-hourly check-ups. Claremont warned of COVID-19 in their Level 1, so after consulting Gilly, I decided, for safety reasons, not to go on Wednesday. We phoned Claremont on Sunday 10th July, and again decided it was safer not to go. On Sunday 17th July, Stephen and I took a taxi to Claremont and "had about forty minutes with Lennie, mostly orchestrated by Stephen with photographs of the family in the past. I was pretty unassuming and didn't really do much more than hold Lennie's hand while Stephen showed her the photographs. Time seemed suddenly up, and we left Lennie with a wave and a smile." On Wednesday 20th July, I slipped and had a fall and so didn't visit Lennie.

On Sunday 24th July, Richard drove Stephen and me to see Lennie, "who looked very pleased to see me. Her face grinned, especially when I tickled her under her neck. Richard gave her a real cuddle and Stephen helped with the chat. In sum, it was one of the most successful visits so far. All the same, it is a pity they don't care for Lennie's hair, and I think she is losing weight quite significantly."

On Wednesday 27th July, Victoria drove me in the wheelchair to visit Lennie. After a short time in the corridor, we followed her back to her room, where Victoria gave her a biscuit and mug of water. We held her hand and Lennie kissed Victoria and responded to my attempts to hold her hand and cuddle.

On Saturday 30th July, Andrew came after a twenty-minute visit to see Lennie. He said that Fr. Tristan had promised to visit Lennie in Claremont after Mass at St. Mary's. On Sunday 31st July, Stephen and I took a taxi to Mass at St. Pius' and in the early afternoon to Claremont. Apparently, Fr. Tristan had taken Lennie Holy Communion and given her the anointing of the sick. Stephen and I had "a very pleasant thirty-to-forty-minute chat with Lennie. Stephen, as usual, was very verbal and helpful, giving Lennie a biscuit and glass of water and putting on her radio player. Lennie was friendly and smiling, holding hands and cuddling Stephen."

On Wednesday 3rd August, Victoria "turned up to drive me to Claremont. Lennie had been walking all morning with her zimmer frame and was lying relaxed on her bed. Victoria pushed me next to her. We held hands and I tried to chat to her and Victoria read a Valentine card and gave her a chocolate biscuit and mug of water." On Saturday 6th August, Andrew called and aimed to go and see Lennie, taking her out into the garden. On Sunday 7th August, "Gilly aimed to go and see Lennie the next morning, but because of the uncertainties about COVID-19 on Floor 2 I decided (with Stephen's agreement) not to go and visit Lennie today."

On Sunday 14th August, I took a taxi to Claremont where "they brought down Lennie pretty quickly. We took her out into the shed in the garden and we spent twenty to thirty minutes enjoying the temperature but also the shade and breeze. Lennie was in great shape, always smiling and happy to hold hands and kiss whenever possible. As always, Stephen was most helpful, keeping the conversation going all the time. Lennie looked happy and cheerful and had a grin on her face. I held her hand and tickled her throat and she was smiling all the time we were there." On our way to visit Lennie on Wednesday 17th August, we met a torrential rainstorm, and as I was in a wheelchair and needed getting out of the car, we decided not to go that day.

On Saturday 20th August, Claremont called to say Lennie had had another fall. "Tom said she was very anxious." On Sunday 21st August, Richard drove us to Mass and afterwards straight up to Claremont to see Lennie, whom we took "out into the garden and had a pleasant chat with her for half an hour. She looked pretty happy and had a good grin on her face and the three of us had a bit of a cuddle with her." On Wednesday afternoon, on 24th August, Victoria drove me to Claremont where "Daniella brought Lennie down to the garden, where we had a good chat". Lennie looked fine, friendly and smiling, and even a little flirty. For the first time, Victoria managed to get us sufficiently close that we were able to kiss each other because our wheelchairs faced each other in opposite directions.

On Sunday 28th August, Gilly drove us to Claremont after Mass. "We managed to go out into the garden and had a very pleasant half an hour with Lennie. I managed to kiss her, and we held hands and eyed each other flirtily. I was surprised at Gilly's relatively quiet session. But they thought it had been a successful visit and Lennie was smiling and happy most of the time ... Gilly suggested I ought to go and speak to the Funeral Directors at Burpham and ask about possibilities." On Wednesday 31st August, Leanne drove us to Claremont, where we had about half an hour's chat with Lennie. "I thought our visit today was a bit disappointing, but Leanne was more positive."

On Sunday 4th September, after Mass, Richard drove us to Claremont, "where the three of us took Lennie out into the garden for about three-quarters of an hour, with her in the hut in the garden. Richard thought she had not been the most voluble since going into the care home." On Wednesday 7th September, Jane drove us between periods of rain to Claremont, where Lennie was taken from a musical concert to her room, "where we had a kiss and chatted for around half an hour. She seemed quite relaxed and chatted a bit."

On Sunday 11th September, after Mass, "Gilly took the three of us and we took Lennie out into the garden for half an hour. Lennie was quite happy and smiling today and she chatted away pretty well. She seemed pleased to see us and waved us 'goodbye' as we left." On Wednesday 14th September, Victoria drove us to Claremont, "where, after quite a while, Lennie joined us in the garden where we had a pleasant half-hour though we were frequently interrupted ... Lennie seemed relaxed, happy and cheerful and quite good at conversing today. We were placed quite near each other by our carers, so I was able to kiss her. She looked relaxed and at ease."

On Sunday 18th September, after Mass, we took a taxi to Claremont, "where we had to wait half an hour before Lennie came down to us in the garden. She was in a bad mood for twenty minutes or so before suddenly cheering up and kissing me as she was taken back to her room by Stephen. It seems she'd 'had an accident' earlier." On Monday 19th September, I recorded that Lennie "was visited by Richard, Luke and Ben this afternoon. I gathered from Richard that it was a bit difficult." On Wednesday 21st September, Victoria drove us to Claremont, where Lennie "seems quite at ease and reasonably happy here". On Thursday 22nd September, it was decided to move Lennie to the ground floor to make access to the garden easier. Gilly had a later call; Lennie had had another fall but had seen the doctor and was apparently OK.

On Sunday afternoon, 25th September, Richard drove Stephen and me to Claremont where Andrew joined us. "I thought our chat wasn't as lively as it has been. We had about half an hour with Lennie and the boys were helpful in putting on music, which she danced to with Andrew a bit, clearly enjoying the cuddles." The boys brought her bags of clothes and toiletries. On Wednesday 28th September, Victoria drove me to Claremont where we joined Lennie in her room. She'd had a 'hair do' "and looked livelier, though her hair was thinning. She was smiling and affectionate and we managed to keep chatting. I couldn't think of much to talk about, but somehow, we had a friendly half-hour."

After Mass on Sunday 2nd October, Gilly drove us to Claremont, "where we visited Lennie for half an hour or a bit more. Unfortunately, I was parked (in my wheelchair) in such a way that I couldn't kiss Lennie. But we held hands and the three of us chatted away fairly aimlessly. Lennie had a grin on her face, though she wasn't able to tell us about her everyday life. As always, I felt I was pretty incompetent in introducing topics."

On Wednesday 5th October, "Rebecca drove me to Claremont, where Lennie was brought along with a lovely smile on her face. Rebecca wasn't much help with conversation, but we kept going for about an hour. Rebecca distributed water and liquorice allsorts." On Thursday 6th October, "Claremont phoned me during the day to inform us that Lennie's medications had been modified again to cope with her anxieties". Andrew visited Lennie on Saturday 8th October.

On Sunday 9th October, Richard drove us to Claremont after Mass, where we went into Lennie's new ground-floor room. We took her "outside into the garden, where we sat within some flower beds. We had a chatty and an amiable three-quarters of an hour with a cheerful Lennie, who enjoyed cuddles with her two sons and spoke flirty comments about me. I hope she wasn't too upset when we went off for our lunch." On Wednesday 12th October, Marie took me to see Lennie, "who looked quite happy and friendly. But after half an hour she'd had enough and Marie took her back to her community room."

On Sunday 16th October, Stephen and I caught a taxi to Claremont to see Lennie. "She was very warm and friendly and kissed me and told me 'I love you.' Andrew unexpectedly joined us and pretty well took over the rest of the conversation for the rest of the afternoon. Stephen and I had to leave to take the taxi back home, so Andrew and Lennie had a quarter of an hour or so to themselves." On Tuesday 18th October, Claremont phoned to inform me that "Lennie had hit another client". On Wednesday 19th October, in the afternoon, Jade drove me to Claremont where "we took Lennie out into the garden, where we enjoyed a chat for half to three-quarters of an hour. We managed quite well with Andrew's music disc. She was clued up enough to resist giving me the power of voting on her behalf."

On Sunday 23rd October, in the afternoon, Stephen and I took a taxi to Claremont, "where we had about three-quarters of an hour's chat with Lennie. Most of the time Stephen led the conversation with family photos. Then Andrew joined us and he is never short of talk." He then spent some time with Lennie on his own before joining us back at home. On Wednesday 26th October, Louise took me to visit Lennie. "I found today's visit hard going because I had no obvious issues to raise, and Lennie couldn't recall anything that had happened this week."

On Sunday 30th October, after Mass, "Richard drove Stephen and me to visit Lennie in her room at Claremont. I sat in the wheelchair next to her and we held hands but Richard and Stephen chatted to her all the time, and offered her chocolate biscuits and liquorice allsorts, and Stephen had brought her a recent edition of his painting, which we hope they will put up in her room. On Wednesday 2nd November, "Louise drove me to Claremont, and I thought it was one of the least successful visits so far. Lennie kept getting up to go for a walk along the corridor. She didn't answer a single question and seemed rather disorientated."

On Sunday 6th November, after Mass, "Andrew turned up to drive Stephen and me to visit Lennie. She smiled and was friendly, but I thought our three-quarters of an hour's session fell rather flat. Andrew wasn't as lively as usual, but in fact he had a small dance with Lennie and tried to get her chatting before she went off for lunch." On Wednesday 9th November, "Ralph drove me to Claremont, where we found Lennie sitting on a chair at the end of a corridor. We sat there trying to chat to her for about three-quarters of an hour. It was all quite pleasant though Lennie didn't respond to any of our questions."

On the afternoon of Sunday 13th November, after Mass, Richard drove Stephen and me to visit Lennie. Andrew joined us a quarter of an hour later, "so Lennie was able to cuddle her three boys. Lennie smiled and seemed contented but didn't really take part in any conversation. I merely sat next to her and managed to hold her hand and only managed to kiss the top of her head." On Wednesday 16th November, Vicky drove me to Claremont for "one of the most satisfactory visits". She wheeled me close to Lennie, where we managed to hold hands, but had difficulty kissing.

On Sunday 20th November, Andrew drove Stephen and me to Claremont, "where the three of us ended up with Lennie in her room for about three-quarters of an hour. Andrew had a bit of a dance with her and Stephen was very helpful in getting a mug of water and a straw for her to drink. During our visit, Lennie twice wet herself, which probably annoyed the nurse. We tried to sing with her and managed a couple of Christmas carols or those we could remember."

On Wednesday 23rd November, Louise drove me to Claremont to see Lennie. "She wasn't very cheerful today. She hardly smiled today, but Louise and I tried to chat with her. She was rather difficult to chat to, but we struggled on."

On 27th November, Richard drove us to Claremont, where "they wheeled me in to see Lennie and I was put next to her and held her hand. She wouldn't answer any questions I put to her about life in Claremont, but we both kept on chatting with her. But after half an hour, we said our goodbyes. Andrew arrived and popped in to see Lennie for a short time." On Wednesday 30th November, Jane B. came "and drove Stephen and me to Claremont, where we spent an hour with Lennie. She looked reasonably happy and her hair looked nicely washed. But, as usual, there was virtually no conversation or response to any questions about her life, games and fun over the past few days." On Thursday 29th November, "I'm stuck in my wheelchair, so it is difficult to just hold her hands and practically impossible to cuddle or kiss her."

On Saturday 3rd December, I declined to go with Andrew to visit Lennie because I had a heavy cold and also didn't go on Sunday or the following Wednesday. I couldn't visit her on her birthday, 8th December, because of Covid restrictions. A strange period followed. My diaries listed failures of sleep and possibly heavy cold or illness until Tuesday 20th December, when Shawn "left me with Lennie for about an hour. Lennie had no conversation and didn't answer any queries about her life." On the following day, I was told that Lennie had tested positive for COVID-19 and this determined our inability to visit her for much of the time over Christmas.

On Wednesday 28th December, I was going to visit Lennie with Louise but fell down by the car and when a neighbour or visitor helped me sit up, she badly damaged my arm before an ambulance took me to A&E. On Thursday 29th December, Lennie's and my wedding anniversary, "Gilly, bless her, visited Lennie and apparently had a pleasant session with her going through our wedding photographs." I was going through a terrible time with writing my diaries but as far as I could see, I first visited Lennie around Saturday 7th January, when Andrew drove us to see her after several weeks of the COVID scares. "Lennie was fast asleep but the two boys were brilliant and kept talking to her, and got her to swallow a tasty ball of chocolate. After half an hour, the two boys and I were not able to do much other than occasionally hold her hand. It was my first contact with Lennie since before Christmas."

On Sunday 8th January, Richard kindly drove us to Claremont. "The three of us spent just over half an hour with Lennie, who was lying in bed asleep. She smiled at us and the two boys. Richard and Stephen chatted non-stop with her." On Wednesday 11th January, Jane B. came with me in a wheelchair taxi to Claremont, where "we saw Lennie for about forty minutes. Sadly, I wasn't able to get close enough" to cuddle her. On Saturday afternoon, 14th January, Andrew drove me "to Claremont Court, where we spent a half to three-quarters of an hour enjoying each other's company A little to my surprise, Andrew thought she was very good today. She was smiling a bit and we held hands and even had a kiss. She danced a little with Andrew and particularly seems to enjoy cuddling and being close to him."

On Wednesday 18th January, the wheelchair taxi took me to see Lennie. "She had a cheerful grin on her face but didn't contribute much conversation. I was so tired that I dozed off." On Sunday 22nd January, Richard drove Stephen and me to Claremont, "where we saw a smiling Lennie for about three-quarters of an hour. We had a pleasant time. I had a small cuddle with Lennie and held her hand, while the boys showed her some of Andrew's calendar with family photos. I thanked the Lord for the gift of seeing Lennie with our three boys." After my recent fall, there seems to have been pressure that I take a wheelchair taxi to go to Claremont.

On Wednesday 25th January, "a wheelchair taxi to Claremont, where we spent about forty minutes with a smiley Lennie, whom I actually managed to kiss today. We made pleasant eye contact and I managed to feed her with three chocolates. Bless her, Lord. At the entrance they told us she had been asking about Mike and her husband." On Stephen's birthday, Friday 27th January, Gilly visited Lennie. I was unable to visit on Sunday because there was no wheelchair taxi.

However, on Wednesday 1st February, Dawn drove my carer and me to see Lennie at Claremont. We had quite a pleasant three-quarters of an hour there with Andrew, who was grateful that Claremont had on Sunday replaced his stolen CD player. So, he and Lennie had some dancing while I largely sat next to Lennie holding her hand, but not able to kiss her while I brushed her hair back. On Sunday 5th February, Richard, after Mass and taking Will and Iris to his ex-wife, Carole, drove Stephen and me to Claremont, where we had a pleasant three-quarters of an hour with Lennie, who had a pleasant smile on her face all the time. Richard cuddled her and Stephen showed her a range of family photos.

On Wednesday 8th February, we didn't get to Claremont because Everycare wouldn't drive me anywhere and there was no available wheelchair taxi. Early on Saturday 11th, "a consultant at the Royal Surrey phoned us to let us know that Lennie was in the hospital with a fractured hip and asking for my approval for an operation. I agreed and later in the day Gilly took us to the Ewhurst Ward at the Royal Surrey, where Lennie didn't look too bad, though she didn't respond to questions about her life. This issue rather dominated the day ... Be with Lennie, Lord." Gilly phoned on Sunday 12th February to say that Lennie had had her operation.

On Monday 13th February, Andrew drove me to see Lennie in the Ewhurst Ward in the Royal Surrey Hospital. "They had operated on her hip yesterday and couldn't get her to eat or drink anything. Andrew spoon-fed a very slow Lennie for well over an hour. Lennie looked a bit run-down and her eyes rarely made contact with us. I managed once or twice to hold and cuddle her hand." On Thursday 14th February, Richard "drove us to the Royal Surrey, where Lennie was very heavily asleep. We stayed around three-quarters of an hour, but hardly got any response from her, though I kept on encouraging Richard to keep on kissing and talking to her." On Wednesday 15th February, it became apparent that the hospital aimed to return Lennie to Claremont before the end of the week. Lennie's carer at Claremont, Tom, phoned on Thursday 16th to confirm she had been delivered back.

On Saturday 18th February, Gilly drove Stephen and me to Claremont. "There we found a rather disturbed Lennie, who wasn't able to respond to our queries. Gilly found out what she could about Lennie's refusal to have her medication and tried to arrange that she would be given appropriate pain killers, etc." On Sunday 19th February, after Mass, Richard took Stephen and me to Claremont, "where we spent about forty minutes with Lennie. She was kissed by her boys and seemed generally to be less stressed than yesterday." When we visited her on Wednesday 22nd February, she was fast asleep, and I didn't have any clear eye contact. Andrew turned up on Saturday 25th February and drove me to Claremont. We were both quite shocked to "find Lennie shaking uncontrollably. Both of us felt she was either having a stroke or was on her death bed. Andrew managed to get help from the nurse, and I managed to hold Lennie's hand quite a bit, though she didn't seem to respond all that clearly to me. But the two of us, plus a friendly nurse, all said the 'Our Father' before we left after nearly an hour with her."

After driving us to Mass on Sunday 26th February, "Gilly drove Stephen and me to see Lennie in Claremont. On Monday morning, 27th February, just after Stephen had left, we received a phone call from Claremont that Lennie seemed to be on the way to death. I phoned Gilly and she informed the boys. Doug even drove to Cranleigh to try and pick up Stephen. So, I was driven to Claremont Court by Richard, and we were joined there by Gilly and Andrew. I held Lennie's hand while the boys kissed her and stroked her hair. But she never woke up and was clearly showing signs of a big loss of weight. The nurse came and told us how little food or drink she'd managed to swallow. We were there for about an hour and ended by praying for her together.

On Tuesday 28th February, Gilly phoned to tell us that Claremont had warned that Lennie was probably on her 'last legs'. All our four children and I drove to Claremont along with Alison. "I sat in the wheelchair holding Lennie's arm but getting no response while the children took it in turns to go to the top of the bed, kiss her on her forehead and stroke her hair. I tried to pray a bit but didn't think I was very successful. In the evening, Andrew drove Stephen and me to Claremont where we sat and quietly prayed for Lennie, who slept non-stop."

On Wednesday afternoon, 1st March, Andrew drove Stephen and me to see Lennie for around three quarters of an hour. "Lennie was a little more open than yesterday. Her eyes were open, and Andrew and Stephen took it in turns to kiss her forehead and stroke the hair on her head. I sat in the wheelchair and held her hand, but I didn't feel there was any response from her." There were no signs that Lennie could swallow anything, and she looked as if she was losing weight. In the evening, I continued to write a draft Requiem for Lennie. We also visited Claremont on Thursday 2nd March, where Lennie didn't open her eyes and the boys took it in turn to kiss her. Unfortunately, I couldn't from the wheelchair. Richard and Ben were in tears. "Strangely, I didn't feel like that but seemed to be dominated by a belief in life everlasting with the Lord for Lennie."

On 3rd March 2023, I noted: "Dear Lennie died around midday and by the grace of God managed to get the three of us, Andrew, Stephen and me, for final strokes of hair, kisses and frequent prayers. Andrew washed her mouth and lips and he and Stephen cuddled and chatted to her while I sat in the wheelchair next to the bed and held her left hand, though she didn't respond at all. After only twenty minutes she stopped breathing and was confirmed dead in a quarter of an hour by a medic. The three of us were very grateful to the Lord for allowing us to be with her when she died in a time of peace. Thank You, Lord, for your kind gift and for the sixty-two years of our married lives together."

EPILOGUE

The following text was written by the author and delivered as a eulogy at Lennie's funeral.

Margaret Mary Leonide Early was born on the Feast of Our Lady's Immaculate Conception, 8th December 1935 in West Hartlepool. She was always called Leonide after her much-loved aunt who was a nun in Ireland. I was responsible for her nickname, Lennie. I thought the abbreviation Leo, might help. Then I recalled that Leo was Latin for Lion and that reminded me of the Television programme 'Lennie the Lion' and it has been generally used ever since.

Lennie had quite strong memories of the war years. In particular she remembered hiding under the dining room table terrified during the blitz early in the war. When she was five years old she had to say in a play in front of her priest uncle: 'I've never heard anything so disgraceful in all my life!' Her parents were both teachers and their school was evacuated to Whitby where they spent the rest of the war years.

After the end of the war, her father was appointed headmaster of the Catholic school just south of the river in Berwick-On-Tweed. Lennie suffered from discrimination against her from her father who didn't want to be seen to give his daughter special treatment. When she went to the local convent at first, she was the subject of anger from the nuns because her older sister, Maureen, had left to go to the local grammar school. Things improved when she showed she was a great hockey player and scored some fine goals. She became captain of the team and they even beat the local grammar school. In her teen years she had a deep friendship with 'Malcolm' who is said to have been identified in a window in Durham Cathedral. She was devastated when told at her 21st birthday celebration that the friendship had ended.

Lennie had a struggle after leaving school. She spent a year at Hexham studying domestic science but for some reason got on the wrong side of the notorious Hetty, probably because she had not had any basic teaching in domestic science while at the convent, and was not allowed to proceed into the second year. Lennie's father helpfully arranged for her to become an assistant teacher at a school a dozen miles from Berwick and he used to drive her there and back each day. This proved helpful when he persuaded the formidable Mother Ward at Fenham College, Newcastle, to accept her training as a primary school teacher. Lennie quickly managed to satisfy her and completed her training in the late fifties. In retrospect it was providential that she ended up at Fenham and as a primary school teacher where her skills and personality were so widely appreciated.

I understand that Lennie's mother advised her to get a job away from Berwick because she would have been too closely controlled by her father. So it was then that she ended up doing her first two years teaching at the primary school in Charlbury near Oxford. It was during this time that I first met Lennie and was flirtingly rude on a slope after Mass at St. Marie's in Sheffield when I told her to 'stick her bum in'! About four years later her sister, Maureen, asked me to make up a foursome at a dance in Senate House, London. We 'hit it off' and had a delightful night. Lennie was such fun, pretty, lively and flirty. Four days later I remembered her birthday. I had just started teaching at Battersea College of Technology and we used to meet regularly in Oxford Street. We got engaged at the Easter Vigil service in Berwick and the first photograph on today's programme was taken a couple of days later in Edinburgh. Neither of our parents were helpful in encouraging us to get married during the summer vacation and I think we insisted on the Christmas break, getting married on 29th December 1960.

Lennie taught briefly in Walton then a full year at St. Dunstan's, Woking. Our oldest son, Andrew, was born eleven months after our marriage. We then had three more children at roughly eighteen-month intervals i.e. four children in six years. Somewhat desperately we discussed our concerns with Canon Gordon Albion who was our parish priest at St. Mary's, Burpham and he was very helpful. It was around this time that I was following up the suggestion of a colleague at Battersea to do a degree in Sociology by night study at what was then the Regent Street Polytechnic. In effect I was changing my career direction. But I only managed this because of the support of my wife who on three or four days each week had to cope with four lively children with my going to night classes when I didn't get home until well after 10 o'clock. Lennie often found this very hard going as a neighbour testified. But it was an indication of her great support and love and I will always be grateful that she supported me so well during the five years of the degree.

When Richard was three, she started part-time jobs. For a brief time, she served as Head of a Nursery in Godalming, then for some time at Holy Trinity School and Pewley Down School. After our return from my sabbatical in Australia in 1986 she became a reception and first year teacher at St. Thomas's in Guildford. In 1995 she was exhausted and unwell and decided it was time to retire shortly before her sixtieth birthday. In all she worked the equivalent of 20 years full-time mainly as a reception or year 1 teacher. She clearly was a much liked teacher as was obvious when former parents of children she had taught used to make a point of expressing their gratitude for what she did for their children, now in their 20s, when they bumped into each other in Guildford High Street or

Sainsbury's. In our parish she, for several years, ran the First Holy Communion programme with sensitivity and skill and she was a member of the choir and a Eucharistic Minister for many years.

We were married 62 years ago. For the first decade or so we were quite stressed financially. Nowadays when we see young families having a meal out we reminisce that we were unable to afford to do this and for the first decade of our marriage only managed to take the children in a camper van on camping holidays near Newquay in Cornwall. In order to cope, Lennie used to start saving tins of food every week from the New Year. Lennie was always great and in the early 1970s we steadily expanded our visits to camping holidays in Brittany, the Dordogne, and Mediterranean coast with journeys back via Chartres and Paris. Thanks to Lennie, our holidays were always fun. For a good part of a year, we looked after two grandchildren, and they have always appreciated her love and care during this time.

Early in the twentieth century I remember our oldest grandson coming out of the kitchen saying that Nana had asked him about six times whether he would like a drink. I was in complete denial for several years and even wrote to our GP in 2014 saying that I ought to know because I lived with her all the time. It took me some time to realise that there had been a steady development and that the problem was Lennie's denial and strong resentment about being encouraged to go for medical check-ups. Eventually we managed to get her to have a brain scan in Mt. Alvernia and the Farnham Road consultant confirmed she had 'mixed dementia'.

Since my early adult years I have kept a daily diary and around a year ago it occurred to me that it would be helpful to write a book along the lines of 'Coping with Dementia: Reflections of a Catholic Layman' based on the nearly two million words I had written in my diaries over the ten years from 2013 to 2022 when Lennie went into the Claremont Court Care Home. Reading my diaries confirmed my denial in the first year or so. Secondly, in 2018/9 following my fall in the garden and broken hip and later knee replacement, we started having Everycare Surrey carers to help us in a way that I was too immobile to do. Thirdly, we then had the COVID-19 pandemic and had to come to terms with the lockdown. During this period especially, Lennie was in total denial or awareness of the pandemic or lockdown and days became ever more difficult with Lennie getting dressed and wanting to go on walkabouts in the middle of the night. In the mornings, we used to read the day's Mass readings and the 'Bible Alive' commentaries on them plus prayers for the living and the dead members of our families and fellow parishioners. During this period there would be sudden shifts from her accusing me of being a liar and the carers only being concerned about 'money; money; money' to 'I do love you, darling; I always have'. This period of such dramatic twists and turns and broken nights led the children eventually to arrange a fortnight's respite care or 'holiday' for Lennie. We all agreed afterwards that it was best if she remained in Claremont Court.

In this fourth period we have all visited Lennie regularly and have been aware that while she seemed to have been quite happy in Claremont Court where the staff have been very friendly and helpful, her health has steadily declined. She used to wheel her zimmer frame up and down the corridors and had numerous falls until she broke her hip earlier this year, was quickly discharged from the Royal Surrey to Claremont Court and steadily became unable to eat or drink. Members of the family used to visit her regularly. Nearly every person who has sent me a condolence card has drawn attention to Lennie's smile and helpfulness. Andrew, Stephen and I were gifted by the Lord on Friday 3rd March because I was able to hold her hand and the boys to stroke her hair and kiss her head for twenty minutes before she stopped breathing and we prayed for her that she would have eternal peace.

I feel lacking in the gift of summarising what Lennie has done for all our family over the 62 years of our married lives. As far as I am concerned, she was always faithful and supportive and I'll always remember the five years when she enabled me to study for a radical change of career. She was always warm, loving and flirty, an excellent cook and knitter of jumpers, and totally committed to caring for her family. I am grateful to the Lord for giving me such a lengthy life's gift. I know she was a natural, highly gifted teacher of the youngest children in a primary school, and she was much loved by her four children and six grandchildren. She was a committed Catholic and always used her God-given gifts in our parish and elsewhere. God bless her and welcome her into eternal life.

We are delighted that you have all been able to come today to express our love and gratitude to Lennie for all she has done for us in our lives. Andrew will now offer an outline of the memories of our four children and six grandchildren and of Lennie's kindness, understanding, support and encouragement. She was always there with love and concern for all of us.

MPHS

12th March 2023.

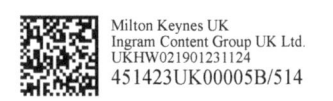

Milton Keynes UK
Ingram Content Group UK Ltd.
UKHW021901231124
451423UK00005B/514

9 781835 633281